Penguin Health

Sense and Nonsense in

Dr Jack Yetiv graduated from the Ohio State University
College of Medicine in 1979 and received his doctorate in
Pharmacology from the same institution in 1981. He is the
author of numerous medical articles.

JACK ZEEV YETIV

Sense and Nonsense
in Nutrition

PENGUIN BOOKS

Penguin Books Ltd, 27 Wrights Lane, London W8 5TZ (Publishing and Editorial)
and Harmondsworth, Middlesex, England (Distribution and Warehouse)
Viking Penguin Inc., 40 West 23rd Street, New York, New York 10010, USA
Penguin Books Australia Ltd, Ringwood, Victoria, Australia
Penguin Books Canada Ltd, 2801 John Street, Markham, Ontario, Canada L3R 1B4
Penguin Books (NZ) Ltd, 182–190 Wairau Road, Auckland 10, New Zealand

First published in the USA by Popular Medicine Press 1986
Published in Penguin Books 1988

Printed and bound in Great Britain by
Richard Clay Ltd Bungay, Suffolk

Table of Contents

Section Two: Nutrients—The Good, the Bad, and the Ugly

Acknowledgments

A book such as this depends to a large extent on knowledge transmitted to me by past tutors. I would therefore like to thank most of all the many teachers and mentors to whom I was exposed during various phases of my education. They all demanded of me, and themselves demonstrated, the supreme effort. To these role models, who had confidence in me when the going was rough, and who provided that nod of encouragement when I needed it most, I owe a great debt. Dr. Hutchison ("Hutch") Williams, Dean of Students at the Ohio State University College of Medicine, is especially gratefully acknowledged in this regard.

I would also like to thank many friends and medical colleagues, who gave of their time, and reviewed various portions of the manuscript. They are, in alphabetical order: Jill Bronson, Phyllis Crapo, R.D., Alfred E. Harper, Ph.D., David Jensen, M.S., Ken Mullé, Daniel O'Meara, J.D., Paul Saltman, Ph.D., Daniel Steinberg, M.D., Ph.D., Michael Sullivan, M.S., Gopi Tejwani, Ph.D., Patti Tveit, R.D., Elizabeth Whalley, Ph.D., Leslie White, M.D., F.R.A.C.P., and Isaac Yetiv, Ph.D.

I would especially like to thank William Norcross, M.D., Associate Clinical Professor of Community and Family Medicine, University of California, San Diego; and Robert Baron, M.D., Assistant Clinical Professor of Medicine, University of California, San Francisco, for extensive review and helpful comments on various drafts of the manuscript.

Thanks must also go to the following dietitians at The Toledo Hospital, Toledo, Ohio, for reviewing the manuscript and making helpful comments: Lynn Brookfield, R.D., Carol Fahle, R.D., Vivian Kiraly, R.D., Anita Minard, R.D., and Lillian Peluso, R.D. I would also like to thank Susan Filkins, M.S., R.D., Clinical Coordinator, Nutrition Services, St. Vincent Medical Center, Toledo, Ohio, for her critical review and comments. Heartfelt thanks must also go to Tammy Beard for designing the cover and preparing the illustrations in the book.

Last but not least, I would like to thank the staff of the medical library at the San Diego Kaiser Permanente Medical Center for their help in literature review: Sheila Latus, Laurel Windrem, Bonnie Tarantino, and Nancy Milligan.

Preface

This book is not meant as a panacea—a cure-all for the world's ills, a recipe to make fat melt off overnight, a magic bullet to banish all disease and confer immortality upon mankind. Books which promise the above can't possibly deliver. What this book will do, however, is review the scientific research on the value of various supplements in "Life Extension", the usefulness of some herbal remedies, the medical aspects of weight reduction, the need for vitamin supplements, the nutritional adequacy of vegetarian diets, the value of chelation therapy, the hazards of liquid protein diets, the dangers of salt, saturated fat and cholesterol, and many other topics.

One may question the need for such a book in view of the plethora of "diet" books on the market. I myself have wondered about the need for such a book. However, while researching the topics in this book, I had the occasion to discuss this project with many people, including physicians, paramedical professionals, and nonmedical individuals. I was *awestruck* by the lack of nutrition knowledge among these individuals, physicians included. Perhaps of greatest concern was not the lack of information but the amount of *mis*information. For instance, after describing some vague symptoms, including episodic shortness of breath, to his physician, a 54 year old acquaintance of mine was told that he had hypoglycemia, one of the most common and usually erroneous "wastebasket" diagnoses. This is despite the fact that the symptoms were easily consistent with ten other diagnoses, and that the appropriate kind of tests to diagnose hypoglycemia had not even been done. What is even more disconcerting is the advice given to this acquaintance—he was told to eat more red meat and other protein, and decrease his carbohydrate intake. This is especially shocking since this person's serum cholesterol was over 300 mg% and his triglycerides were almost 350 mg% (tests obtained *after* he was told that he had hypoglycemia). This person should *decrease* his intake of red meat and *increase* his intake of complex carbohydrates.

This is only one example, and many more could undoubtedly be offered. No wonder the public is having a difficult time knowing what to eat if this physician (an internist) could give such erroneous advice.

Books and articles in the popular literature often advise the patient to "consult your physician for further details". Unfortunately, since nutrition continues to receive short shrift in medical school curricula (1), your physician is unlikely to be a very enlightening source of nutrition information, unless he has a special interest in the field. Nutritional biochemistry and physiology are taught in medical school, as well they should, but the questions that patients ask their physicians, such as whether vegetarian diets are nutritionally adequate or whether megavitamin therapy has any benefits, are not addressed in most medical schools. Organized medicine has to a large extent swept many of these concepts under the rug as "fads". For instance, acupuncture sounded pretty weird to Western medicine a decade ago, but at least some of its capabilities now seem to be well-based in scientific fact, and who knows what "crazy" concepts of today will be the mainstay of therapy tomorrow? It is sometimes the revolutionaries of today that are tomorrow's conservatives.

This haughty attitude of some medical professionals has not helped their credibility with the public, and has induced many people to turn to less-established, non-traditional forms of therapy, sometimes with disastrous results (see Laetrile discussion, Ch. 1). Thus it is small wonder that many consult the *National Enquirer* for their nutritional information, or follow a papaya and pineapple diet for weight loss. I am now more convinced than ever that there is a dire need for such a book, both for medical personnel and for an information-yearning lay public. I quote Dr. Albert Stunkard, one of the leading medical experts in the obesity field:

> "Failures of nutrition education do not stop at the elementary school level. The poor state of nutrition education in higher education, *notably in medical school*, [emphasis mine] is undoubtedly one of the many factors contributing to the nutrition problem—including obesity—of our nation" (2).

In view of the foregoing discussion, this book has two specific goals:

1) To inform the medical student, physician or paramedical professional (dietitian, nurse, nurse practitioner, physician's assistant, etc.) of the medical facts that will equip them to respond appropriately to patients' nutritional questions. Each chapter is extensively referenced, so that the evidence from which conclusions are drawn can be critically examined and so that these chapters can serve as a springboard for further study. It is also hoped that the motivated medical professional may use this volume for self-study, since various medical curricula may not have sufficient space to incorporate such a course as yet.

My goal in writing this nutrition handbook has been to depart from the shortcomings of "textbooks" while retaining a comprehensive, though not encyclopedic, volume. I have found textbooks often to be dry, voluminous, expensive works which are overly detailed in some areas and insufficiently detailed in others. In contrast, the style and tone of this volume are more toward the conversational and the practical. It is hoped that this is the type of book that the reader may care to peruse during lunch hour as well as in preparation for class.

It should be emphasized that this book is not meant to replace standard nutrition texts, if any, that are used in medical or paramedical training programs; this book builds upon those texts and picks up where those texts leave off. For the medical professional already in practice, it is likely that this book will be sufficient to answer most patients' nutritional questions.

Finally, although a thorough understanding of biochemistry (body's chemistry) is important, it is not required in order to understand this book. Consequently, I also envision this volume as a useful core text, with suitable amplification from the instructor, in undergraduate nutrition courses, even for students with little scientific background.

2) The second purpose of this book is to inform the layperson who is interested in learning more about nutrition. Having two such seemingly dissimilar target audiences (medical professional and layperson) demands several modifications in style and content. To facilitate the layperson's efforts in understanding the concepts and language, parenthetical phrases explain terms or concepts which may not be familiar to the non-medical person. Appendix A presents a simple explanation of the scientific method, which will help the reader (including the medical reader) to better appreciate the studies quoted in the text, while Appendix B is a glossary of all medical terms used in this book. There are some sections that the non-medical reader may find difficult to follow; these may be skipped without losing the continuity of the book. Such sections were included for the benefit of the interested medical reader. Friends without a medical background have read and understood this book without any difficulty, and have made suggestions, many of which have been incorporated into the book.

The reader who is not interested in the scientific analysis can still benefit from this volume. Most chapters are summarized in a section entitled "The Bottom Line", which presents recommendations which I believe are substantiated by the scientific data. However, this section is obviously subject to my own biases in interpretation of the studies, and the reader will ultimately benefit more by considering the scientific data for himself.

As can be noted from the table of contents, this book is divided into two sections. The first section, along with Appendix A, discusses the concept of how we know what we know, and how to separate fact from fiction. In order to illustrate these concepts, a review of some questionable regimens is undertaken, including starch blockers, Laetrile, herbal remedies and various "Life Extension" regimens. The point is made that many regimens often become very popular without any proof at all that they are either safe or effective.

The second section of the book discusses the "bread and butter" nutritional topics, like cholesterol and fats, salt and high blood pressure, vitamins, minerals, vegetarian diets and fiber. The latest, and sometimes surprising data on these topics, is reviewed.

Chapter 13 in the second section deals with obesity, perhaps the most common nutrition-related disease. This chapter builds upon the concepts developed in earlier chapters and extends them to the obesity field. The many facets of obesity, from etiology (cause), pathogenesis (how it develops) and harmful effects, to the medical and popular approaches to its management, are briefly reviewed. Finally, several of the more popular "popular" diets are described and discussed, using scientific literature to support or refute various claims.

I have searched the medical literature for scientifically well-designed studies which are relevant to the topics of this book. This volume is a distillation of many scientific and some lay books, and more than 5000 scientific articles were reviewed during the preparation of this volume. More than 1000 references are cited in this book. Most references are very current; about two-thirds of the references have been published since 1980, and almost half were published in 1984 and 1985.

The reader should realize, however, that although this book is up-to-date in 1986, the nature of medical research is such that new facts continuously appear, although the basic principles often don't change. This is the reason that principles, and not only selected facts, are stressed in this book. In this way, the reader will be able to evaluate new information as it comes along. This flux in knowledge should not be a cause for concern but should be taken into account as the book is read. The nature of science is that of a dynamic living creature, and that, to me, is one of its greatest attributes. I sincerely hope that the reader will share with me in this adventure as he reads the following pages.

I apologize to readers of this book for using "he" when "he or she" would be more accurate. The reader should rest assured that such use was adopted strictly for ease of composition and reading, and is not meant to be sexist. Indeed, the first draft of this book did contain "he or she" but was found extremely cumbersome.

Finally, I invite comments from all readers. The reader may contact me c/o Popular Medicine Press, P.O. Box 12607, Toledo, OH 43606. All comments and suggestions will be carefully considered during the preparation of future editions.

REFERENCES

1. Editorial. Nutrition in medical education. Lancet 1:1422, 1983.
2. Stunkard AJ: Obesity and the social environment: Current status, future prospects. In Bray GA (Ed.): Obesity in America, NIH publication #80-359, 1980.

SECTION ONE

WHOM SHOULD YOU BELIEVE?

"We should have our minds open, but not so open that our brains fall out"

Allen Ross Anderson
eminent philosopher

CHAPTER 1

The Laetrile and Starch Blocker Stories

The question as to whom you should believe is becoming progressively more crucial with the passage of time. A century ago, the physician's word and opinion were viewed as incontrovertible, and to doubt your physician was almost sacrilegious. This same doubt is encouraged these days (witness the encouragement of second opinions prior to surgery) and for good reasons, a full discussion of which is beyond the scope of this book. However, the more practical question of whom to believe is not only within the scope of this book—it is the heart of this book.

Nutrition has probably stimulated more discussion and controversy in the lay media than any other medical topic. Much has been made of the role of diet in degenerative diseases such as heart disease, cancer, diabetes, and stroke. These diseases are epidemic in the United States and other developed countries, and thus are of great public concern.

The widespread interest in nutrition and other "popular medicine" topics, like homeopathy, exercise, and chiropractic, is a two-edged sword. On the plus side, this interest makes the public more aware and educable about concepts that may greatly affect the quality and quantity of their life. On the other hand, a gullible public can be easily persuaded to pursue forms of therapy that may either be of little value, or even harmful, and in some unfortunate cases, lethal.

Many diets and "nutritional" programs pandered to the public include high doses of various substances. In most cases, this is recommended by the seller without scientific evidence to support the recommendation. It is often argued that since the substance is "natural", it cannot be harmful, even in megadoses. As will be clearly demonstrated in Chapters 2 and 3, nothing could be further from the truth. Plain water and oxygen, two substances essential for life, can, in excess, both cause death. Even chicken soup, the venerable remedy, can be harmful (1).

To a large extent, one's approach to such claims is based on a philosophical difference, although it is rarely recognized as such. Proponents say that substance X (e.g., vitamin C, or selenium, or Laetrile, etc.) is "innocent until proven guilty"; they put the burden of proof on opponents of that regimen to show that the approach is ineffective and/or harmful. The scientific approach, on the other hand, is based on the null hypothesis, which states that substance X is useless and probably harmful until proven otherwise. Please consult Appendix A for a more in-depth discussion of the scientific method. It may be appropriate to read Appendix A at this time since appreciation of the material which follows will be enhanced if the concepts presented in Appendix A are understood.

Each person has to choose which of the two philosophies discussed above he adheres to. In some cases, e.g., terminal cancer, even scientists may require little proof before trying a certain therapy; however, most scientists would require considerable proof of efficacy *and* safety before suggesting an unusual nutritional therapy with purported future benefits to people that are currently healthy. In other words, if substance X offers both risks and benefits, which *all* substances do, the terminal cancer patient has little to lose, whereas the healthy patient has much to lose. Although the substance is the same, the cost-benefit analysis is quite different for the two individuals. What makes this analysis difficult is that often neither the long-term benefits nor risks are known, but it is assumed that since the person is healthy to begin with, he has more to lose than gain. Since most readers of this book will be presumably healthy (and in view of the author's scientific background), the bias in this book will be toward the scientific method, i.e., that a regimen must show both efficacy and safety prior to its use. In many cases, seemingly benign treatments (e.g., thyroid irradiation [x-rays] in the 1950s or thalidomide in the 1960s) are found to be harmful only years later (causing thyroid cancer and birth defects, respectively).

Let's now consider two more recent examples of this sort.

STARCH BLOCKERS

An example of a dietary fad with no apparent benefit is the recent craze of taking starch blockers as a diet aid. Phaseolamin, a substance in raw kidney beans, was shown to inhibit the action of amylase in 1945 (1a). Amylase is an enzyme made in the body which digests starch. It was noted that rats fed uncooked kidney beans grew poorly, and this was attributed to the amylase-inhibiting actions of phaseolamin (2). Phaseolamin was purified 30 years later (3), at which time it was proposed, logically, I think, that eating phaseolamin could block the digestion (and thus absorption) of ingested carbohydrate. Figure 1-1 is a diagrammatic representation of this hypothesis.

This hypothesis was never tested in humans, although a related amylase inhibitor was shown to decrease postprandial serum glucose (blood sugar level after a meal)—a response which should probably be further studied. It was also shown that although this related amylase inhibitor did slow starch absorption

Figure 1-1

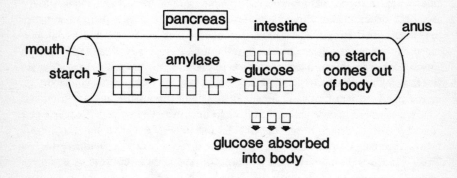

NORMAL SITUATION

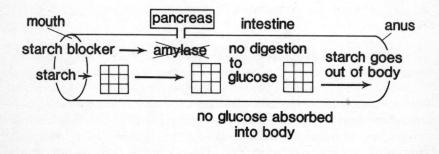

WITH STARCH BLOCKER

Proposed mechanism of action of starch blockers
Starch blocker (lower panel) supposedly block the action of amylase. If amylase action is inhibited, it cannot digest starch and the starch leaves the body in the stool.

(which probably accounted for the decrease in postprandial serum glucose), *total* starch absorption was unchanged—no undigested starch was found in the stool. In addition, the serum-glucose-lowering effect of this amylase inhibitor was markedly diminished when cooked (as opposed to raw) starch was fed to rats, a more realistic test (4).

Despite the lack of evidence for clinical efficacy (evidence that a substance does what it's supposed to do) of phaseolamin, nor any testing of its side effects, over 200 different starch blocker preparations were widely sold in pharmacies and health-food stores in 1982 (5). The question of safety is not a trivial one, since many natural substances can be quite toxic, especially when taken in high doses. However, since starch blockers were initially marketed as dietary aids, the Food and Drug Administration (FDA) could not (or so it was assumed by the starch blocker manufacturers) regulate the sale of these substances.

In the advertising (Figure 1-2), it was claimed that each starch blocker tablet was capable of "inactivating" the 600 calories in 150 grams of starch (6). This "having your cake and eating it too" (or having your cake and not absorbing it either) so appealed to an overweight public always looking for an easy fix that in early 1982, over one million starch blocker tablets were estimated to be consumed daily in the United States (5). Indeed, due to widely publicized news stories that the "bad" FDA was going to take these great treats off the market, the public started stockpiling these tablets. In July 1982, the FDA classified starch blockers as drugs (and therefore within its jurisdiction) and insisted that sales be stopped until safety and efficacy had been shown. Some of the manufacturers sued, but their suit was denied, and in October, 1982, a federal court in Chicago upheld the right of the FDA to designate the products as drugs and thus to control their distribution.

The reader should note that the public and starch blocker manufacturer uproar to retain starch blockers on the market occurred in the absence of any scientific evidence that these products *were either efficacious or safe*.

A study which carefully and thoroughly investigated the alleged starch-blocking and calorie-sparing claims was recently published in the New England Journal of Medicine (7). The starch blocker purveyors claim that by blocking amylase activity in the small intestine, carbohydrate digestion will be prevented, and thus, the undigested carbohydrate (and its calories) will pass out in the stool. This idea can be simply tested by measuring the calories in the stool of a person eating two identical meals, one with starch blockers and one without. If the meal contains 400 starch calories, one would expect that, if starch blockers actually work, the stool following the meal containing starch blocker should contain approximately 400 more calories than the stool following the meal eaten without starch blocker.

Well, this is the exact experiment that Bo-Linn and colleagues performed (7). They studied five healthy volunteers. Before the test meal, a tube was passed into

Figure 1-2

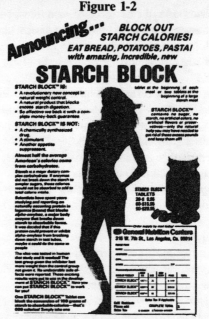

Starch blocker advertisement
See text (ref. 6).

the stomach, and the gastrointestinal tract (tract from mouth to anus) was washed clean. After the washout, the subjects consumed a placebo (fake) starch blocker with the test meal (spaghetti, sauce, bread, margarine, water) containing 19g protein, 14g fat and 108g carbohydrate (97g starch), totaling 680 calories (388 starch calories). The gut was then washed out and the calories in the washing measured. The identical meal was then eaten again, except that this time *real* starch blocker was taken, and the gut was washed out again.

Two types of starch blockers were tested. One (Carbo-Lite) was chosen because it is manufactured under the supervision of Dr. Marshall, who first purified and characterized phaseolamin (3), and because this brand has been shown by *in vitro* (test tube) tests to produce the stated amount of anti-amylase activity. In addition, *three* tablets were given, two at the beginning of the meal and one half-way through the meal, even though only one would be needed according to the starch blocker claims.

The results were interesting. The gut washings after the placebo starch blocker averaged 80 calories, while after the 3 actual starch blocker tablets, the washings averaged 78 calories in the five volunteers. There was absolutely no difference in starch digestion or absorption from the same meal in the same people with and without starch blockers!

Thus, this extremely carefully performed study showed that starch blockers do not decrease the absorption of carbohydrate, and thus couldn't be expected to decrease body weight. As discussed in an editorial in the same issue of the New England Journal of Medicine (NEJM), this lack of efficacy raises questions about marketing, consumer response, and the proper role of regulatory agencies in controlling the availability of such quasi-nutritional products.

Two other studies, utilizing different techniques, have also demonstrated the ineffectiveness of starch blockers (8,9). The authors of this study (7) speculated that the human pancreas could secrete so much amylase that even if a little was blocked by the starch blocker, there was plenty of reserve. An analogous situation is that pancreatic secretion of lipase, a fat-digesting enzyme, must be reduced by more than 90% before malabsorption (poor absorption) of fat occurs (10). Other possible explanations include insufficient time for the blocker to bind and inactivate the amylase, and the possible digestion of the starch blocker (it is itself a type of protein) by the enzymes in the gut. Interestingly, an editorial in the Lancet (11) postulated that even if starch blockers *were* able to block starch absorption in the GI tract, they wouldn't result in weight loss because the person would probably increase his food intake to compensate for the poorly absorbed starch.

The point of this discourse was both to show that starch blockers do not perform as their proponents claimed, and to raise the reader's suspicion the next time that he is presented with poorly-substantiated claims.

LAETRILE

The unwary public is frequently duped into spending money for worthless miracle cures, but beyond the loss of a little money and the disappointment following lack of benefit, little harm is done. Starch blockers were presented as an example of this. Sometimes, however, such misinformation leads to a dangerous, or even lethal, practice. Two examples of this are the liquid protein diets (discussed in Chapter 13) and Laetrile. Let us consider the latter in some detail because I think the take-home message of this chapter, namely, the inadvisability of following unsubstantiated claims, should be firmly established before going on to the rest of the book.

Amygdalin (Laetrile, "vitamin" B_{17}), a substance derived from raw bitter almonds and apricot pits, has been employed medically for many centuries. Ancient herbal pharmacopeias (books of drugs) recommended the bitter almond for the treatment of a variety of illnesses, including drunkenness and hemorrhoids. Current amygdalin use dates from the 1950s, when it was initially marketed as a remedy for cancer (12). The legislatures of over half the states had legalized its use by 1982 (13).

In 1978, the National Cancer Institute (NCI) solicited over 400,000 medical professionals and pro-Laetrile groups to submit cases of patients thought to have benefited from Laetrile (14). Although it is estimated that over 70,000 Americans have used the drug, only 93 cases were submitted for evaluation, of which only 68 were sufficiently complete to evaluate. Twelve oncologists (doctors specializing in cancer) evaluated these 68 cases and compared them to 68 conventional chemotherapy patients and 24 no treatment control cases. The oncologists, who did not know who had received Laetrile and who had received conventional chemotherapy, judged Laetrile to have produced two complete responses and four partial responses. As had been previously predicted by some, "These results allow no definite conclusions supporting the anticancer activity of Laetrile" (14).

Prior to this NCI review, there had been suggestions both for (15-18) and against (19) legalization and/or a full-scale clinical trial of Laetrile. The reason that some highly respected physicians (15-18) recommended legalization of Laetrile or the performance of a clinical trial is best explained by Dr. Ingelfinger, former editor-in-chief of the NEJM,

> "If any agent offers but a glimmer of hope, the denunciation or prohibition of such an agent—Laetrile in this case—by the FDA, the AMA or any other organization, will only swell the ranks of those clamoring for this extract of apricot pits. Forbidden fruits are mighty tasty . . ." (16).

The NCI chose first (20) to conduct the survey of Laetrile effects (described above), but after the inconclusive results (14), the decision to perform a prospective trial was made; this definitive study is described below. Many proponents of antiestablishment "popular" medicine complain about the lack of interest among practitioners of Western medicine in potentially promising but unconventional treatments. In this regard, the study by Mayo Clinic investigators Moertel et al (21), of the efficacy and safety of Laetrile, deserves particular mention. This was a study performed under the auspices of organized medicine which was responsive to some very unconventional, unproven, but widespread quasi-medical practices. Indeed, many physicians felt that it was unethical to conduct a prospective trial of a substance without any evidence of efficacy (19). Moertel and his colleagues (21) bent over backwards to anticipate and accommodate any possible objections that proponents of Laetrile might have about the study.

The study selected patients with terminal cancer in whom conventional chemotherapy was not expected to prolong survival. Thus, any response that would have been noted would have been ascribed to the Laetrile. Furthermore, to blunt criticism from Laetrilists that sick patients had been chosen, the Laetrile recipients in this study were otherwise healthy, and fully a third had never received chemotherapy or radiation therapy. These individuals would consequently have the greatest chance of responding to Laetrile, since patients unresponsive to previous therapy often have more "resistant" forms of cancer. No patient had undergone surgery, radiotherapy, or chemotherapy—which could confuse interpretation of the study—during the month prior to study. Disabled or bedridden patients were not eligible to participate in the study.

The Laetrile was supplied by the Pharmaceutical Resources Branch of the NCI, made to correspond to the product distributed by the major Mexican supplier. The identity and potency of the Laetrile were established by no less than six analytic techniques at the NCI, and each drug lot was also studied for purity by the Mayo Clinic investigators.

The route, dosage and schedule of administration were chosen after consultation with Laetrile practitioners. Laetrile was even combined with the so-called "metabolic" therapy (megavitamins and a "natural" diet) so enthusiastically touted by Laetrile therapists. The Mayo investigators had difficulty in obtaining a consensus among the Laetrile practitioners on what constituted appropriate metabolic therapy. Some Laetrilists felt that such therapy was not needed while others urged megadoses. The investigators compromised and used high but not massive doses in most patients. To meet anticipated objections of some Laetrilists, some patients received higher doses of both Laetrile (50% higher than the regular dose) and of vitamins. For instance, standard dose therapy included 4.5 $g/m^2/d$ of Laetrile, 25,000 U of vitamin A, 2 g of vitamin C, and 400 U of vitamin E; the high dose regimen utilized daily doses of Laetrile of 7.0 g/m^2, 100,000 U of vitamin A, 10 g of vitamin C, and 1200 U of vitamin E.

The patients were put on diets currently recommended by most Laetrile proponents, which restrict eggs, dairy products, refined-flour products, refined sugar and sugar-coated cereals, salt, coffee, tea, cola and all alcoholic beverages. The consumption of fresh fruit and vegetables, whole grain breads and cereals, seeds, nuts, raisins, dates and figs was encouraged.

Beyond the special concessions in study design mentioned above, this study was conducted in a manner entirely comparable to that in other studies testing a new anticancer drug. This study was designed to provide the maximum opportunity for Laetrile to display anticancer activity if any existed.

A total of 175 patients with cancer received Laetrile and could be evaluated for response. Tumor types included a preponderance of colorectal, lung and breast cancers.

Not even one of the 175 Laetrile recipients had a total response to Laetrile. Only *one* met the established and widely accepted criteria for partial response. The partial response (a temporary decrease in tumor size) was maintained for 10 weeks, but was then followed by clear progression of the cancer and death of the patient after 37 weeks of Laetrile therapy. For unclear reasons, such partial responses also occur spontaneously on occasion.

Of 178 patients entered at the beginning of the study, 152 had died at the time of publication of the article (21), and average survival was 4.8 months from the start of therapy. The survival times were similar to those that would be anticipated in comparable patients receiving no treatment. The results for the 14 high-dose therapy recipients were very similar. No responses were noted, and average survival was 5 months.

In reviewing these data, one might say that although Laetrile was obviously of no benefit, at least it did no harm. Unfortunately, this was not the case, because commercial Laetrile has been shown to release cyanide, especially when it is taken with raw almond or apricot pits. Several patients receiving Laetrile experienced nausea, vomiting, headache, dizziness and mental obtundation (being "out of it"). These symptoms were associated with high blood levels of cyanide in several patients, and subsided promptly when the Laetrile was discontinued. One patient receiving the high-dose regimen had episodes of tachycardia (fast heart rate) and dyspnea (difficulty breathing) two hours after her morning dose of Laetrile. Her blood cyanide level during one of these episodes was 2.9 ug/ml, a dangerous level.

Eleven patients had worrisome cyanide levels. The highest level recorded was just under 4 ug/ml, which is of concern since levels >3 ug/ml are considered potentially fatal (22). One patient had symptoms typical of cyanide toxicity when she took large amounts of raw almonds with her Laetrile—an unwise practice since raw almonds contain an enzyme (glucosidase) which increases the release of cyanide from Laetrile.

Since several deaths from cyanide toxicity have been reported in people taking Laetrile (23-25), special precautions to avoid fatal cyanide reactions were a vital component of this study. Who knows how many Laetrile recipients have died from cyanide poisoning and not cancer (as was probably assumed) in Laetrile regimens where technically demanding cyanide levels were not as carefully monitored as in this study?

This study demonstrates that Laetrile is clearly both ineffective and dangerous. Particular attention was paid to current methods of Laetrile practitioners. Despite this, Laetrile proved ineffective, and dangerous cyanide levels were recorded. Since many Laetrilists recommend the ingestion of raw almonds with Laetrile, one wonders how familiar these practitioners are with the dangers of Laetrile. Add to this the hazards associated with the administration of a drug from questionable sources (indeed, Laetrile from the major Mexican supplier has been found to have a high frequency of germ contamination (26)) and one becomes even more concerned about the claims of Laetrile practitioners.

In his editorial on this topic in the same issue of the NEJM (13), Dr. Arnold Relman (current editor-in-chief of the NEJM), made the following comments:

"Laetrile, I believe, has now had its day in court. The evidence, beyond reasonable doubt, is that it doesn't benefit patients with advanced cancer . . .some undoubtedly will remain unconvinced, but no sensible person will want to advocate its further use and no state legislature should sanction it any longer. The time has come to close the books on Laetrile and get on with our efforts to understand the riddle of cancer and improve its prevention and treatment".

One wonders how many lawsuits a drug manufacturer would be facing if the FDA had approved Laetrile as an official drug and then all of its toxic effects were discovered. The consumerist uproar that the FDA hadn't done its job would be deafening.

THE BOTTOM LINE

These well-documented examples—of starch blockers and Laetrile—should help the reader, whether medical professional or lay person, to put widely-touted but poorly-substantiated claims in perspective. It will arm the medical professional with sufficient information to convince a patient not to readily accept everything he hears. At the same time, the intelligent lay person will be equipped with some healthy skepticism which may enable him to easily ferret out the next charlatan.

REFERENCES

1. Fujiwara P, et al: Chicken-soup hypernatremia. N Engl J Med 313:161,1985
1a. Bowman DE: Amylase inhibitor of navy beans. Science 102:358, 1945
2. Jaffe WG, Lette CL: Heat-labile growth inhibiting factors in beans (Phaseolus vulgaris). J Nutr 94:203, 1968
3. Marshall JJ, Lauda CM: Purification and properties of phaseolamin, an inhibitor of alpha-amylase, from the kidney bean, Phaseolus vulgaris. J Biol Chem 250:8030, 1975
4. Puls W, Keup U: Influence of an alpha-amylase inhibitor (BAYd 7791) on blood glucose, serum insulin and NEFA in starch loading tests in rats, dogs and man. Diabetologia 9:97, 1973
5. Rosenberg IH: Starch blockers—still no calorie-free lunch. N Engl J Med 307:1444, 1982
6. Los Angeles Times, June 20, 1982, Part IV, p.19
7. Bo-Linn GW, et al: Starch blockers—their effects on calorie absorption from a high-starch meal. N Engl J Med 307:1413, 1982
8. Garrow JS, et al: Starch blockers are ineffective in man. Lancet 1:60, 1983
9. Carlson GL, et al: A bean alpha-amylase inhibitor formulation (starch blocker is ineffective in man. Science 219:393, 1983
10. DiMagno EP, et al: Relations between pancreatic enzyme outputs and malabsorption in severe pancreatic insufficiency. N Engl J Med 288:813,1973
11. Editorial: The starch blocker idea. Lancet 1:569, 1983
12. Moertel CG, et al: A pharmacologic and toxicologic study of amygdalin. JAMA 245:591, 1981

13. Relman AS: Closing the books on laetrile. N Engl J Med 306:236, 1982

14. Ellison NM, et al: Special report on Laetrile: The NCI Laetrile review. Results of the National Cancer Institute retrospective Laetrile analysis. N Engl J Med 299:549, 1978

15. Ashai S, et al: Legalization of Laetrile—a suggestion. N Engl J Med 295:116, 1976

16. Ingelfinger FJ: Laetrilomania. N Engl J Med 296:1167, 1977

17. Moertel CG: A trial of Laetrile now. N Engl J Med 298:218, 1978

18. Relman AS: Laetrilomania—again. N Engl J Med 298:215, 1978

19. Lipsett MB, Fletcher JC: Ethics of Laetrile clinical trials. N Engl J Med 297:1183, 1977

20. Newell GR: Clinical evaluation of Laetrile: Two perspectives. Why the National Cancer Institute chooses a case-record review of Laetrile. N Engl J Med 298:216, 1978

21. Moertel CG, et al : A clinical trial of amygdalin (Laetrile) in the treatment of human cancer. N Engl J Med 306:201, 1982

22. Graham DE, et al: Acute cyanide poisoning complicated by lactic acidosis and pulmonary edema. Arch Intern Med 137:1051, 1977

23. Herbert V: Laetrile: the cult of cyanide. Promoting poison for profit. In Cunningham JJ (Ed.): Controversies in Clinical Nutrition. George Stickley Co., Philadelphia, 1980, pp. 190-227

24. Sadoff L, et al: Rapid death associated with Laetrile ingestion. JAMA 239:1532, 1978

25. Humbert JR, et al: Laetrile intoxication: report of a fatal case. N Engl J Med 300:238, 1979

26. Davignon JP, et al: Pharmaceutical assessment of amygdalin (Laetrile) products. Cancer Treatment Rep 62:99, 1978

CHAPTER 2

Homeopathy, Herbal Medicine and the Medical Establishment

This chapter is, in a sense, a continuation and expansion of the concepts presented in the previous chapter. However, whereas Chapter 1 was restricted to the claims of Laetrile and starch blocker enthusiasts, this chapter will evaluate other quasi-medical approaches to disease. These quasi-medical and some frankly-fraudulent modalities have recently attracted the attention of the FDA, leading to the creation of a new fraud branch in the Center for Drugs and Biologics. Fighting health fraud has become one of the top priorities in the FDA's new action plan, and the FDA, in collaboration with several other interested groups, is mounting a national ad campaign to educate the public about health fraud.

What makes things difficult for the consumer is the fact that while many (probably *most*) unconventional approaches have failed the tests of both science and time, some alternative remedies have shown promise in initial scientific experiments. It is unfortunate that proponents of such therapies rarely subject their claims or practices to objective scientific evaluation; fortunately, enough studies have been done to give us a scientific bird's-eye view of these regimens.

EVALUATING ALTERNATIVE HEALTH CARE STRATEGIES

In a recent editorial, two scientists made several observations on alternative health systems that are germane to this book (1). They noted that Western physicians presumably do what they do (prescribe medicine, recommend surgery, etc.) because they believe that these recommendations are based on scientific evidence that has shown them to be effective. It is true (as demonstrated in Appendix A) that this not always the case, and that scientific evidence is fallible, but when possible, recommendations are made on the basis of scientific evidence. Lack of scientific support for a certain regimen does not necessarily imply lack of value of that regimen, but if presented with two choices, the Western, scientifically-trained physician should always choose the one with the better *documented* benefit-to-risk ratio. If the reader does not agree with this premise, then this book will be meaningless to him because that is the central premise from which this book evolved.

Thus, therapeutic decisions should be guided by scientific evidence. This is not to say, however, that the personal aspects of the doctor-patient relationship must be lacking. The fact that some doctors don't take the time to comfort and console their patients should not imply that Western medicine is inadequate. There is *nothing* mutually exclusive between adhering to the scientific precepts noted above and also taking the time to consider the non-physical (psychological, social,situational, etc.) causes of ill health. Indeed, many medical schools are now emphasizing the more humanistic aspects of the doctor-patient relationship. Thus when a holistic practitioner offers to evaluate the "whole" patient ("Fundamental to holistic medicine is the recognition that each state of health and disease requires a consideration of all contributing factors: psychological, psychosocial, environmental and spiritual" (2)), he is not offering anything that a good conventionally-trained physician can't offer. What only the holistic practitioner will offer are treatments like psychic healing, tai chi, chiropractic, iridology, herbs and homeopathic remedies, clairvoyant diagnosis, human auras, etc. Most of these techniques are unrelated to nutrition and will therefore not be considered in this book. However, it may be instructive to examine a few of these (e.g., iridology and chiropractic) since they are commonly employed and because the concepts of this chapter can be illustrated utilizing these examples. Prior to considering these specific examples, some general comments about alternative health care systems may be warranted.

Alternative medicine has recently received significant attention in the scientific literature, especially in England. A recent survey (3) was undertaken to explore the attitudes of British doctor trainees to alternative medicine. Of the 86 physicians responding, 18 were already using at least one alternative treatment in their practice, while 70 wanted to train in one or more. Twelve of these doctors had referred patients to non-medically-qualified practitioners and 22 had been themselves treated by an alternative practitioner.

Both this article and the accompanying editorial (4) generated significant correspondence (5). The editorial took a balanced view of alternative medicine, calling for controlled clinical trials to either support or refute the validity of various alternative therapies. The letters to the editor were much more polarized, one suggesting that alternative medicine has flourished due to the failures of conventional physicians in addressing the "whole" person, while another stated that before these young doctors embrace alternative medicine, they should ask for controlled clinical trials. Another editorial (6) in the British literature made the very important point that since the term alternative medicine has come to embrace every practice from the frankly fraudulent to the probably useful, each individual modality must be examined in its own right.

Although the above references suggest a polarization between orthodox and alternative medicine, some authors have argued that the two modalities are in fact *complementary* (6a-c). In these surveys, patients appeared to be satisfied with both types of medicine, and did not appear to abandon orthodox medicine while embracing heterodox, or alternative, modalities. This finding has not been universal, however; in a study of cancer patients, 40% of patients abandoned conventional care entirely after adopting alternative methods (6d). It is this abandonment of orthodox medicine, rather than the pursuit of complementary methods, that concerns most physicians, especially those dealing with cancer patients.

For unclear reasons, it appears that the American literature has been somewhat less accepting of alternative medicine. In an article entitled "Science and Scam: Alternative Thought Patterns in Alternative Health Care" (7), Dr. Fitzgerald divides proponents of alternative modalities into three types: (a) the *true believer*, who does not respond to scientific reason and is reminiscent of a religious zealot, (b) the *mercantilist*, the basic con artist who's out to make a fast buck, (c) the *audience*, the American people, whose allegiance is to efficacy (i.e., does it *work*?) rather than to logic (i.e., maybe a placebo would work just as well?). During her media appearances, Dr. Fitzgerald was impressed that members of the audience believed (erroneously) that science had or could easily obtain the answers to all medical problems, and that if orthodox medicine didn't provide the answer, it (e.g., the AMA, FDA, etc.) was concealing it for commercial reasons.

She also found that the audience believed that well-being is normal and that if one does not exude health and happiness from every pore perpetually, therapy is required. Perhaps medicine (and the media, too) are at fault here. We in medicine have often been accorded (and played along with) the notion that medical science is omnipotent and that failures, if not non-existent, are rare. I remember being recently confronted by an incredulous patient who didn't believe me when I told him that we didn't have any medicine to cure the common cold. He retorted, "Do you mean to tell me, Doc, that you guys can keep a guy with an artificial heart alive for several months but can't cure the common cold?" Perhaps this book will enable the reader to understand both the methods and the capabilities of science. Other references on alternative medicine (8-10) should be consulted by the interested reader.

Another unscientific concept in several alternative health care systems is the common thread, especially in holistic thinking, that "*all* states of ill health and *all* disorders are considered to be psychosomatic" (2) (emphasis mine). This seems a bit extreme; being hit by a car while crossing the street or contracting rabies after being bitten by a rabid animal would hardly qualify as psychosomatic conditions.

It is often stated that alternative health care has not been properly investigated, and that funds ought to be made available for evaluating such practices; meanwhile, it is recommended that we keep our minds open about unconventional approaches to disease. There are several answers to this:

1. It is customary for proponents of new, untested regimens to present at least preliminary evidence supporting the efficacy and safety of the regimen. Much research could be easily and cheaply done by alternative health practitioners themselves (see some of the articles in the latter portion of this chapter). Unfortunately, many alternative health care practitioners do not believe that such evaluation is necessary or that they are obliged to participate. Skeptics have said that proponents of alternative health practices have no interest in conducting such studies because if the studies show the practice to be worthless, they have nothing to gain, and a lot to lose.

2. In medical research, funds are rarely assigned to a research project unless preliminary evidence suggests a reasonable chance for success. Without such preliminary research, it is difficult to support grant applications for money to investigate alternative health practices. Indeed, in the majority of instances when research of alternative health care practices has been done, it has shown them to be either ineffective or less effective than standard medical practice. Negative preliminary research is hardly supportive of further financial outlay for research.

3. Western medicine has often investigated popular medical practices *despite* the lack of positive preliminary evidence or even in the presence of negative initial studies (see Chapter 1). In most such instances, when practices without preliminary supportive evidence were investigated, negative results were obtained. In view of this, how should society decide when to expend rare and limited resources? Is the current evidence against Laetrile and iridology good enough to discount these modalities? Was it good enough before the latest studies? Could the funds expended on these studies have been applied to more promising therapies? Since society's resources for research are not unlimited, it behooves us to assign research funds to those projects which are most promising. Certainly, "we should leave our minds open, but not", in the words of the eminent philosopher, Alan Ross Anderson, "so open that our brains fall out" (1).

It has often been said that even if alternative modalities don't truly work, they should still be available to individuals who request them, even if only for their placebo benefits. Proponents of alternative health care systems often say that no harm can be done, and that some good may ensue. As was shown with Laetrile, this is certainly not true. In this chapter, we will briefly consider another example of this type—Christian Science (on occasion derogatorily referred to as Christian *non*-Science)—wherein the availability of an alternative modality can be fatal.

CHRISTIAN SCIENCE

Christian Science, which depends entirely on the healing powers of prayer, teaches that its approach to healing is exclusive, i.e., it "cannot be combined with medical treatment" (11). This has resulted in the death of many children, who died from infectious diseases while being treated with prayer only (instead of antibiotics). Rita Swan, a former devout Christian Scientist whose son recently died of meningitis, is president of Children's Healthcare Is a Legal Duty (CHILD), an organization devoted to the protection of children's health.

In an article in the NEJM (12), Mrs. Swan notes that the entire training of Christian Science healers consists of two weeks of religious instruction. Christian Science rejects not only drugs, but even the simplest actions of a healer such as hot packs, ice packs and backrubs. Its nurses cannot take a temperature or pulse or recognize communicable diseases which must legally be reported. It is shocking that such care qualifies as a tax-deductible expense (which means that the federal government is subsidizing Christian Science "healing") and that Medicare and many insurance companies reimburse recipients of such care. It seems inconsistent for the government to require mandatory reporting of *suspected* child abuse, while allowing children to die of meningitis because their parents deny them readily available and effective medical care, which in my opinion is *clear* child abuse. Mrs. Swan cites a case in 1973 wherein California obtained a manslaughter conviction against parents whose Fundamentalist beliefs directed them to deny their son insulin, while simultaneously recognizing the prayers of a "duly accredited" Christian Science practitioner as proper health care of children. I quote Mrs. Swan:

> "In my opinion, the state has no business determining which churches are 'well recognized' and passing out special privileges to them. The state should not be giving Christian Science practitioners special authority on the basis of accreditation by their church."

In rebuttal to Mrs. Swan's commentary, Nathan Talbot, a senior Christian Science church official in Boston, says that the Church speaks of its care as "scientific" because "its truth has been demonstrated through practical healing experience time and time again" (13). Mr. Talbot says that there are approximately 50,000 published "testimonies of healing" in the denomination's periodicals. I'm afraid that anecdotal experience by biased parties, however extensive it may allegedly be, is hardly what a true scientist would consider "scientific".

Many letters to the editor condemning Christian Science were received (14). One correspondent described the poor care her husband received in a Christian Science facility, which she believed resulted in his death. Another suggested that although Fleming discovered penicillin, God created it, and that therefore, using drugs can be properly considered part of spiritual healing. One writer suggested a scientific trial comparing the efficacy of Christian Science healing against antibiotics in, for instance, meningitis. Although the interested reader should review these articles carefully, even a cursory analysis of the discussion should readily reveal that the Christian Science argument is not scientific, and that is one of the points of this chapter.

Several popular alternative modalities which have been examined in reasonably scientific fashion are discussed below. Unfortunately, only a few such studies are available, and consequently, this chapter must, of necessity, be more eclectic than comprehensive.

IRIDOLOGY

Iridology is the analysis of health and disease based on examination of the iris. Iridologists believe that each part of the iris represents a different organ in the body. Though iridology has been much criticized (15), it has never been scientifically studied. One reason for the criticism, no doubt, is the lack of an even remotely credible hypothesis to explain how pathology in a distant corner of the body may be expressed in the iris. Secondly, no scientific evidence has come from iridologists to support their practice. Therefore, this is the sort of practice that probably doesn't even merit the expenditure of scarce research funds. Due to the popularity of the technique, however, and the ability to mount such an experiment without any danger to the patients, such an experiment was performed (16).

Three iridologists were asked to evaluate iris photographs of 143 subjects. Some of the subjects were healthy, while others had kidney disease, including 21 in whom disease was severe enough to require dialysis. One of the iridologists (observer A) is world-renowned and the author of what is considered to be the definitive text on iridology. All three iridologists felt, prior to conducting the study, that it was within their ability to discriminate levels of kidney function from the iris photographs. The camera used to take the photographs belonged to one of the iridologists, so that the pictures obtained were of a quality to which he and most iridologists were accustomed.

The slides were presented to the iridologists in their offices in random order. They were given the option of rejecting any slides that were of a quality rendering analysis impossible or errant.

Observer A, the best screener, correctly identified kidney disease 57% of the time and correctly identified no disease 57% of the time. The other iridologists did even worse. A coin toss (i.e., mere chance) would correctly identify disease or health 50% of the time. Thus, iridology did no better statistically than flipping a coin.

Several points could be made by iridologists in response. One is that they are used to evaluating the "whole" patient, not just the iris in a photograph. If the iridologists felt this to be the case, they should have so stated, and the study wouldn't have been done this way. The iridologists believed, however, that this was within their capability. Another possible objection is that iridology could do better with another disease, but again, the iridologists were consulted prior to choosing kidney disease as the disease to study, and they felt comfortable with this choice. Thus if iridologists believe that they can ascertain disease and are in reality unable to do so, it casts serious doubts on their modality, suggesting that iridology is a practice without scientific merit.

HOMEOPATHY

Homeopathy is defined by the Merriam-Webster dictionary as a "system of medical practice that treats disease with minute doses of a remedy that would in healthy persons produce the symptoms of the disease treated." For instance, ipecac is a drug which induces vomiting. A homeopathic physician might use a million-fold dilution of ipecac to *treat* vomiting (16a). This is the homeopathic phenomenon of "aggravation," wherein the symptoms often become worse immediately after initiation of treatment, but allegedly, improvement follows. Although homeopathy is quite popular and is even covered under the British National Health Service, only a few scientific studies have investigated this modality.

The first, published in 1978 (17), showed some benefits of the homeopathic treatment. It was charged (18), however, that the design of that study was inadequate and that therefore the conclusions were not warranted. In an attempt to answer these criticisms, a double-blind trial was conducted comparing rheumatoid arthritis patients being treated by a combination of orthodox and homeopathic means to a similar group being treated by orthodox medications and placebo (19). Small but statistically significant improvements in pain, articular index, morning stiffness and grip strength were noted in the patients receiving the homeopathic remedies. No side effects or changes in blood tests were noted in patients receiving the homeopathic remedies. This study therefore suggested that a good benefit/risk ratio existed for homeopathic remedies and inspired a call for more such scientific trials of homeopathy (20). It should be recognized that since 20 different homeopathic herbs were used in this study, it is not clear which one(s) was(were) responsible for the improvement. In addition, the results from this study, though encouraging, can't be generalized to all homeopathic remedies.

Only one other scientific study evaluating homeopathy has been published (21). The investigators, composed of both homeopaths and conventional physicians, evaluated *Rhus tox 6x*, a common homeopathic remedy, against fenoprofen, a standard anti-arthritic drug, in double-blind placebo-controlled fashion in patients with osteoarthritis. The homeopathic remedy was judged by the patients to be no better than placebo, while fenoprofen was judged significantly better than placebo. Despite more side effects with fenoprofen, 21 of 31 patients preferred it, whereas 5 preferred the homeopathic remedy (and 5 preferred the placebo!).

In an editorial (22), this study drew praise due to the coooperation of homeopathic and allopathic ("regular") physicians, which the editor thought would preclude criticism of the trial. Such, however, was not the case. Several letters to the editor (23) were published; one correspondent charged that the study was biased in favor of fenoprofen, while another proclaimed that this study only confirmed the lack of efficacy of homeopathic remedies.

In response, the homeopathic authors of the paper said they were dismayed by the overreaction to their study findings. They noted that the study only showed that *Rhus* had no therapeutic effect in osteoarthritis when taken for 2 weeks, and that one could not logically extrapolate from this study to other doses or duration of treatment of *Rhus*, to other homeopathic remedies, or homeopathy in general. Although I would agree with this statement, the fact that this trial, which was conceived with the input of homeopathic practitioners, was unable to confirm the efficacy of a very commonly administered remedy, makes me skeptical about similar claims.

Perhaps the most logical approach to this quandary is that recently described in an article which stated that two-thirds of pediatric rheumatology (arthritis) patients had tried one or more unconventional treatments while receiving conventional care (24). Specific treatments included ointments, liniments, vitamins and minerals, faith healing, metal bracelets, aloe vera, DMSO, chiropractic, and elimination diets. Most patients reported that the unconventional treatments did not provide the degree of relief they had anticipated. The investigators felt, however, that since most of these therapies were of low cost and low side effect risk, that denial to their patients of these alternative therapies was unreasonable, as long as conventional therapy was also continued.

HERBAL AND "NATURAL" REMEDIES

Herbal remedies have become extremely popular in the last decade. Many health-food and several supermarket-type stores sell herbs for medicinal purposes, as do many chiropractors and other alternative health care personnel. Physicians, who may often see the herb recipients for other reasons, may be totally unfamiliar with the purported and *actual* effects of the herbs. A book by Tyler (25) is a good reference for health care professionals who are confronted with unfamiliar herbs.

It is often assumed by patients that herbs have only benefits and no side effects; physicians often adopt the opposite point of view. The truth is probably somewhere in between. The majority of herbs (indeed, the majority of *all* substances) are probably placebos and have minimal good and bad effects. Some herbs (and drugs) are more beneficial than harmful, while others have the opposite benefit-to-risk ratio. Harm can befall herbalists in other ways as well. One way is when the harmless herb that is bought is contaminated with poisonous substances (25a). Another is when the herbalist gathers a poisonous herb, mistaking it for a harmless one, with occasional fatal results (25b). The latter situation often occurs with wild mushrooms.

Usually derived from a plant, an herb is basically an aggregation of many chemical compounds. Some of the most potent drugs in our Western medical arsenal were initially used in the form of "herbal" remedies, e.g., digitalis from the foxglove plant, morphine and other strong painkillers from the poppy seed (opium). Although both morphine and digitalis are extremely useful, they are also both potentially fatal. Thus, the fact that a remedy is found in a plant says nothing about its potential for good or bad. This also applies to homeopathic remedies; thus, in the experiment which found that homeopathic remedies were of benefit in arthritis (17), it is quite possible that one or more of the 20 herbs used has medicinal properties in the Western sense.

These concepts seem fairly self-evident, but it is only recently that this sort of reasoning was accepted even in the medical community. Many in the medical community still do not accept it, but others are pursuing herbs as potential sources for Western medicines. As recently noted (26), a hybrid of Western and traditional Chinese medicine has been evolving in China since 1949. An international scientific meeting entitled "The Interaction of Traditional Chinese Medicine and Western Medicine: Impact on Immunology" was held recently at the new Cancer Institute in Beijing, China to discuss these topics. Scientists in both countries are using contemporary research procedures and controlled clinical trials to evaluate the efficacy of the most commonly used Chinese medicinal herbs.

For instance, a mixture of 11 herbs was found to prolong the lifespan of mice with leukemia. When each of the 11 herbs was tested individually, it was discovered that only *Indigo naturalis*, which itself contains many compounds, significantly prolonged the lifespan of the mice. When one of the compounds (indirubin) derived from this herb was tried in clinical trials, complete remission was observed in 82 of 314 patients with a type of leukemia (all data quoted here are from the article [26] mentioned above; no original references were cited in that article). This finding should not be surprising because some of the most potent anticancer drugs currently used in the United States are derivatives of natural products (e.g., vinca alkaloids, bleomycin, Adriamycin—see ref. 27 for further details).

The interested reader should also consult reference 28, a review article on herbs which appeared recently in the FDA Consumer, a magazine which the FDA publishes for the general public. Table 2-1 is a list of unsafe herbs which should not be used in foods or beverages and is reprinted from the article in the FDA Consumer.

In order to discuss the diverse effects of herbs, I have searched the medical literature for herb-related publications. Most of the citations are of a negative nature, showing the potential side effects of herbs, although some beneficial effects are also discussed.

Herbal Tea and Bleeding

A 25-year-old woman consulted her gynecologist about abnormally heavy menstrual bleeding (29). History revealed that she had been drinking large amounts of an herbal tea containing tonka beans, melilot, and woodruff, among other ingredients. These three herbal ingredients all contain natural coumarins, potent compounds that interfere with blood clotting and are on occasion prescribed by physicians as "blood thinners". The patient's abnormal bleeding stopped after she ceased to drink the tea.

Ginseng and Vaginal Bleeding

A 72-year-old woman experienced vaginal bleeding and a moderate estrogen effect after ingesting one tablet daily of a Swiss-Austrian geriatric formula containing 200 mg of ginseng (30). Ginseng has been reported to produce a physiological estrogenlike effect on the vaginal mucosa (resulting in vaginal bleeding in this woman) and breast pain with diffuse breast nodules in postmenopausal women.

Cryptic Illness from Herbal Remedy

An 80-year-old woman had had diarrhea for two months, became dehydrated and pale, lost weight and felt very weak and ill (31). Her serum potassium was low, she was anemic, and blood tests showed kidney function to be depressed (increased BUN and creatinine). She had been taking an alcoholic extract of herbs which was said to "help you become 100 years old in full health". The recipe included laxative herbs like senna, aloe, rhubarb and jalap (these would cause dehydration), and diuretic herbs like juniper berry and radix ononidis (these would exacerbate the dehydration and lower the blood potassium level). After stopping this "remedy" and increasing her intake of fruits and vegetables

Botanical Name of Plant Source	Common Names	Remarks
Arnica montana L.	Arnica. Arnica Flowers. Wolf's-bane. Leopard's Bane. Mountain Tobacco. Flores Arnicae.	Aqueous and alcoholic extracts of the plant contain choline, plus two unidentified substances that affect the heart and vascular systems. Arnica, an active irritant, can produce violent toxic gastroenteritis, nervous disturbances, change in pulse rate, intense muscular weakness, collapse and death.
Atropa belladonna L.	Belladonna. Deadly Nightshade.	Poisonous plant that contains the toxic solanaceous alkaloids hyoscyamine, atropine and hyoscine.
Solanum dulcamara L.	Bittersweet twigs. Dulcamara. Bittersweet. Woody Nightshade. Climbing Nightshade.	Poisonous. Contains the toxic glycoalkaloid solanine; also solanidine and dulcamarin.
Sanguinaris canadensis L.	Bloodroot. Sanguinaria. Red Puccoon.	Contains the poisonous alkaloid sanguinarine and other alkaloids.
Cytisus scoparius (L) Link.	Broom-tops. Scoparius. Spartium. Scotch Broom. Irish Broom. Broom.	Contains toxic sparteine, isosparteine and other alkaloids; also hydroxytyramine.
Aesculus hippocasteranum L.	Buckeyes. Aesculus. Horse Chestnut.	Contains a toxic coumarin glycoside, aesculin (esculin). A poisonous plant.
Acorus calamus L.	Calamus. Sweet Flag. Sweet Root. Sweet Cane. Sweet Cinnamon.	Oil of calamus, Jammu variety, is a carcinogen (causes cancer). FDA regulations prohibit marketing of calamus as a food or food additive.
Heliotropium europaeum L.	Heliotrope.	A poisonous plant. It contains alkaloids that produce liver damage. Not to be confused with garden heliotrope (*Valeriana officinalis* L.).
Conium maculatum L.	Hemlock. Conium. Poison Hemlock. Spotted Hemlock. Spotted Parsley. St. Bennet's Herb. Spotted Cowbane. Fool's Parsley.	Contains the poisonous alkaloid coniine and four other closely related alkaloids. Often confused with water hemlock (*Cicuta maculata* L.). Not to be confused with hemlock, hemlock spruce, etc. (*Tsuga canadensis* (L). Carr.).
Hyoscyamus niger L.	Henbane. Hyoscyamus. Black Henbane. Hog's Bean. Poison Tobacco. Devil's Eye.	Contains the alkaloids hyoscyamine, hyoscine (scopolamine) and atropine. A poisonous plant.
Exagonium purga (Wenderoth) Bentham. *Ipomoea jalapa* Nutt, and Coxe. *Ipomoea purga* (Wenderoth) Hayne. *Exagonium jalapa* (Wenderoth) Baillon.	Jalap Root. Jalap. True Jalap. Jalapa. Vera Cruz Jalap. High John Root. (Possibly also known as High John the Conqueror. John Conqueror. St. John the Conqueror Root. Hi John Conqueror.)	A large twining vine of Mexico, this plant has undergone many name changes. The drug is a powerful, drastic cathartic. Purgative powers of jalap reside in its resin. In overdoses, jalap may produce dangerous hypercatharsis.
Datura stramonium L.	Jimson Weed. Datura. Stramonium. Apple of Peru. Jamestown Weed. Thornapple. Tolguacha.	Contains the alkaloids atropine, hyoscyamine and scopolamine. Illegal drug for nonprescription use. A poisonous plant.
Convallaria majalis L.	Lily of the Valley. Convallaria. May Lily.	Contains the toxic cardiac glycosides convallatoxin, convallarin and convallamarin. Poisonous plant.

(continued on next page)

Unsafe herbs
List compiled by FDA of some herbs that should not be used in foods, beverages or drugs (ref. 28).

Botanical Name of Plant Source	Common Names	Remarks
Lobelia inflata L.	Lobelia. Indian Tobacco. Wild Tobacco. Asthma Weed. Emetic Weed.	A poisonous plant that contains the alkaloid lobeline plus a number of other pyridine alkaloids. Overdoses of the plant or extracts of the leaves or fruits produce vomiting, sweating, pain, paralysis, depressed temperatures, rapid but feeble pulse, collapse, coma and death.
Mandragora officinarum L.	Mandrake. Mandragora. European Mandrake.	The plant is a poisonous narcotic similar in its properties to belladonna. Contains the alkaloids hyoscyamine, scopolamine and mandragorine.
Podophyllum peltatum L.	Mandrake. May Apple. Podophyllum. American Mandrake. Devil's Apple. Umbrella Plant. Vegetable Calomel. Wild Lemon. Vegetable Mercury.	A poisonous plant, it contains podophyllotoxin, a complex polycyclic substance, and other constituents.
Phoradendron flavescens (Pursh.) Nutt. *Viscum flavescens* (Pursh.)	Mistletoe. Viscum. American Mistletoe.	Poisonous. Contains the toxic pressor amines B-phenylethylamine and tyramine.
Phoradendron juniperinum Engelm.	Mistletoe. Viscum. Juniper Mistletoe.	May be poisonous. Little is known about its properties.
Viscum album L.	Mistletoe. Viscum. European Mistletoe.	Poisonous. Contains the toxic pressor amines B-phenylethylamine and tyramine.
Ipomoea purpurea (L) Roth	Morning Glory.	Contains a purgative resin. In addition, morning glory seeds contain amides of lysergic acid but with a potency much less than that of LSD.
Vinca major L. and *Vinca minor* L.	Periwinkle. Vinca. Greater Periwinkle. Lesser Periwinkle.	Contains pharmacologically active, toxic alkaloids such as vinblastine and vincristine that have cytotoxic and neurological actions and can injure the liver and kidneys.
Hypericum perforatum L.	St. Johnswort. Hypericum. Klamath Weed. Goatweed.	A primary photosensitizer for cattle, sheep, horses and goats. Contains hypericin, a fluorescent pigment, as a photosensitizing substance.
Euonymus europaeus L.	Spindle-tree.	Violent purgative.
Dipteryx odorata (Aubl.) Willd. *Coumarouna odorata* (Aubl.) and *Dipteryx oppositifolia* (Aubl.) Willd. *Coumarouna oppositifolia* (Aubl.)	Tonka Bean. Tonco Bean. Tonquin Bean.	Active constituent of seed is coumarin. Dietary feeding of coumarin to rats and dogs causes extensive liver damage, growth retardation, and testicular atrophy. FDA regulations prohibit marketing of coumarin as a food or food additive.
Euonymus atropurpureus Jacq.	Wahoo Bark. Euonymus. Burning Bush. Wahoo.	The poisonous principle has not been completely identified. Laxative.
Eupatorium rugosum Houtt. *E. ogeratoides* L.f. and *E. urticaefolium*	White Snakeroot. (Also called Snakeroot, Richweed.)	Poisonous plant. Contains a toxic, unsaturated alcohol called *tremetol* combined with a resin acid. Causes "trembles" in cattle and other livestock. Milk sickness is produced in humans by ingestion of milk, butter, and possibly meat from animals poisoned by this plant.
Artemisia absinthium Linné	Wormwood. Absinthium. Absinth. Absinthe. Madderwort. Wermuth. Mugwort. Mingwort. Warmot. Magenkraut. Herba Absinthii.	Contains a volatile oil (oil of wormwood) that is an active narcotic poison. Oil of wormwood is used to flavor *absinthe*, an alcoholic liqueur illegal in this country because its use can damage the nervous system and cause mental deterioration.
Corynanthe yohimbi Schum. *Pausinystalia yohimbe* (Schum.) Pierre	Yohimbe. Yohimbi.	Contains the toxic alkaloid yohimbine (quebrachine) and other alkaloids.

rich in potassium, she recovered, gained weight, and kidney function normalized.

The author stated: "Patients do not always realize that herbal remedies, which can be bought in any drugstore, can produce side effects as other drugs do, and many do not tell their doctors that they are taking such preparations. The doctor should always ask about herbal remedies, otherwise he could overlook unwanted effects of these natural (and therefore 'healthy') treatments".

Folk Remedies and Lead Poisoning

A Laotian folk remedy widely used to cure fevers within the Hmong refugee community in St. Paul, Minnesota, contains up to 8% lead (32,33). The red powder, called "pay-loo-ah" appears to be responsible for many cases of lead poisoning in children in the Hmong community. It appears that Mexican folk remedies, called azarcon and greta, also contain lead, some samples containing up to 90% lead by weight! It is suspected that azarcon (which is actually lead tetroxide) is responsible for the death of at least one child (34). Until recently, these Mexican folk remedies were readily available at herb shops and from folk healers on both sides of the Mexican-American border. A recent letter to the editor also reports 34 cases of lead poisoning which were traced to contaminated stoneground flour (35).

Poisoned by Licorice

A man who was advised to stop drinking alcohol drank an alcohol-free beverage that curbed his drinking behavior. He was admitted to the hospital with history of progressive fatigue and was noted to have a very high blood pressure of 200/110 mm Hg (36). His serum potassium was 1.6 (normal is 3.5-5.5). It turned out that this was due to glycyrrhizinic acid, a substance found in this beverage and in licorice. After treatment, his blood pressure and serum potassium returned to normal. A similar case of hypokalemia (low serum potassium) due to the same beverage was more recently reported (37), except that in the latter case, the patient had a cardiac arrest and died, probably due to the hypokalemia. A third case of hypokalemia and hypertension, this one due to excessive licorice intake, has also been reported (38). In this case, a 20-year-old woman who had been eating up to one-half pound of licorice per day was admitted to the hospital paralyzed from the waist down and had a serum potassium of 0.8! All abnormalities resolved after administration of large amounts of potassium and cessation of licorice ingestion.

Although low serum potassium as can be caused by licorice is dangerous, high serum potassium can also be life-threatening. A recent letter reports the case of a 63-year-old gentleman whose potassium increased dangerously due to excessive intake of a salt substitute (39). Other substances readily available around the house which might be thought of as innocuous, such as baking soda (40) and epsom salts (41), can also be life-threatening if taken in excess.

Datura Poisoning from Hamburger

On October 18, 1983, a husband and wife collapsed after eating hamburger (42). Within 24 hours, the couple regained consciousness and explained what had happened. In preparing the hamburger, the wife added what she thought was seasoning but turned out to be seeds of Angels' Trumpets (*Datura suaveolens*). Having realized this before they ate the hamburger, they removed most of the seeds and proceeded to eat one patty each. Within an hour, they started to hallucinate and had severe tachycardia (fast heart rate) and diarrhea. *Datura* species, all of which are poisonous, contain a significant percentage of anticholinergic alkaloids such as atropine, hyoscyamine and scopolamine. These substances were responsible for the symptoms which the couple experienced. These anticholinergic alkaloids are very potent drugs which are often prescribed by physicians for certain serious conditions.

Raw Milk Ingestion and Disease

In 1983, 123 cases of *Salmonella dublin*, an invasive type of bacterium, were reported in California (43). Sixty percent of these individuals had ingested either certified raw milk (CRM) or consumed raw-to-rare beef or liver. It was calculated that the risk of contracting this disease was 158 times greater in CRM-drinkers than in non-CRM drinkers! A dangerous form of bacteria from raw milk which was resistant to all conventional antibiotics has caused an outbreak of disease which was fatal to one victim (43a). Many other types of diseases have been associated with drinking raw milk (see the bibliography in ref. 43). Indeed, in recognition of this fact, Scotland banned its sale in 1983. Incidentally, there is *no* evidence that CRM has any advantages over homogenized milk. Indeed, low-fat and non-fat milks, which must be processed to remove the fat, are much healthier than raw milk. Recognizing these facts, several articles have called for the mandatory pasteurization of milk (43b-d).

It has been said that acidophilus milk is beneficial in lactase-deficient individuals or those with irritable bowel syndrome. A recent double-blind randomized study investigated acidophilus milk in "correcting the imbalance of bacteria in the gut" in such individuals. Irritable bowel syndrome patients were not helped by the ingestion of acidophilus milk, and lactase-deficient patients were as intolerant of acidophilus milk as of unaltered milk (44).

Raw Fish Can Contain Parasites

Several reports of parasite infestation have been traced to raw fish (sushi) (44a-c). Although this occurs more frequently in Japan where raw fish is common fare, it is becoming more common in the states where a return-to-natural-food movement encourages the consumption of raw foods. In the United States, consumption of raw salmon seems to have been implicated, although other freshwater fishes can also carry the parasites.

Pangamic Acid and Athletic Prowess

Pangamic acid, often erroneously referred to as vitamin B-15 (there is no such vitamin), is frequently recommended in the lay press as an aid to athletic performance. Many of these recommendations are based on old Russian studies, only a few of which have involved human subjects. The human studies are interesting, but the scientific method is not well-documented in these studies. Therefore, not much confidence is placed in these studies by American scientists.

Part of the confusion is due to the fact that there seems to be no consensus as to *what pangamic acid is*! Many different compounds on the market are identified as pangamic acid, but the compound most frequently studied (the so-called "Russian formula", U.S. patent #3,907,869) and used widely by American athletes, is composed of 61.5% calcium gluconate and 38.5% N,N-dimethylglycine.

A double-blind experiment investigating the effects of pangamic acid on maximal treadmill (athletic) performance in 16 male track athletes was recently published (45). Subjects were paired according to best-mile-run performance; members of each pair were randomly assigned to either the experimental (E) or control (C) group. Members of the E group ingested 300 mg of pangamic acid daily for 3 weeks, whereas the C group members took identical-appearing placebos. Subjects were treadmill tested before and after treatment. No significant differences between the two groups were noted in any monitored parameters (e.g., maximal heart rate, treadmill time, recovery heart rate, blood glucose and lactate levels before and after exercise). It was concluded that short-term pangamic acid intake does not produce any changes in maximal treadmill performance in male athletes. Nothing definitive can be said about the effects of pangamic acid over a longer period of time, or in women or non-athletic men. This study does, however, put the burden of proof on proponents of pangamic acid to demonstrate in scientific fashion that pangamic acid has beneficial effects.

Bee Pollen

Bee pollen has been widely promoted an a panacea for all ills as well as an enhancer of athletic prowess. There is essentially no evidence to support these claims. This topic has been well addressed in a recent FDA Consumer article (45a). In addition, some individuals may suffer life-threatening allergic reactions after ingesting bee pollen.

"Tanning" Pills

"Tanning" pills are said to tan the skin without exposure to the sun. Tanning pills don't tan the skin in a conventional sense. True tanning is due to increased deposition of the skin pigment, melanin, usually stimulated by exposure to sunlight but can also occur secondary to exposure to artificial light (tanning lamps). Most of the so-called tanning pills contain canthaxanthin, a food color. Some also contain beta carotene, a natural food color and precursor of vitamin A (see also Ch. 7). High doses of either substance dye the blood, and consequently, the skin. The color of beta carotene is more of an orange color than a tan one, and may even be mistaken for jaundice (although it is said that carotene does not color the white of the eye). To my knowledge, no scientific studies evaluating either the safety or efficacy of tanning pills have been performed. Therefore, an individual taking them is experimenting on his own.

Ginger Root Seems To Work Against Motion Sickness

Up to this point in this chapter, the lack of value and possible risks of several quasi-medical nostrums have been discussed. It was mentioned in the introduction, however, that there are some preliminary data that suggest the efficacy of some herbal-type remedies. Ginger root, at least with respect to anti-motion-sickness actions, seems to fall in this category.

Powdered ginger root (940 mg in capsules) was compared to 100 mg of dimenhydrinate (Dramamine) and a placebo in the ability of each to decrease symptoms of motion sickness (46). The capsules were taken 20 minutes before the highly motion-sickness-susceptible students were spun in a tilted chair, which induces motion sickness in normal untreated subjects. None of the 24 subjects taking either Dramamine or placebo were able to last the six minute spinning test without vomiting or experiencing severe symptoms, whereas 6 of the 12 who took the ginger root were able to last the full six minutes in the chair. Thus, ginger root was statistically significantly better than either Dramamine or placebo in suppressing motion sickness.

Good Effects of Garlic

Unlike other studies discussed in this chapter which have dealt with humans, this study deals with the effects of garlic in animals (47). Although there have been some studies of the effects of garlic in humans (see the bibliography in ref. 47), this animal study is the most detailed study to date. Lyophilized (freeze-dried) garlic decreased plasma cholesterol level in cholesterol-fed and lard-fed rats. Garlic supplementation decreased VLDL and increased HDL (see Ch. 6 for an explanation of these terms); both of these effects are presumed to be beneficial. It was speculated that garlic decreases these plasma fats by increasing their excretion in the stool. A recent letter-to-the-editor provides corroboration that garlic lowers blood cholesterol (47a). In this group of 10 hypercholesterolemic individuals, average cholesterol levels decreased about 10% with garlic supplementation, as did plasma viscosity.

Hot Pepper Might Be Good for You

Capsaicine, found in several types of hot pepper (e.g., chili, cayenne, long yellow peppers) significantly decreased serum cholesterol in turkeys eating a high cholesterol diet (48). Turkeys were studied because they share with man the tendency to atherosclerosis. Capsicum, a related hot condiment, has been found to increase fibrinolytic activity (tendency to break down blood clots) and thus to decrease the tendency of blood to clot (49). Thai subjects, who ingest large amounts of dietary capsicum, had significantly ($p<0.001$) higher fibrinolytic activity than American whites. It was speculated that this may account for the rarity of thromboembolism (tendency to form blood clots) among Thais.

Aloe Vera for Frostbite and Burns?

All but 1 of 44 patients with frostbite injuries (3 third degree, 19 second degree, 22 first-degree injuries) given topical aloe vera and aspirin orally healed without major tissue loss (50). The investigator said: "The results are startling: a much greater amount of tissue loss is usually associated with frostbite injuries". It is not clear to me, however, how much of the improvement might have been due to the aspirin, which blocks the production of prostaglandins that may cause tissue damage. In addition, this was not a controlled double-blind study, so bias is much more likely, as discussed previously.

CHIROPRACTIC

Although this topic is even more outside the scope of this chapter than the other topics discussed, I was asked many questions about chiropractic while writing this book. Therefore, I'll discuss it briefly and direct the interested reader to the references below.

Most scientific studies that have examined the value of manipulation for low back pain have shown chiropractic to give some short-term relief but no real cure (51-54). Some reports have suggested chiropractic to be dangerous (55-58). Several cases of lumbar disc rupture, all of which followed manipulation and all of which required urgent surgery, were recently reported (56,57). It was suggested by the authors that favorable results claimed by chiropractic are more likely to be related to the self-healing tendencies of most low back pain problems rather than the manipulation itself. Brain stroke following manipulation has also been reported (58). In all fairness to chiropractors, and as was pointed out in a letter to the editor (59), it is unclear how common these complications are, in view of the many manipulations which are performed daily. I am unaware of any study or reasonably scientific estimate of the true incidence of these complications.

Although chiropractors have used the lack of such information as supportive of their practice, my opinion is exactly the opposite. I believe that when someone offers you a therapy, they must be able to give you at least a ballpark estimate of major risks (like stroke). Once the prospective patient knows this information, he can make an intelligent decision of whether to undergo that therapy. Such information, to my knowledge, is unavailable for the major risks of manipulation, so I believe someone is taking a risk (how big of a risk I can't honestly say) when undergoing manipulation. The reader interested in low back pain is referred to an excellent paperback by Dr. Augustus White on this topic (60).

A brief word may be in order about gravity boots, a fad that literally swept millions of Americans off their feet in the early 1980s, but appears to have faded away. A recent report has shown that hanging upside down can cause alarming increases in blood pressure, heart rate, central retinal arterial pressure (blood pressure in the back of the eye), and pressure within the eye (61,62). In the latter study (62), 20 college students ranging in age from 22-33 years had these parameters measured both in the sitting position and after three minutes in the inverted position. The measurements were repeated 1 minute after cessation of inversion. Systolic blood pressure increased 30 points, heart rate increased from 67 to 78, and retinal artery pressure increased from $45/26$ to $105/62$! Intraocular pressure rose from 19 to 35. Since these changes occurred within 3 minutes of inverting, it is not known what would happen if measurements are taken after 15-30 minutes (not unusual "hanging" times for aficionados of inversion). The authors concluded that inversion could be "potentially dangerous" for those with glaucoma, high blood pressure, heart failure, atherosclerosis in arteries leading to the brain or patients on "blood thinners".

THE BOTTOM LINE

It is hoped that this chapter has demonstrated, with multiple examples, the concept that calling something "herbal" does not make it either safe or effective.

It could potentially be both safe and effective or it could just as easily be ineffective and dangerous (or any other combination). The only way to differentiate these conditions is by unbiased experiments, and these are generally lacking in the herbal and alternative health care arena. On the other hand, we should be careful not to embrace all ideas and therapies just because they have been developed by scientists (e.g., a recent report demonstrates that diathermy, a technique commonly used for back pain by Western physicians, is no better than placebo [63]), or to reject novel ideas just because they sound crazy, such as:

1) Yoga for bronchial asthma (64)

2) Rectal infusion of feces for relapsing *Clostridium* enterocolitis (65)

3) Treatment of severe life-threatening infection (mediastinitis) with supermarket-bought granulated sugar in the wound (66)

4) Injection of botulinum toxin (one of the most potent toxins known to man) in eyelids to treat involuntary blinking (67)

The principle of unbiased scientific evaluation applies not only to herbs but also to various practices such as chiropractic and gravity boots. Although the majority of such practices are probably ineffective and safe (i.e., they are equivalent to placebos), it is hard to know which one might be dangerous. In the final analysis, the patient should realize that in participating in these practices, he is experimenting on himself. Thus, it is my opinion that such remedies should not be practiced casually, and should be reported to one's physician since they may prove to be the cause of medical problems.

REFERENCES

1. Glymour C, Stalker D: Engineers, cranks, physicians and magicians. N Engl J Med 308:960, 1983

2. Pelletier KR: Holistic medicine: from stress to optimal health. Dell, New York, 1979, pp. 13

3. Reilly DT: Young doctors' views on alternative medicine. Br Med J 287:337, 1983

4. Smith T: Alternative medicine (editorial). Br Med J 287:307, 1983

5. Letters to editor. Alternative medicine. Br Med J 287:494, 1983

6. Editorial: Alternative medicine is no alternative. Lancet 2:773, 1983 ˙

6a. Fulder SJ, Munro RE: Complementary medicine in the UK: Patients, practitioners and consultations. Lancet 2:542, 1985

6b. Donnelly WJ, et al: Are patients who use alternative medicine dissatisfied with orthodox medicine? Med J Aust 142:539, 1985

6c. Moore J, et al: Why do people seek treatment by alternative medicine? Br Med J 290:28, 1985

6d. Cassileth BR, et al: Contemporary unorthodox treatments in cancer medicine. Ann Int Med 101:105, 1984

7. Fitzgerald FT: Science and scam: Alternative thought patterns in alternative health care. N Engl J Med 309:1066, 1983

8. Lister J: Current controversy on alternative medicine. N Engl J Med 309:1524, 1983

9. Letters to editor: Alternative health care. N Engl J Med 310:790, 1984

10. Letters to editor: Alternative medicine. N Engl J Med 310:1195, 1984

11. Relman AS: Christian science and the care of children. N Engl J Med 309:1639, 1983

12. Swan R: Faith healing, Christian science, and the medical care of children. N Engl J Med 309:1639, 1983

13. Talbot NA: The position of the Christian science church. N Engl J Med 309:1641, 1983

14. Letters to editor: Christian science and the care of children. N Engl J Med 910:1257, 1984

15. Relman AS: Holistic medicine. N Engl J Med 300:312, 1979

16. Simon A, et al: An evaluation of iridology. JAMA 242:1385, 1979

16a. Anonymous: Riding the coattails of homeopathy's revival. FDA Consumer, March, 1985, p.30

17. Gibson RG, et al: Salicylates and homeopathy in rheumatoid arthritis: preliminary observations. Br J Clin Pharmac 6:391, 1978

18. Huston G: Salicylates and homeopathy (letter). Br J Clin Pharmac 7:529, 1979

19. Gibson RG, et al: Homeopathic therapy in rheumatoid arthritis: evaluation by double-blind clinical therapeutic trial. Br J Clin Pharmac 9:453, 1980

20. Turner P: Clinical trials of homeopathic remedies. Br J Clin Pharmac 9:443, 1980

21. Shipley M, et al: Controlled trial of homeopathic treatment of osteoarthritis. Lancet 1:97, 1983

22. Editorial. The trial of homeopathy. Lancet 1:108, 1983

23. Letters to the editor. Homeopathy. Lancet 1:482, 1983

24. Hoyeraal HM, et al: Most pediatric rheumatology patients try unconventional therapy. Ped News, 1983

25. Tyler VE: The honest herbal. Philadelphia, George F. Stickley Co., 1982

25a. Bryson PD, et al: Burdock root tea poisoning. Case report involving a commercial preparation. JAMA 239:2157, 1978

25b. Haynes BE, et al: Oleander tea: Herbal draught of death. Ann Emerg Med 14:350, 1985

26. Macek C: East meets West to balance immunologic yin and yang. JAMA 251:433, 1984

27. Neidhart JA: New anticancer agent development: "Dirt to drugs". In Yetiv JZ, Bianchine JR (eds.): Recent Advances in Clinical Therapeutics, vol. 3, New York, Grune & Stratton, 1983, pp.79-84

28. Larkin T: Herbs are often more toxic than magical. FDA Consumer 17(#8): 4, 1983

29. Hogan RP: Hemorrhagic diathesis caused by drinking an herbal tea. JAMA 249:2679, 1983

30. Greenspan EM: Ginseng and vaginal bleeding. JAMA 249:2018, 1983

31. Eichler I: Cryptic illness from self-medication with herbal remedy. Lancet 1:356, 1983

32. Folk remedy linked to poisoning. Am Med News, June 17, 1983, p.16

33. Folk-remedy-associated lead poisoning in Hmong children. JAMA 250:3149, 1983

34. Lead poisoning from Mexican folk remedies. JAMA 250:3149, 1983

35. Eisenberg A, et al: Stoneground flour as source of lead poisoning. Lancet 1:972, 1984
36. Cereda JM, et al: Liquorice intoxication caused by alcohol-free pastis. Lancet 1:1442, 1983
37. Haberer JP, et al: Severe hypokalaemia secondary to overindulgence in alcohol-free "pastis". Lancet 1:575, 1984
38. Nielsen I, Pedersen RS: Life-threatening hypokalaemia caused by liquorice ingestion. Lancet 1:1305, 1984
39. McCaughan D: Hazards of non-prescription potassium supplements. Lancet 1:513, 1984
40. Levin T: What this patient didn't need: A dose of salts. Hosp Prac July, 1983, pp.95.
41. Garcia-Webb P, et al: Hypermagnesemia and hypophosphataemia after ingestion of magnesium sulfate. Br Med J 288:759, 1984
42. Leads from MMWR: *Datura* poisoning from hamburger—Canada. JAMA 251: 3075, 1984
43. Leads from MMWR: *Salmonella dublin* and raw milk consumption. JAMA 251: 2195, 1984
43a. Tacket CO, et al: An outbreak of multiple-drug-resistant *Salmonella* enteritis from raw milk. JAMA 253:2058, 1985
43b. Potter ME, et al: Unpasteurized milk. The hazards of a health fetish. JAMA 252:2048, 1984
43c. Sharp JC, et al: Pasteurization and the control of milkborne infection in Britain. Br Med J 291:463, 1985
43d. Howie J: The case for compulsory pasteurization. Br Med J 291:422, 1985
44. Newcomer AD, et al: Response of patients with irritable bowel syndrome and lactase deficiency using unfermented acidophilus milk. Am J Clin Nutr 38:257, 1983
44a. Ching HL: Fish tapeworm infections (diphyllobothriasis) in Canada, particularly British Columbia. Can Med Assoc J 130:1125, 1984
44b. Sugimachi K, et al: Acute gastric anisakiasis. Analysis of 178 cases. JAMA 253:1012, 1985
44c. Goldmann DR: Hold the sushi. JAMA 253:2495, 1985
45. Gray ME, Titlow, LW: The effect of pangamic acid on maximal treadmill performance. Med Sci in Sports & Exercise 14:424, 1982
45a. Larkin T: Bee pollen as a health food. FDA Consumer, April, 1984, p.21
46. Mowrey DB, Clayson DE: Motion sickness, ginger and psychophysics. Lancet 1:655, 1982
47. Chi MS, et al: Effects of garlic on lipid metabolism in rats fed cholesterol or lard. J Nutr 112:241, 1982
47a. Ernst E, et al: Garlic and blood lipids. Br Med J 291:139, 1985
48. Negulesco J: Pungent research adds zest to "sheltered lives". Ohio State Univ Coll of Med J 33(1):13, 1982
49. Visudhiphan S, et al: The relationship between high fibrinolytic activity and daily capsicum ingestion in Thais. Am J Clin Nutr 35:1452, 1982
50. Robson M: ASA, aloe vera Rx vs. frostbite? Med Tribune, ⅔/83, p.3
51. Doran DM, Newell DJ: Manipulation in the treatment of low back paina— multi-centre study. Br Med J 2:161, 1975

52. Sims-Williams H, et al: Controlled trials of mobilization and manipulation for patients with low back pain in general practice. Br MedJ 2:1338, 1978

53. Glover JR, Morris JG, Khosla T: Back pain. A randomized clinical trial of rotational manipulation of the trunk. Br J Industr Med 31:59, 1974

54. Kane RL, et al: Manipulating the patient: A comparison of the effectiveness of physician and chiropractor care. Lancet 1:1333, 1974

55. Hooper J: Low back pain and manipulation paraparesis after treatment of low back pain by physical methods. Med J Aust 1:549, 1973

56. Malmivaara A, Pohjola R: Cauda equina syndrom caused by chiropraxis on a patient previously free of lumbar spine symptoms. Lancet 2:986, 1982

57. Gallinara P, Catesegna, M: Three cases of lumbar disc rupture and one of cauda equina associated with spinal manipulation (chiropraxis). Lancet 1:411, 1983

58. Daneshmend TK, Hewer RL, Bradshaw, JR: Acute brain stem stroke during neck manipulation. Br Med J 288:189, 1984

59. Letters to editor: Acute brain stem stroke during neck manipulation. Br Med J 288:641, 1984

60. White AA: Your aching back: A doctor's guide to relief. New York, Bantam, 1983, pp.135-142.

61. Friberg TR, Weinreb RN: Ocular manifestations of gravity inversion. JAMA 253:1755, 1985

62. Klatz RM, et al: The effects of gravity inversion procedures on systemic blood pressure, intraocular pressure and central retinal arterial pressure. J Am Osteopathic Assoc 82:853, 1983. Also discussed in Hosp Prac, Sept. 1983, pp. 196

63. Gibson T, et al: Controlled comparison of short-wave diathermy treatment with osteopathic treatment in non-specific low back pain. Lancet 1:1258, 1985

64. Nagaratha R, Nagendra HR: Yoga for bronchial asthma. Br Med J 291:1077, 1985

65. Schwan, et al: rectal infusions of bacterial preparations for intestinal disorders. Lancet 2:845, 1983

66. Trouillet JL, et al: Use of granulated sugar in treatment of open mediastinitis after cardiac surgery. Lancet 2:180, 1985

67. Elston JS, Russel RW: Effect of treatment with botulinum toxin on neurogenic blepharospasm. Br Med J 290:1857, 1985

CHAPTER 3

Natural Foods, Food Additives and Food Intolerance

With the current craze of natural foods (and natural everything else, e.g., childbirth) sweeping the country, it is noteworthy that most food additives used in the United States *are* natural, and many are essential to the food supply. When most people think of food additives, they think of the tongue-twisting chemical names of artificial additives; in reality, these account for less than 2%, by weight, of all the additives used in the United States (1). The other 98% is made up of salt, sugar, corn sweeteners, and other naturally-derived substances.

That some additives are unnecessary (e.g., food colors), and that some may even be harmful, is not in question. The goal of this chapter is to evaluate the necessity and safety of food additives in general, and then discuss some individual additives which have been implicated in certain medical conditions. The rest of this chapter deals with food intolerance ("allergy"), cytotoxic testing and other (often questionable) ways of assessing food allergies, food-induced migraine, defined diets (e.g., Feingold's), and the effect of food on mental function. Before delving into that, however, a brief discussion of natural foods is in order.

NATURAL FOODS

There is no legal definition of "natural food". The term is usually taken to mean that no chemical fertilizers or pesticides were used and if the product is processed, that no artificial substances were added. Instead, it is assumed that natural fertilizers (cow manure) or natural additives (corn sweeteners or honey) were used. Natural foods are often touted as being "better", although it's not clear how the latter adjective is defined. Does better mean bigger, tastier, fresher, lasts longer, or what? One thing it almost always means is more expensive, often more than double the price of conventional foods. This might be acceptable if natural foods were superior to conventional ones. In a recent study, however, a taste panel judged 25 natural and conventional foods on the basis of odor, texture, color, and flavor, and found absolutely no difference between the two (2).

51

It is often assumed that naturally-cultivated produce is different in composition from its conventionally-grown counterpart. This assumption is largely incorrect, because the composition of a plant depends on its genetic make-up and not on the environment within which it grows. For instance, a cherry tomato will not become a beefsteak tomato regardless of where it grows. To some extent, however, the environment can influence the composition of the plant. For instance, the selenium content of the plant will depend on the selenium content of the soil. If we assume that the selenium content of a vegetable can affect the color, taste, texture or other property of the vegetable, plants grown in different soils may have somewhat different properties. It doesn't follow, however, that the organically-grown food will always be superior to its conventionally grown counterpart. To pursue our example, if the soil is deficient in selenium, a properly selected artificial fertilizer is much more likely to contain the necessary selenium than is manure derived from cows which forage on plants growing in the selenium-deficient soil. An excellent review article which assesses "health foods" should be consulted by the interested reader (2a).

Another important point to consider is that once a substance (e.g., calcium) enters the human body and is absorbed from the intestine, the body does not know or care if the substance came from an artificial (e.g., calcium pill supplement) or a natural (e.g., milk) source. This is not to imply that these sources of calcium (or whatever example one chooses) are always equivalent. The important phrase here is "once it is absorbed from the intestine". For instance, iron in meat (heme iron) is much better absorbed by the human body than iron in plant foodstuffs (non-heme iron) (3). Thus, 10 mg of iron in meat represents much more iron to the human body than 10 mg in soybeans. This is also true of zinc in human breastmilk (which is almost totally absorbed) compared to zinc in most other foods (poorly absorbed) (4). In other words, the source of a nutrient is of some relevance, but it can't be assumed that the natural is always better than the artificial. The sources must be individually studied in order to determine which one is better. Thus, it is possible that some organic foods are better than conventional ones, although the opposite is equally likely. Most likely, however, is that in most cases, the differences are sufficiently small as to render them inconsequential.

Another point that has only recently become widely appreciated is that many natural substances contain poisons or carcinogenic (cancer-causing) chemicals, or both. Indeed, the National Academy of Sciences has published a whole book on this topic, entitled "Toxicants Occurring Naturally in Foods". Dr. Bruce Ames, a noted biochemist, opines in a recent article (5) that naturally occurring chemicals may play a much greater role in carcinogenesis than artificial chemicals. Dr. Ames believes that "the human dietary intake of 'nature's pesticides' is likely to be several grams per day—probably at least 10,000 times higher than the dietary intake of man-made pesticides". It is not only the quantity but also the potency of these natural carcinogens and pesticides that may surprise the reader. For instance, aflatoxin, produced by a fungus that grows on alfalfa and other plants, is one of the most potent carcinogens known to man.

The number of toxin-containing foods on Dr. Ames' list is rather long, and includes the burnt material produced during frying and barbecuing; cocoa, tea and chocolate—which contain the carcinogen theobromine; celery, okra, parsnips, parsley, mushrooms, rhubarb, potatoes, certain herbs and herbal teas, oil of mustard, horseradish, black pepper, fava beans and figs. Dr. Ames believes that these substances are second only to cigarette smoking as important factors in the development of cancer. In an accompanying editorial, it was predicted that as further research accumulates, it should be possible to intelligently select a diet which minimizes exposure to these potential carcinogens (6).

Another recent editorial (7) refers to the inadvisability of equating "natural" with good and "artificial" with bad. The author points out that "What may at first glance seem unnatural is the human capacity to prevent the natural from occurring. Yet human beings are part of nature, too; so in that sense, whatever we do becomes natural . . ."

As noted above, natural foods are probably not substantially different from their conventional counterparts. Some natural foods, however, expose the consumer to unnecessary risks. For instance, several recent papers describe parasitic and bacterial infections due to ingestion of sushi (raw fish) (8), raw goat's milk (9) and unpasteurized cow's milk (10). Indeed, as was mentioned in Chapter 2, the risk of Salmonella infection was>150 times greater in individuals drinking certified raw milk than in those drinking regular pasteurized milk.

FOOD ADDITIVES

In order to discuss food additives, their role in the food supply must be appreciated. Additives are used for various reasons, which are detailed below (this section is a summary of reference 1):

1) To maintain or improve nutritional value—many foods are fortified with vitamins and minerals that have been lost in processing (e.g., B vitamins in breads and cereals, vitamin C in fruit drinks) or to supplement the normal diet with nutrients that are often deficient (e.g., vitamin D in milk, iron in infant formulas, iodine in table salt, fluoride in drinking water). With the exception of, perhaps, fluoridation, there is not much controversy on this application for food additives. This use of additives is credited with the near-total eradication in the United States of vitamin deficiency diseases like rickets, pellagra, and scurvy.

2) To improve flavor or appearance—this use of additives is more controversial, especially the use of coloring agents. Many consumers would accept the use of artificial flavors; fewer would endorse the addition of colors. Although the

addition of artificial food colors and flavors is ubiquitous, these substances account for less than 2%, by weight, of all additives. The other 98% is made up of sugar, salt and corn syrup (by far the most common additives), plus citric acid, baking soda, vegetable colors, mustard and pepper. Thus, although artificial colors and flavors are found in many prepared foods, daily per capita intake of these substances is only a few milligrams. Some people, however, seem to be exquisitely sensitive to certain colors (e.g., tartrazine, discussed later in this chapter). Others have even hypothesized, without much scientific proof to support it at this time, that some food additives cause hyperactivity and other behavioral problems in some children (see p. 75 for a discussion of this topic). An allergic-type syndrome—dubbed the "Chinese restaurant syndrome"—has been observed in some individuals after ingestion of the flavor enhancer monosodium glutamate (MSG). This is discussed in more detail later in this chapter.

3) To maintain freshness—many of the strange chemicals on food labels such as BHT, BHA, sodium benzoate and sodium nitrite, belong in this category. The oldest preservatives—salt (used to cure meats) and sugar (in jams, etc.)—are also still commonly used for this purpose. These additives facilitate the preservation and transportation of food from the producing to the consuming areas. The food distribution system in the United States is largely dependent on the ability to preserve various foods. It is interesting to note that while some purists shun preservatives like BHT and BHA, others recommend taking *supplements* of these chemicals in the belief that this will "preserve" the human body and delay the aging process (see Chapter 5).

4) To help in food processing—many natural (e.g., lecithin) and artificial substances are added to foods to enhance their texture, evenly distribute particles (emulsifiers), enable baked products to rise, retain moisture in some foods and prevent moisture in others. Thickeners enhance the smoothness of foods and prevent the formation of ice crystals in foods like ice cream.

These are the four major categories of food additives. The reader may wonder how additive use is regulated. Before 1906, additive use was totally uncontrolled and toxic materials containing lead and arsenic, for instance, were used to color candy. In 1906, and more comprehensively in 1938, the Food, Drug and Cosmetic Act gave the government authority to remove poisonous additives from the marketplace. In 1958 and 1960, lawmakers shifted the burden from the government—to prove that an additive was unsafe—to the manufacturers, who had to prove that an additive was safe. This act also had a special provision, called the Delaney Clause, which stated that a substance which, in *any* dose, causes cancer in man or animals cannot be added to food. It is this clause which led to the FDA proposal to ban saccharin in 1977 (more on that below).

Substances already in use at the time that these laws were passed were placed in the *generally recognized as safe* (GRAS) category, which meant that they would be allowed to remain in foods because they had presumably stood the test of time. Any GRAS substance, however, could be removed from the list if new evidence suggested it to be toxic or carcinogenic (this is what happened with saccharin).

In addition, the FDA started a formal review, which continues to the present, of 450 GRAS substances. This review included a search of the world medical literature as far back as 1920. As a result of this review, the FDA banned the food color Red No. 2 in 1976, then the most widely used coloring agent, because animal studies suggested it may cause cancer. In 1973, evidence suggested that BHT causes liver enlargement in laboratory animals. The GRAS review is continuing (11); to date, the FDA has reaffirmed the GRAS status of 6 preservatives out of more than 2 dozen undergoing review (11a). These six are benzoic acid, methylparaben, propyl gallate, propylparaben, sodium benzoate, and stannous chloride. The two most widely used preservatives—BHT and BHA—are still under review.

As mentioned previously, the Delaney Clause would have required the banning of saccharin when it was discovered that this sweetener caused cancer in animal studies. The FDA did issue a ban, but had to rescind it due to public outcry. Thus, despite supposed public concern about the unnecessary use of artificial additives (indeed, in a recent survey, respondents cited chemical additives as their most common nutritional concern (12)), public outcry forced the continued widespread use of a potentially carcinogenic food additive! Furthermore, despite a great push toward natural foods, additive-laden convenience foods continue to be bought in large quantities. Thus, it appears that the consuming public is voting with its pocketbook to keep additives in our food.

As mentioned previously, some food additives have unique side effects in sensitive individuals. Some of these have been recently reviewed (13), and are briefly discussed below.

Tartrazine

Tartrazine (FD&C Yellow No. 5) is used in foods, beverages, drugs and cosmetics. It has been estimated by the FDA that 50,000 to 100,000 persons in the United States are sensitive to this substance. Signs and symptoms of allergy include generalized urticaria (hives), angioedema (swelling, often of the face and lips), rhinitis (runny nose), and on occasion, even life-threatening asthma (14-18). About 15% of patients who react to aspirin also react to tartrazine. Avoiding tartrazine may be easier said than done, however, because it is found in a large number of products. A list of tartrazine-containing drugs (19) and a partial list of foods (20) have recently been published. The latter is reproduced in Table 3-1. Since tartrazine is contained in so many products, tartrazine-sensitive individuals are advised to read labels and avoid foods containing "FD&C Yellow No. 5".

Table 3-1

Beverages
 Orange drinks (Tang, Daybreak, Awake)
 Other drinks: Gatorade (lime flavored), imitation lemonade mix (Jewel)
Ice cream and sherbets
 New York ice cream (Hillfarm)
 Rainbow sherbet (Hillfarm)
Desserts
 Gelatin (Jell-O, Royal)
 Instant pudding and pie filling (Jell-O, Royal)
Salad dressings
 Presto Italian dressing (Kraft)
 Zesty Italian (reduced calorie) dressing (Kraft)
Bakery products
 Cake mix (some—Duncan Hines, Pillsbury)
 Cake icing (Cake Mate, Dec A Mate)
Confections
 Imitation butter, banana flavoring (McCormick, Durkee)
 Imitation pineapple extract (McCormick, ?Durkee)
 Seasoning salt (French's)
Other products
 Macaroni and cheese dinner (Kraft, Golden Grain)
 Egg noodle and cheese dinner (Kraft)
 "Cheez" curls and balls (Planters)
 Fruit chews (Skittles)
 Candies (lemon drops), butterscotch, candy corn (Brach's)

Tartrazine-containing foods
Some food products containing tartrazine (FD&C Yellow No. 5)
This is not an all-inclusive list. A tartrazine-sensitive individual must check the ingredients list to be sure that a food does not contain this food color.
Modified from ref. 20.

Sulfite Preservatives

Sulfites are commonly used preservatives which can cause asthmatic attacks in susceptible individuals, usually within an hour of ingestion. They have been used in restaurants and supermarkets to keep salad bar fare looking fresh. One serving of treated lettuce can precipitate asthma in a susceptible individual (13). Many cases of asthma have been reported from orange soft drink, and in one soft drink factory, there was enough sulfur dioxide in the air to cause wheezing in a sensitive asthmatic (13,21,22). In addition, 13 deaths have been possibly associated with sulfite-treated foods (22a).

Many medications, including, paradoxically, the drug (epinephrine) that is used to combat severe allergic reactions, are preserved with sulfite additives. One author described her own sensitivity to sodium bisulfite, found in the commonly-used local anesthetic, Xylocaine (23). Her symptoms included generalized hives, itching, severe abdominal pain and diarrhea. This author believes that sulfite preservatives should be removed from the FDA's GRAS list. In fact, after review of health hazards associated with sulfites, the FDA proposed banning all use of sulfites on raw fruits and vegetables in August, 1985 (22a), and the ban was reported to have been passed the following month (22b). The ban does not affect the use of sulfites in processed foods, such as frozen potato products, seafood, dried fruits, wine or beer. By law, however, additives must be listed in the ingredients list of such processed foods; thus, sulfite-sensitive individuals are encouraged to read labels.

Monosodium Glutamate (MSG)

MSG is a flavor enhancer commonly used in gram amounts in Chinese cooking and in smaller amounts in Western cooking and soup cubes. The Chinese restaurant syndrome, due to MSG, was first described in 1968 (24), and consists of headache and nausea one to two hours after a Chinese meal (classically) or any meal containing a large amount of MSG. Occasionally, flushing and warmth of the upper body, and abdominal pain, are also experienced. A recent report described the case of a three-year-old girl who had three 45-minute episodes of inappropriate behavior, confusion and slight ataxia (unsteady gait), each following the ingestion of wonton soup and a cola (25). One of her parents has classic Chinese restaurant syndrome which is precipitated by wonton soup. A recent study suggests the reason why the Chinese restaurant syndrome seems to follow the ingestion of soup (26). In this study, eating a large amount of MSG (150 mg/kg) with a meal resulted in a peak serum glutamate concentration of 10.8 micromole/dl. In contrast, ingesting the same amount of MSG in water (or one would suppose, soup) resulted in peak glutamate concentration of 71.8! It therefore appears that ingesting MSG with a meal (as opposed to soup) significantly retards its absorption, and consequently, is less likely to result in adverse symptoms.

It appears that large amounts of MSG (as in Chinese cooking) are needed to cause the Chinese restaurant syndrome, and that small amounts, found in Western cooking, are probably without much risk. In view of this syndrome, some Chinese restaurants have stopped using MSG, and many others will leave it out at the request of a customer.

Life-threatening asthma after ingestion of Chinese food has also been reported (27). Both patients were eating additive-free diets for suspected or documented additive sensitivity when their reactions occurred. Both patients developed severe asthma 11 to 14 hours after eating Chinese food on several occasions (one wonders why they kept going back several times for more!). Single-blind challenge tests performed in both patients resulted in severe asthma 11-12 hours after taking 2.5 g of MSG in capsule form, and repeat challenge in one patient produced the same response. One of the patients experienced severe unresponsive asthma (requiring ventilatory support) following one of the challenge tests.

The 11 to 12 hour time delay after MSG ingestion is rather curious, since an asthmatic response suggests an immediate hypersensitivity reaction, but that is inconsistent with such a long delay. It may be that this asthmatic response is not of the immediate hypersensitivity type; the authors speculate that MSG may cause asthma by release of hypothalamic-pituitary hormones, which could also explain the delay.

Whereas the Chinese restaurant syndrome appears fairly benign, Chinese restaurant asthma may be life-threatening, as noted above (28,29). It may be that the mechanism of action of these two syndromes is different. It is unknown whether individuals with a history of the Chinese restaurant syndrome are also more likely to suffer the asthmatic reaction. Caution would appear to be advised, especially if challenge tests are undertaken. It is suggested that if a challenge test is deemed appropriate, that it be initiated with 1 g of MSG, and that the test be performed under extremely close supervision.

Unintended Additives (Contaminants)

Genuine food allergies are often difficult to document because many foods may be ingested simultaneously and the specific components of all the foods are usually unknown. This becomes even more complicated when unknown contaminants such as the antibiotics streptomycin in beef (29a) and penicillin in the meat portion of a frozen dinner (29b,c), are implicated as the allergy-causing agents. Most adverse reactions to foods have been blamed on the proteins in the ingested food, but in these three cases, the patients did not react to the pure meat on various occasions. The investigators believed that the allergic reaction was due to these antibiotic contaminants. This type of reaction (i.e., to contaminants) may explain the puzzling situation wherein patients react to a food on some occasions but not on others.

Smoked Foods

Some have suggested that Icelandic mothers ingesting smoked meat at about the time of conception are more likely to have diabetic children (30). Although no such effect has been observed in another study (31), feeding this meat has been shown to cause diabetes in mouse offspring (32), and smoked foods are now suspected to be one of the environmental causes of juvenile (Type I) diabetes. More recently, no significant difference was observed in the smoked food intake of mothers with diabetic children compared to control mothers (33). It may be that smoking methods in various countries account for these differences. In view of these findings and those of Dr. Ames (5), it may be wise to restrict the intake of smoked/cured foods.

EXERCISE- AND ASPIRIN-DEPENDENT FOOD SENSITIVITY?

In the preceding sections, specific substances which are thought to elicit various reactions in susceptible individuals have been discussed. Some reports suggest that two factors operating in concert may be necessary to induce allergic symptoms in some individuals. A recent report, for instance, described a 24-year-old woman who was able to exercise or eat peaches without difficulty. On two occasions, however, when eating a peach was followed by exercise, she experienced episodes of itching, hives, facial swelling, abdominal distress and diarrhea. This reaction was duplicated during treadmill testing in hospital, which followed ingestion of a peach. This reaction was accompanied by an 8-fold increase in plasma histamine (34). One correspondent thought this case report was unconvincing, and was more likely due to ragweed inhalation (35). It is difficult to ascertain, from one case report, whether the peach ingestion was incidental or actually played a role in the development of the reaction.

Another recent case report is conceptually similar (36). A 14-year-old boy had taken aspirin in the past without difficulty. When he had eaten peanuts on three occasions in the past, he experienced tingling and dryness of the lips and mouth followed by swelling of the lips and face with a sensation of choking. In the past, this all passed within five minutes. On the day of admisssion, he had taken 600 mg (an adult dose) of aspirin for a headache. Five minutes later, he ate a piece of cake containing peanuts, and suffered his usual reaction, which subsided totally in five minutes. Thirty minutes after eating the cake, he felt generalized itching, a choking sensation, and extreme shortness of breath, and then collapsed. On admission to the hospital, he was unconscious, cyanotic (blue), and covered with hives. His pH was 6.85, pCO_2 110 mm Hg, and pO_2 41 mm Hg (i.e., he was near death). After vigorous treatment with epinephrine, sodium bicarbonate, aminophylline, steroids and antihistamine, he made a dramatic recovery, and was completely well within 45 minutes.

The authors believe (and cite several studies to support this view) that aspirin increased the gastrointestinal absorption of antigenic material in the ingested peanuts. They further speculate that aspirin may potentiate the effect of food allergens in man, and may result in a life-threatening reaction, concluding that "Patients who suffer even mild immediate hypersensitivity reactions to foods should be warned that they could suffer a dangerous reaction if they take the offending allergen together with aspirin" (36).

Conceptually similar to these reports is a recent letter to the editor describing a case of food allergy following cobalt-60 radiation therapy (36a). The authors speculated that the radiation therapy caused an increased permeability of the gut to allergenic molecules, increasing the absorption of offending substances and consequent sensitization of the individual. It must be remembered that none of the case reports described in this chapter (and indeed, this book) can prove a cause and effect relationship. They are merely presented to stimulate critical thought on the part of the reader, and perhaps lead to the performance of controlled studies.

FOOD INTOLERANCE AND CYTOTOXIC TESTING

Cytotoxic testing has received much attention in the lay press in recent years. Especially in California, many ads for cytotoxic and "food allergy" testing appear in newspapers, magazines and other popular media. In these ads, food allergy is held to be responsible for nervousness, fatigue, depression, and many other ills. Separating the "wheat from the chaff" in this area is very difficult, and food allergy is a controversial topic even among respected physicians.

Food Allergy

One fact which is clear is that some individuals are exquisitely sensitive to certain foods, the exposure to which can result in a fatal reaction (37). Among food reactions, peanuts seem to be especially deadly for a few individuals. For instance, a severe illness resulted in a peanut-sensitive individual who simply inhaled near an open jar of peanut butter. Another individual died after he mistakenly ate a small amount of peanut butter, even though he immediately spit it out, knowing of his reactivity to peanut.

Such immediate and severe reactions are easily ascribed to food allergy. Milder reactions, especially those of a psychologic nature, are more difficult to associate with a specific food. In a recent study (38), Pearson and colleagues sought objective evidence for food allergy in 23 patients who attributed a wide variety of symptoms to food allergy. In addition to allergy testing, the subjects also underwent psychiatric examination, the results of which were witheld from the investigating physicians. To establish the presence of food allergy, patients were given double-blind provocation tests. These tests consisted of giving the food(s) to which the subject thought he was allergic in opaque capsules, alternating randomly with an inactive placebo enclosed in identical capsules. Each test consisted of three "active" and three placebo preparations. For allergy to be considered present, the subject had to correctly identify 5 of the 6 administrations as being active or placebo.

The results were interesting. Food sensitivity was confirmed by double-blind challenge in 4 of the 23 subjects. These four initially complained of what are classically considered real allergic symptoms—asthma, eczema, allergic rhinitis ("stuffy nose")—but had no psychological symptoms. Food allergy could not be confirmed in the remaining 19 patients. They were unable to distinguish, by their symptoms, the real from the placebo capsules; in 5 patients, this was partially due to poor cooperation. These 19 patients all had multiple (largely psychiatric) symptoms which would not normally be considered due to allergy. Of the patients in whom food allergy could not be confirmed, none had a positive skin test to any food. Of the 19 patients, 7 accepted the doctors' opinion that it was unlikely that their symptoms were due to allergy. Of these 7 subjects, 6 had significant improvement in their symptoms (without altering their dietary habits). Only 2 of the 7 who did not accept this opinion improved.

All patients were psychiatrically evaluated. A score of 12 or more was regarded as indicative of psychiatric problems. All the (four) patients in whom food allergy was confirmed had scores below 12 (remember that the psychiatrists administered this test without knowing which category the subjects were in). All of those in whom food hypersensitivity could not be confirmed and who were fully assessed had scores greater than 12! In these patients, the most common psychiatric diagnosis was neurotic depression.

In the four patients with confirmed food allergy, testing with the allergy-producing food did not induce psychological symptoms. In contrast, among the patients in whom food allergy could not be confirmed, psychiatric symptoms accompanied many of the food challenge tests, but were as frequently associated with placebo as they were with the alleged allergy-inducing food. Many subjects were quite adamant that their symptoms occurred every time they ate a particular food, but were unable to identify that food when it was given in a double-blind manner. Some even became hostile when asked to make a decision as to whether or not they had reacted to the individual food challenges.

The origin of the subjects' beliefs that they had food allergy differed between the patients with confirmed and unconfirmed allergies. Most of those whose allergy was confirmed by double-blind tests had been aware since childhood of a particular food sensitivity (true food allergies are much more common in childhood than in adulthood). Of the patients with unconfirmed allergies, 6 became convinced that they had a food allergy after reading the book *Not All In The Mind*.

The fact that several patients were able to resume normal diets (which included the "allergy-inducing" food(s)) after psychiatric treatment suggests that psychological factors were the cause rather than the result of the food "intolerance".

The authors of this study concluded that psychopathology can often play a role in false impressions of food allergy, and that double-blind testing is the only certain means by which food allergy can be diagnosed. In a letter to the editor, it was charged (39) that this study was biased, but the authors responded (40) that dietary changes resulting from improper diagnosis of food allergy are often potentially harmful, and shouldn't be carried out in the absence of double-blind testing.

A recent review article on food allergy is less definitive than the Pearson paper (41). This article emphasizes the controversial nature of this field, even among respected physicians. The most obvious explanation for the opposing viewpoints is the difference in the type of evidence accepted as indicative of food sensitivity. Most physicians (including me) require double-blind, placebo-controlled food challenges as proof, while others are satisfied with anecdotal reports. For instance, Bock evaluated the role of foods suspected to cause health disorders in infants (41). Of a total of 98 suspected food reactions, only 11 were confirmed by double-blind food challenge. Parental report of a food reaction in their child was experimentally verified only 12% of the time. Documented food allergy symptoms were limited to conventional ones like skin rashes, respiratory problems, and gastrointestinal problems. Behavioral symptoms could not be objectively related to food ingestion.

In summary, it appears obvious that allergies to many foods exist, and that the signs and symptoms are quite variable. Food allergies are much more common in children, and can even be life-threatening on occasion. If we accept the double-blind food challenge as the "gold standard" for establishing the presence of food allergy, only 10-15% of all food allergies suspected by patients or their parents can be confirmed. It appears that in adults, psychiatric difficulties are more often the *cause* than the result of presumed food allergy symptoms. The interested reader is encouraged to consult several recent excellent reviews on food allergy (41-44) for further detail and multiple references.

Migraine and Food Allergy

As we have noted, the media have popularized the idea that food allergy can cause a host of psychosomatic problems such as fatigue or depression. There appears to be little scientific documentation of this hypothesis. Physicians may be as skeptical of food allergy causing migraine as they might of such allergy causing fatigue or depression; recent studies suggest that this skepticism may be unwarranted.

Two double-blind trials (45,46) and a review (47) suggest that reactions to food can precipitate migraine in certain sensitive individuals. One study was presented at a meeting of the American College of Allergy and is discussed in the review article quoted previously (41). Forty-one migraine patients referred from neurology clinic were skin-tested against 83 food antigens. Sixteen had positive tests; the number of positive reactions varyied from 1 to 29. Patients were asked to eliminate from their diet foods to which they had had a positive skin test, and record any changes in migraine frequency. The 25 skin-test-negative patients were put on a diet free of eggs, corn, wheat and milk for a month.

During the one-month food elimination period, 10 of the 16 skin-test-positive patients had a significant (more than two thirds) decrease in migraine frequency, whereas only 3 of the 25 skin-test-negative patients had a similar improvement. Thus, a positive skin test appeared to be a good predictor of whether an elimination diet would be beneficial, presumably because the skin test could guide the elimination of specific offending foods.

The 13 patients whose headaches decreased significantly with selective food elimination underwent double-blind food challenge tests. Of the 12 patients completing these tests, 9 developed migraine in response to challenge with the suspect foods. This high (75%) response rate suggests that skin test positivity and subsequent improvement on elimination diet are fairly reliable indicators of true food intolerance (as determined by double-blind tests).

To put these findings in perspective, of the 41 original migraine patients, 9 had positive results on blinded food challenge (the "gold standard"); this yields an incidence of documented food-induced migraine of 22%. These authors speculated that the true incidence in the general migraine population may be much lower because patients were selected for this study because they suspected that food sensitivity played a role in their migraine.

Other investigators, on the other hand, have provided data that suggest an even greater incidence of food-induced migraine. Monro and colleagues (45) found that 23 of 33 (70%) migraine patients were benefited by an elimination diet, with resultant complete relief from migraine in most of these patients. A good correlation was found in this study between clinically relevant foods (i.e., foods that were thought to provoke migraine) and RAST tests (an allergy test) for these foods. Unfortunately, this was not a placebo-controlled or a double-blind study, so the results, though impressive, are hard to interpret.

Egger and colleagues (46) studied migraine in children and obtained results similar to those of Monro. Of 88 children with suspected food-induced migraine, 78 recovered completely and 4 improved greatly (93% response rate!) on an elimination diet. Of these, 40 entered a double-blind, placebo-controlled study of suspected migraine-producing foods. In this experiment, active food produced headache in 26 patients, while placebo caused headache in only 2 (4 had headaches with both active and placebo foods, and 8 had no headache with either food). It is impressive to note that 35 of these 40 patients preferred the placebo (presumably non-headache-producing) food, and 2 preferred the active food (3 had no preference). This double-blind portion of this study is strong evidence for a major role of foods in the migraine of these patients.

Several correspondents criticized this study (48,49). One writer noted that the patients were highly selected and did not represent the average migraine patient—50% had behavioral disorders, 16% had seizures and 7% had permanent neurological signs! Another pointed out that the response was judged only over two weeks, and that placebo response could have accounted for the marked improvement in most of the patients. Although these are valid criticisms, none can explain the ability of the patients to identify with such accuracy the active versus the placebo food. Assuming that this ability was not due to differences in the taste, texture or other properties of the active versus placebo food, this is strong evidence that in some individuals, certain foods can induce migraine.

It seems reasonable to conclude from the above studies that some migraine patients may benefit from an evaluation of the potential role of certain foods in the development of their migraine. RAST and skin testing may be useful, and elimination diet may help confirm suspected intolerance. In my opinion, however, a double-blind, placebo-controlled food challenge test is necessary before certain foods can be unequivocally implicated.

As has been noted previously, the elimination diet is the cornerstone of both diagnosis and treatment of food intolerance. An elimination diet, though easily described, is not so easily implemented. Some allergenic substances may not be listed on food labels, although by law, additives must be listed. Furthermore, the composition of the same food may vary with the brand of the product. Finally, if intolerance to several foods is documented, the resulting elimination diet may be very restricted, and especially for children, very hard to adhere to. Elimination diets may also be nutritionally inadequate unless assistance from a physician and/ or dietitian is obtained and followed.

Although elimination diet is the cornerstone of treatment, two recent studies suggest that sodium cromoglycate (a drug used in the treatment of asthma) can prevent or minimize food-induced allergic reactions. In one (double-blind) study, 24 adults with adverse reactions to foods and food additives took either placebo or 1600 mg sodium cromoglycate prior to food challenge (50). Intake of the active drug minimized but didn't totally abolish symptoms in most patients. Thus, the authors recommended the use of sodium cromoglycate along with elimination diet.

In the other study, 9 patients with food-induced migraine refractory to standard management were given either sodium cromoglycate or placebo in double-blind fashion prior to eating a meal containing the suspected migraine-producing foods (51). Eight of the nine patients preferred the active drug over the placebo pill (p=0.025), suggesting that sodium cromoglycate was significantly better than placebo in preventing the headache. Since sodium cromoglycate is believed to work by preventing the formation of immune complexes, this study strongly supports the hypothesis that some cases of migraine are immunologically mediated. Since this drug is poorly absorbed from the gastrointestinal tract, the authors suggest that "it acts locally on the gut mucosa (lining) to block an immunological 'trigger' for the absorption of antigen (i.e., the offending food)" or formation of immune complexes. It is still unclear as to how prevalent food-induced, immunologically-mediated migraine really is.

Food Allergy and Other Disorders

Food allergy has been implicated in several other disorders in addition to the ones described above. For instance, it has been proposed that irritable bowel syndrome (IBS) may be due to food allergy in some patients (51a,b). IBS is characterized by (usually) abdominal pain in association with alternating periods of diarrhea and constipation. No anatomic causes can be found, and IBS has usually been considered to be a psychosomatic disorder. In one of these studies (51b), 9 of 28 refractory IBS patients responded to a hypoallergenic diet. At one year follow-up, 7 of these 9 patients were still well, provided they avoided the foods to which they were intolerant.

Food sensitivity has also been implicated as causing eczema in infants (51c), and a case of nephrotic syndrome has responded to elimination of pork from the diet (51d). In the former article (51c), exclusively-breastfed infants were studied. Those with eczema were much more likely to have positive skin tests to food antigens than those without eczema. Interestingly, egg protein was found in the mothers' breast milk. The authors hypothesized that babies developing eczema may be sensitized by foods eaten by their mothers.

Cytotoxic Testing

Cytotoxic testing and other means (e.g., skin tests and RAST) of identifying allergies were alluded to previously. Whereas skin tests and RAST are commonly used in allergists' offices, the leucocyte cytotoxic test (LCT) is considered quackery by the FDA and most allergists.

The test consists of taking white blood cells (leukocytes) from a patient who may have food allergies and placing it on a glass slide containing the suspected food. After incubation for an hour or two, the white cells are examined under the microscope. If disintigration (or other changes—e.g., cessation of pseudopod formation) of the white cells are observed, the patient is considered to be allergic to the tested food.

Although several authors have supported the value of the LCT in the diagnosis and treatment of food allergies (52-55), none of these studies are double-blind or placebo-controlled. Indeed, one wonders about the objectivity of some of these studies—especially since one author of reference 55 is the president of a cytotoxic testing laboratory in California! One study which has been quoted as supporting the value of the LCT (56) in actuality presented data that showed little correlation between the results of the test and the clinical diagnosis of food allergy (which is really the bottom line). Due to the likelihood of bias and placebo effect, uncontrolled studies are not useful in supporting the validity of the cytotoxic test. This is underscored by the fact that all the controlled studies of the LCT show it to be useless in the diagnosis and treatment of food allergies (57-59). I am unaware of any scientifically controlled study which has shown the LCT to be valuable in this setting. Recognizing this, the American Academy of Allergy has issued a position paper to this effect (60) and several editorials have reached similar conclusions (61-64).

The two major problems with the LCT are that it is not reproducible from one occasion to another and that test results do not correlate with the presence of food allergy (as determined by elimination diet and then a challenge test with the suspected food). For instance, Lieberman and his colleagues (57) describe one patient who was known to be clinically allergic to buckwheat, but to no other foods. On the first occasion that this patient was tested, the LCT was positive not only for buckwheat (accurately), but also for barley, rye, egg and banana. Even more interesting is that on the second test, the LCT was no longer positive to buckwheat (or for that matter, any of the other foods which were positive on the first occasion). On the third try, a new group of foods were declared to be allergy-producing by the LCT (apricot, lettuce, tomato, egg, and pecan), even though this individual had no trouble eating any of these foods. If this patient had used the LCT to guide him in formulating an elimination diet, he would cease eating 12 foods unnecessarily. It is noteworthy that this problem was not unique to this patient; all five patients who were tested on more than one occasion showed almost no similarity in the lists of foods which were LCT-positive on different occasions, and there was little correlation between LCT positivity and the clinical situation.

One might argue that even if the LCT is useless, that little harm is done by following it, and that people have a right to choose to have the test done (often at a cost of several hundred dollars). Unfortunately, harm can result. A recent correspondent to The Lancet described two patients he had seen in the previous month whose lives had been made miserable by strict elimination diets recommended by a cytotoxic testing laboratory (65). With respect to the freedom-of-choice argument, one could also argue that people ought to be able to buy any medicine they want, without a prescription. It is obvious that one function of society and its institutions is to protect the unwary consumer from fraudulent services. Some have called for the outlawing of laboratories that perform the LCT without physician supervision of patients (64), since such laboratories are alleged to be practicing medicine without a license. In the interim, the reader is encouraged to consider the above evidence before obtaining or recommending the leukocyte cytotoxic test.

THE BOTTOM LINE

The food allergy field at present is as confusing as it is exciting. Only in the past few years have meaningful controlled studies been published. In recognition of this increasing interest is the recent conference which was held on this topic (the reader is encouraged to review the published proceedings of this conference (66) as well as an excellent recent review (67)).

Although the data are preliminary, it appears clear that many adverse organic reactions may occur in response to foods in certain susceptible individuals. Some of these reactions can be lethal. The prevalence and scope of such reactions remains to be determined. Only in a scientific and unbiased fashion will such a determination be reasonably made. Furthermore, medical personnel, who have usually held a dim view of food allergy, are encouraged to keep their minds open when patients relate symptoms which are consistent with food sensitivity.

REFERENCES

1. U.S Department of Health, Education and Welfare: More than you ever thought you would know about food additives. Parts I, II, III. FDA Consumer April, May and June, 1979, U.S. Government Printing Office.

2. Appledorf H, et al: Sensory evaluation of health foods: A comparison with traditional foods. Florida Agriculture Experiment Stations Journal Series #5328, 1974

2a. Gourdine SP, et al: Health foods stores investigation. J Am Dietetic Assoc 83:285, 1983

3. Hallberg L, Rossander L: Effect of soy protein on nonheme iron absorption in man. Am J Clin Nutr 36:514, 1982

4. Casey CE, et al: Availability of zinc: Loading test with human milk, cow's milk and infant formulas. Peds 68:394, 1981

5. Ames B: Dietary carçinogens and anticarcinogens. Oxygen radicals and degenerative diseases. Science 221:1256, 1983

6. Abaelson PH: Dietary carcinogens. Science 221:1252, 1983

7. Hiscoe HB: Does being natural make it good? N Engl J Med 308:1474, 1983

8. Sugimachi K, et al: Acute gastric anisakiasis. Analysis of 178 cases. JAMA 253:1012, 1985

9. Sacks JJ, et al: Toxoplasmosis infection associated with raw goat's milk. JAMA 248:1728, 1982. Also discussed in Infectious Diseases, March 1983, p. 8.

10. Leads from MMWR: *Salmonella dublin* and raw milk consumption. JAMA 251: 2195, 1984

11. U.S. Department of Health and Human Services: Food preservatives: A fresh report. FDA Consumer 18(3):23, 1984.

11a. Lecos C: Food preservatives: A fresh report. FDA Consumer, April, 1984, pp.23

12. U.S. Department of Health and Human Services: Pesticides and food: Public worry No. 1. FDA Consumer 18(6):12, 1984

13. Colllins-Williams C: Intolerance to additives. Ann Allergy 51:315, 1983

14. Juhlin L, et al: Urticaria and asthma induced by food and drug additives in patients with aspirin hypersensitivity. J Allergy Clin Immunol 50:92, 1972

15. Lockey SD: Hypersensitivity to tartrazine (FD&C Yellow No. 5) and other dyes and additives present in foods and pharmaceutical products. Ann Allergy 38:206, 1977

16. Stenius BSM, Lemola M: Hypersensitivity to acetylsalicylic acid (ASA) and tartrazine in patients with asthma. Clin Allergy 6:119, 1976

17. Weber RW, et al: Incidence of bronchoconstriction due to aspirin, azo dyes, non-azo dyes and preservatives in a population of perennial asthmatics. J Allergy & Clin Immunol 64:32, 1979

18. Tan Y, Collins-Williams C: Aspirin-induced asthma in children. Ann Allergy 48:1, 1982

19. Lee M, et al: Tartrazine containing drugs. Drug Intell Clin Pharmacol 15:782, 1981

20. Tse CST: Food products containing tartrazine. N Engl J Med 306:681, 1982

21. Freeman BJ: Sulphur dioxide in foods and beverages: its use as a preservative and its effect on asthma. Br J Dis Chest 74:128, 1980

22. Stevenson DD, Simon RA: Sensitivity to ingested metabisulphite in asthmatic patients. J Allerg & Clin Immunol 68:26, 1981

22a. Updates: Sulfite restrictions proposed. FDA Consumer, November, 1985, pp.3

22b. Newsletter: FDA bans use of sulfites in fresh fruits and vegetables. Am Fam Phys 32:17, 1985

23. Huang AS, Fraser WM: Are sulfite additives really safe? N Engl J Med 311:542, 1984

24. Kwok RHM: Chinese restaurant syndrome. N Engl J Med 278:796, 1968

25. Cochran JW, Cochran AH: Monosodium glutamania: The Chinese restaurant syndrome revisited. JAMA 252:899, 1984

26. Stegink LD, et al: Modulating effect of Sustagen on plasma glutamate concentration in humans ingesting monosodium L-glutamate. Am J Clin Nutr 37: 27. Allen DH, Baker GJ: Chinese restaurant asthma. N Engl J Med 305:1154, 1981

28. Kenny RA, Tidbal CS: Human susceptibility to oral monosodium L-glutamate. Am J Clin Nutr 25:140, 1972

29. Morselli PL, Garattini S: Monosodium glutamate and the Chinese restaurant syndrome. Nature 227:611, 1970 194, 1983

29a. Tinkelman DG, Bock SA: Anaphylaxis presumed to be caused by beef containing streptomycin. Ann Allergy 53:243, 1984

29b. Abstracts: Anaphylaxis to penicillin in a frozen dinner. JAMA 252:1755. 1984

29c. Schwartz HJ, Sher TH: Anaphylaxis to penicillin in a frozen dinner. Ann Allergy 52:342, 1984

30. Helgason T, Jonasson MR: Evidence for a food additive as a cause of ketosis-prone diabetes. Lancet 2:716, 1981

31. Christy M, et al: Diabetes and month of birth. Lancet 2:216, 1982

32. Helgason T, et al: Diabetes produced in mice by smoked/cured mutton. Lancet 2:1017, 1982

33. Symon DNK, et al: Smoked foods in the diets of mothers of diabetic children. Lancet 2:514, 1984

34. Buchbinder EM, et al: Food-dependent, exercise-induced anaphylaxis. JAMA 250:2973, 1983

35. El-Dieb MR: Food-dependent, exercise-induced anaphylaxis. JAMA 251:3224, 1984

36. Cant AJ, et al: Food hypersensitivity made life threatening by ingestion of aspirin. Br Med J 288:755, 1984

36a. Ciprandi G, et al: ⁶⁰Cobalt therapy as an "allergic breakthrough" in a case of food allergy. N Engl J Med 311:861, 1984

37. Fries JH: Peanuts. Allergic and other untoward reactions. Ann Allergy 28:220, 1982. Also discussed in Modern Med, Sept., 1982, p.208.

38. Pearson DJ: Food allergy: How much in the mind? A clinical and psychiatric study of suspected food hypersensitivity. Lancet 1:1259, 1983

39. Rippere V: Food allergy: How much in the mind? Lancet 2:45, 1983

40. Pearson DJ, et al: Food allergy. Lancet 2:160, 1983

41. Check W: Eat, drink and be merry—or argue about food allergy. JAMA 250:701, 1983

42. Editorial: Food allergy. Lancet 1:249, 1979

43. May CD: Food allergy—material and ethereal. N Engl J Med 302:1142, 1980 44. Denman AM: Food allergy. Br Med J 286:1164, 1983

45. Monro J, et al: Food allergy in migraine. Study of dietary exclusion and RAST. Lancet 2:1, 1980

46. Egger J, et al: Is migraine food allergy? A double-blind controlled trial of oligoantigenic diet treatment. Lancet 2:865, 1983

47. Perkin JE, Hartje J: Diet and migraine: A review of the literature. J Am Dietetic Assoc 83:459, 1983

48. Letters to the editor: Is migraine food allergy? Lancet 2:1081, 1983

49. Letters to the editor: Food allergy and migraine. Lancet 2:1256, 1983

50. Ortolani C, et al: Prophylaxis of adverse reactions to foods. A double-blind study of oral sodium cromoglycate for the prophylaxis of adverse reactions to foods and additives. Ann Allerg 50:105, 1983

51. Monro J, et al: Migraine is a food-allergic disease. Lancet 2:719, 1984

51a. Alun JV, et al: Food intolerance: a major factor in the pathogenesis of irritable bowel syndrome. Lancet 1:1115, 1982

51b. Smith MA, et al: Food intolerance, atopy, and irritable bowel syndrome. Lancet 2:1064, 1985

51c. Cant A, et al: Egg and cows' milk hypersensitivity in exclusively breast fed infants with eczema, and detection of egg protein in breast milk. Br Med J 291:932, 1985

51d. Howanietz H, Lubec G: Idiopathic nephrotic syndrome treated with steroids for five years, found to be allergic reaction to pork. Lancet 2:450, 1985

52. Ulett GA, Perry SG: Cytotoxic testing and leukocyte increase as an index to food sensitivity. Ann Allergy 33:23, 1974

53. Updegraff TR: Food allergy and cytotoxic tests. Ear Nose & Throat J 56: 450, 1977

54. Boyles JH: The validity of using the cytoxic food test in clinical allergy. Ear Nose & Throat J 56:168, 1977

55. Hughes EC, et al: Effect of time of blood sampling on in vitro tests of food sensitivities. Ear Nose & Throat 61:34, 1982
56. Ruokonen J, et al: Secretory otitis media and allergy, with special reference to the cytotoxic leucocyte test. Allergy 36:59, 1981
57. Lieberman P, et al: Controlled study of the cytotoxic food test. JAMA 231:728, 1975
58. Benson TE, Arkins JA: Cytotoxic testing for food allergy: Evaluation of reproducibility and correlation. J Allerg Clin Immunol 58:471, 1976
59. Lehman CW: The leucocytic food allergy test: A study of its reliability and reproducibility. Effect of diet and sublingual food drops on this test. Ann Allergy 45:150, 1980
60. American Academy of Allergy: Position statements—controversial techniques. J Allerg Clin Immunol 67:333, 1981
61. Grieco MH: Controversial practices in allergy. JAMA 247:3106, 1982
62. Haddad ZH: Nonacceptable, unproven tests for allergy. JAMA 247:3106, 1982
63. Editorial: Self-referral laboratories. Lancet 1:802, 1983
64. Editorial: The cytotoxic test. West J Med 139:702, 1983
65. Letters to the editor: Cytotoxic test for food intolerance. Lancet 1: 989, 1983
66. Multiple authors: Tenth Annual Marabou Symposium: Food Sensitivity. Nutr Reviews 42:70, 1984
67. Truswell AS: Food sensitivity. Br Med J 291:951, 1985

CHAPTER 4

Psychological and Behavioral Effects of Nutrients

On initial analysis, it may appear ridiculous to theorize that food ingestion can affect brain function. When one realizes, however, that many of the chemicals (called neurotransmitters) which are responsible for normal brain activity are derived from certain nutrients, this concept gains credibility. In support of the importance of neurotransmitters is the fact that most psychoactive medications (e.g., antidepressant and antipsychotic drugs) are believed to work by altering the amount and release of neurotransmitters. There is also much animal (and some human) data which supports the hypothesis that certain nutrients can affect brain function.

WHICH NUTRIENTS AFFECT NEUROTRANSMITTER LEVELS?

Three nutrients act as precursors for 3 important neurotransmitters:

Food Precursor	Neurotransmitter
Tryptophan	Serotonin
Lecithin, choline	Acetylcholine
Tyrosine	Dopamine

The behavioral effects of these nutrients have been recently reviewed by Dr. Richard Wurtman, one of the pioneers in this field (1). The basic biochemistry (2), clinical applications of the cholinergic precursors, choline and lecithin (3), and the role of S-adenosylmethionine (a derivative of an essential amino acid) and folic acid (a B-vitamin) in depression and other mood disorders (4) have also been recently reviewed. The interested reader is encouraged to consult these reviews and their excellent bibliographies.

Tryptophan to Serotonin

Tryptophan, an essential amino acid, is converted to serotonin via two chemical steps. Serotonin is believed to be important in the control of pituitary hor-

71

mone secretion, sleep patterns and perception of pain. A high-carbohydrate, protein-*poor* meal elevates brain tryptophan levels, whereas high protein meals have the opposite effect (5,6). This may seem paradoxical, since tryptophan is an amino acid, which is found in protein, but not in carbohydrate. Protein-rich meals depress brain tryptophan because tryptophan is carried from the bloodstream into the brain by the same transport system which carries other amino acids. These other amino acids are more plentiful than tryptophan in most proteins, so tryptophan "loses the battle" in attempting to cross into the brain. A high carbohydrate meal enhances the entry of tryptophan into the brain by releasing insulin, which lowers the blood level of the competing amino acids, allowing tryptophan unimpeded entry into the brain. As might be expected, brain tryptophan levels can also be increased by ingestion of the amino acid itself, especially if it's taken together with an insulin-releasing carbohydrate.

Carbohydrate consumption or tryptophan administration can have several effects. It can affect the sensation of fatigue and accelerate the onset of sleep in adults (7). A recent study showed this to be true in newborns as well (8). Twenty healthy newborns were randomly assigned to receive a feeding consisting either of tryptophan in 10% glucose or valine (one of the competing amino acids mentioned above) in 5% glucose. Sleep patterns after these feedings were compared to those after a normal formula. Tryptophan hastened the onset of active sleep by 14.1 minutes (compared to formula), while valine delayed sleep by 15.8 minutes ($p < 0.05$). The authors concluded that "variations in the composition of the diet may influence sleep behavior in newborns".

A recent double-blind placebo-controlled study (9) suggests that adding tryptophan to lithium therapy can result in greater improvement in psychiatric (9 bipolar and 7 schizoaffective) patients than lithium alone. Since the number of patients in these studies was small, it is hard to recommend the clinical administration of tryptophan. As more data on the use of tryptophan in clinical circumstances accumulate, it may be possible to recommend it. It should also be realized, however, that even though it is a "natural" compound, tryptophan may also have side effects which are as yet undiscovered. Those will also have to be considered before recommendations can be made.

Lecithin (Phosphatidylcholine) and Choline to Acetylcholine

As is true of serotonin, underactivity of acetylcholine (cholinergic mechanisms) has been implicated in various neuropsychiatric disorders. Animal studies have shown that choline and lecithin (the latter contains choline) administration can increase levels of acetylcholine (ACh) in certain parts of the brain (see reference 3 for the relevant bibliography). Lecithin and choline have also been tried clinically. Of the neuropsychiatric disorders, choline has been most effective in tardive dyskinesia (a disorder of abnormal involuntary muscle movements). Since choline has a bitter taste, and often causes an objectionable body odor, lecithin has also been tried in tardive dyskinesia (TD), with similar success (10). In a double-blind crossover study of lecithin in 6 patients with TD, a progressive improvement was noted in all the patients (11).

Other diseases in which cholinergic precursors have been tried, with variable success, include Huntington's disease (chorea), cerebellar ataxias, Gilles de la Tourette's syndrome, schizophrenia, and affective disorders (depression and mania) (3). A double-blind, placebo-controlled trial (12) showed improvement with lecithin (30 g daily) to be significantly greater than with placebo in 5 of 6 patients with bipolar disorder (manic depressives), during the manic phase ($p = 0.02$). Lecithin ameliorated all the symptoms of mania, including hallucinations, delusions and incoherent speech. This exciting finding needs to be replicated in greater numbers of patients.

Cells from patients with affective disorder (such as manic depressive illness) have more ACh receptors than cells from normal controls (13). Although the cells studied were fibroblasts (connective tissue cells) and not brain cells, one might speculate that receptors in brain cells might be similarly affected. As noted in the accompanying editorial (14), one might expect such individuals to be supersensitive to stimulation with cholinergic chemicals such as lecithin, and this may explain the response observed in the study quoted above (12).

Some evidence suggests a role for cholinergic mechanisms in human memory, and of a cholinergic deficit in Alzheimer's disease. While some studies have shown lecithin or choline administration to be beneficial in these circumstances (15), most haven't (16). The combination of lecithin with a drug that augments the endogenous release of ACh (e.g., piracetam) may be promising (3).

Tyrosine to Dopamine and Other Catecholamines

The conversion of tyrosine to dopamine and other substances in the body has been shown to be related to the availability of tyrosine (17). Brain tyrosine levels are most conveniently increased by ingesting pure tyrosine. Tyrosine has been used to treat endogenous depression with some success (18). Tyrosine is thought to ameliorate depression by increasing the synthesis and release of the neurotransmitter norepinephrine, which is deficient in depression. Indeed, antidepressant drugs currently in use are believed to be beneficial in depression because they enhance norepinephrine synthesis and function.

In an impressive though anecdotal report (19), a 30-year-old female was diagnosed as having endogenous depression. She was given 100 mg/kg (about 5 g/day) of L-tyrosine daily in 3 divided doses for two weeks, followed by three weeks of an identically appearing placebo, after which she resumed tyrosine for an additional five weeks. She rated herself, and was also rated weekly by a psychiatrist who was unaware of her treatment. Her depression improved markedly with the first two weeks of tyrosine, and she said she felt better than she had in years. Within one week of placebo substitution, her depressive symptoms began to return, and by the end of the placebo period, her depressive indices were slightly worse than pretreatment levels. Her depression was again completely alleviated when tyrosine was reinstituted.

It remains to be seen if tyrosine will be similarly effective in other patients suffering from depression, and whether this amino acid will be safe when used in this manner. Since antidepressant drugs currently available are potentially dangerous, tyrosine may be a welcome addition to the physician's armamentarium.

Tyrosine has also been reported to help patients with mild Parkinson's disease (20). It may do so by increasing the amount of biopterin, an important cofactor (like an enzyme) which is deficient in patients with Parkinson's disease (21).

VITAMINS AND MENTAL FUNCTION

Nutrients do not affect brain function only by altering neurotranmitters. It has been theorized, with some experimental support, that vitamin and other nutritional deficiencies can also result in neuropsychiatric difficulties, which respond to appropriate supplementation. Little research has been done in this area, perhaps due to the understandable tendency of scientists to avoid topics which have been the object of popular press attention. By avoiding this area, however, scientists are only making it easier for poorly qualified, self-designated "experts" to prey on a gullible public.

It has been known for quite some time that *severe* vitamin deficiencies can result in certain deficiency syndromes. These syndromes, all of which manifest cognitive dysfunction (poor mental function), include (vitamin responsible is in parentheses) pellagra (niacin), Wernicke's (thiamine), scurvy (vitamin C), and pernicious anemia (vitamin B_{12}). What isn't clear is whether *mild* deficiencies of these vitamins, which don't cause the full-blown deficiency disease, might also be accompanied by cognitive dysfunction. Such dysfunction is probably often attributed to "old age".

A recent paper (22) suggests that the answer to this question might be "yes". Goodwin and colleagues found an association between nutritional status and cognitive functioning in 260 noninstitutionalized men and women older than 60 years who were in good health. Subjects with low blood levels of vitamins B_{12} or C scored worse on two tests of cognitive ability (one of abstract thinking and the other of memory) than the rest of the group.

This observation is one that may be significantly misinterpreted by biased parties (e.g., vitamin salesmen). For instance, one way to interpret these findings would be to conclude that vitamin deficiency causes cognitive dysfunction. In fact, the data do not allow such an interpretation, because an equally likely explanation is that poor cognitive function leads to inadequate dietary intake, which consequently results in low blood vitamin levels. Upon reflection, it becomes apparent that this study only showed a *relationship* between low vitamin levels and cognitive dysfunction, and it cannot differentiate between these two interpretations of the data.

The accompanying editorial (23) called for efforts to determine whether a cause-and-effect relationship exists by ascertaining whether nutrient supplementation will improve cognitive dysfunction. Only one such double-blind placebo-controlled study has been performed to date (24), with marginally significant results. In this study, the effect of oral vitamin C or placebo on daily living activities, interest in the surroundings, and appetite, was examined in elderly inpatients in two geriatric hospitals. After 4 weeks of supplementation with 1 g of vitamin C daily, these three parameters were re-evaluated by the charge nurse. Although most patients did not show changes in these parameters, more patients improved and fewer deteriorated in the vitamin C group than in the placebo group (marginal significance, $p < 0.10$). The variable which showed change most frequently was daily living activity. Weight change also differed between the groups, increasing in the vitamin group, while decreasing in the placebo group ($p < 0.05$).

Although both of these studies showed a positive relationship between vitamin supplements and cognitive function, the study populations are very different. The patients in the previous study (22) were ambulatory healthy outpatients, whereas those in the vitamin C study (24) were elderly inpatients with little interest in their environment, most of whom were only partly mobile. Although the improvement in the latter trial was marginal, the trial only lasted 4 weeks, and the patients were such that any improvement was distinctly unexpected.

Another conclusion to be drawn from these studies is that subclinical vitamin deficiency, as determined by blood levels, is very common, epecially in the institutionalized elderly. This may be due to poor dietary intake, intercurrent diseases, inadequate medical supervision, etc. Additional longer-term controlled studies testing the cognitive effects of vitamin supplements would certainly be in order. In the meantime, *multivitamin* supplementation, especially of the institutionalized elderly, might be reasonable. The potential for benefit is illustrated by unexplained cases of neuropathy and psychiatric symptoms which turned out to be due to folate deficiency, and which responded to folate supplements (25,26). Interestingly, contrary to classical teaching, half of these folate-deficient patients did not have megaloblastic anemia.

FOOD ADDITIVES AND BEHAVIOR— FEINGOLD AND OTHER DEFINED DIETS

This topic is in a sense a hybrid of the topics in Chapter 3 (food additives and intolerance) and this chapter (behavioral and psychological effects of nutrients).

Feingold, a pediatric allergist, proposed in 1973 the theory that the ingestion of food additives and natural compounds (salicylates) in various fruits and vegetables can cause hyperactivity in susceptible children. Even though more than a decade has passed, this hypothesis remains controversial, having been neither proved nor disproved in the intervening years. Although many papers have appeared on this topic, most have been anecdotal and unscientific, and have consequently not added to our understanding of the relationship (if any) between food additives and hyperactivity. Several excellent randomized, double-blind studies have also been carried out; most of these have not supported Feingold's hypothesis. A few, however, have yielded data which preclude the outright dismissal of the hypothesis. Thus, perhaps in a modified form, the hypothesis that certain food substances can exacerbate hyperactive tendencies in a subset of children seems reasonable. A recent conference reviewed the data on this topic (27).

The syndrome of hyperactivity has undergone several, often confusing, changes in terminology. Some of the terms that have been applied to this syndrome include hyperkinetic reaction of childhood, hyperkinetic syndrome, hyperactive child syndrome, minimal brain damage, minimal brain dysfunction, and minor cerebral dysfunction. The current official term is the attention deficit disorder with hyperactivity. Whatever the term used, the essential features are developmentally inappropriate inattention, impulsivity and hyperactivity. Its etiology is likely to be multifactorial (i.e., it has many causes), including organic factors such as trauma, infection, lead intoxication, perinatal hypoxia (poor oxygen supply in the first few weeks of life), and psychosocial factors such as anxiety, inadequate parenting, and environmental stresses. In most cases, the specific etiology is unknown.

One of the problems that has plagued research into this topic is that the Feingold hypothesis was popularized on the basis of anecdotal data in a trade book (28) and in the absence of controlled trials. This dissemination to the public without controlled data or scientific review made many scientists (rightly or wrongly) very skeptical about the hypothesis. The popularity of the hypothesis also made it difficult to carry out a controlled trial to evaluate this theory.

Most of the studies supporting the Feingold hypothesis suffered from scientifically inadequate methodology, including unblind conditions, lack of objective measures, inadequate detail, absence of statistical analysis, and absence of controls (29-32). In view of the likelihood of bias in such studies, they will not be further discussed here.

Several high-quality, randomized, double-blind, placebo-controlled studies of the Feingold hypothesis have been published. Some investigators have studied specific substances (e.g., tartrazine, sugar), while others evaluated a blend of food additives. Others still have examined the effect of an elimination diet based on the Feingold hypothesis. Since the designs of these studies are so different, the studies are hard to compare.

In one of the earliest double-blind trials (33), the effects of a Feingold elimination diet were assessed by parents and teachers of 15 hyperactive kids. Teachers noted a significant reduction of symptoms on the elimination diet but parents did not. Improvement, however, occurred only when the elimination diet *followed* the control diet (but not when the order of the diets was reversed!). As was noted in the accompanying editorial (34) this significantly weakens the validity of the results.

It is difficult to maintain double-blind conditions when advising parents on diet in these studies. It is very likely that the parents will be able to figure out when their child is eating the defined diet. How do you hide the fact that the child isn't supposed to eat foods with additives while they are on the experimental study?

One way to do it is to remove all food from the house at the beginning of the study and have the investigators supply all the necessary (either Feingold or control) foods during the whole study. In addition, by preparing certain identical foods (e.g., cookies) with and without additives, one can further mask which diet the child is eating. Although this may sound like a lot of bother (and it probably was), this is exactly what Harley and his colleagues did (35). This is probably, at least scientifically speaking, the best-designed study in this area, and thus the results are especially important.

In this study, 36 hyperactive boys were studied under experimental (Feingold elimination diet) and control diet conditions. Teacher and parental ratings were employed, as were objective classroom and laboratory observational data, and objective psychological measures. For the majority of the hyperactive subjects, there was no improvement with the Feingold diet. For the 10 preschoolers in the group, however, parental observations indicated a positive response to the experimental diet—10 out of 10 mothers and 4 of 7 fathers of the preschoolers rated their children's behavior as improved on the Feingold-type diet.

Williams and colleagues (36) addressed this question by placing *all* children on a modified Feingold diet, and then giving them either additive-free or additive-containing specially-prepared cookies. These investigators also studied stimulant medications against placebo in this trial. Stimulant medications (e.g., methylphenidate—Ritalin) are often used to control hyperactivity, and have been shown to be very effective. This double-blind study found the stimulant medications to be much more effective than elimination diet in reducing hyperactive behavior. Of 26 hyperactive children, however, the behavior of three to eight seemed to be diet-responsive, depending on the criteria used.

In a study of similar design (37), 22 *normal* children on elimination diet were challenged intermittently with a blend of seven artificial colors. Parents' observations were the criteria used for evaluating response. Two children responded to the challenge. An accompanying article (38) supported that finding. In this study, 20 hyperactive and 20 normal children were placed on elimination diet for 5 days.

The children were then challenged with large doses of either a blend of 9 food dyes or identically-appearing placebo, after which a learning test was administered. The performance of the hyperactive children on the learning test was impaired at 1.5 and 3.5 hours after receiving the food color blend, compared to placebo, whereas the performance of the nonhyperactive kids was unaffected.

This is not entirely surprising, since tartrazine, a component of the blend, has been shown to cause allergic effects (see Chapter 3) and exacerbation of hyperkinetic symptoms in some individuals (39). A recent study (40) suggests that erythrosine, a red food dye that was also a component of the nine-dye blend, can produce a dose-dependent increase in the release of acetylcholine (a neurotransmitter) in isolated frog muscles. It has been proposed that some food dyes may have similar neurotransmitter-releasing effects in the human brain, and that this may explain their effects on behavior and activity.

It isn't only artificial food colors that have been studied for their potential effects on hyperkinesis. One study found a correlation between amount of sugar consumed and extent of certain hyperkinetic behaviors (41), although most of the evidence is against such a relationship. It has also been proposed that megavitamins may ameliorate the symptoms of the attention deficit disorder. A recent double-blind trial, however, found no support for this hypothesis (42). One investigator has also suggested that serotonin levels in hyperkinetic children are lower than normal (43), and that pyridoxine (vitamin B_6) can increase them and suppress the hyperactive symptoms (44); another researcher found similar serotonin levels in normal and hyperkinetic children (45). Finally, nitrogen excretion and other aspects of nitrogen metabolism in some hyperkinetic boys were found to be markedly different from normal boys (46).

THE BOTTOM LINE: FOOD AND HYPERKINESIS

Much data on the Feingold hypothesis has been reviewed above, and a summary of the occasionally-contradictory findings may be in order. Feingold originally indicted all artificial flavors and colors, as well as some preservatives and natural salicylates, as etiologic in hyperactivity. Despite that initial wide-ranging focus, the available double-blind studies have dealt almost exclusively with artificial colors. It is therefore impossible to comment here on the other aspects of the elimination diet recommended by Feingold. There is little evidence to support the elimination of fruits and vegetables from the diet; it would be necessary to eliminate these items in order to eliminate natural salicylates from the diet. Fruits and vegetables should not be arbitrarily eliminated from children's diets, since they constitute important low-calorie sources of vitamins and fiber.

What also seems to emerge from this literature review is the conclusion that the Feingold hypothesis finds much more support in unblind studies than in the double-blind placebo-controlled studies. The latter have been largely unable to support the Feingold hypothesis. Since these studies are much less subject to bias than unblind studies, more attention was paid to them in this review. It should be noted, however, that in almost every study quoted above, there seemed to be a small subset of children who did benefit from the elimination diet. This subset was usually 10-15% of the confirmed hyperactive children studied.

It seems clear, therefore, that while most hyperactive kids are not sensitive to the substances implicated by Feingold, some do seem to be affected by them. Hyperactivity is probably multifactorial in etiology, and it seems reasonable to conclude that in some children, certain substances can exacerbate the hyperactive tendency. Unfortunately, it remains unclear which substances are primarily implicated. Most studies used a blend of food colors, and it is unclear whether a single component of these blends (e.g., tartrazine or erythrosine) may be responsible for the effects. The studies of tartrazine and erythrosine (as potential neurotransmitter releasers) certainly make this hypothesis attractive.

In view of the lack of definitive evidence at this time, what recommendations would be reasonable? First, one must consider the potential benefits vs. harm in an elimination diet. For instance, there may be little harm in eliminating sugar-laden products from the diet, if it is believed that they exacerbate hyperactive behavior (although there is little evidence at this time to support this view). Elimination of all fruits and vegetables is not indicated without confirmation of the specific food (by blind challenge) which exacerbates the hyperactivity. In addition, nutritional advice from a physician or registered dietitian should be sought to ensure that all necessary nutrients are obtained in the diet. Thus, although it is too early to close the books on the Feingold hypothesis (as a recent article proclaimed [47]), skepticism is in order, and one must always remember that the cure (elimination diet) can sometimes be worse than the disease.

REFERENCES

1. Wurtman RJ: Behavioural effects of nutrients. Lancet 1:1145, 1983
2. Blusztajn JK, Wurtman RJ: Choline and cholinergic neurons. Science 221: 614, 1983
3. Rosenberg GS, Davis KL: The use of cholinergic precursors on neuropsychiatric diseases. Am J Clin Nutr 36:709, 1982
4. Reynolds EH, et al: Methylation and mood. Lancet 2:196, 1984
5. Fernstrom JD, Wurtman RJ: Brain serotonin content: increase following ingestion of carbohydrate diet. Science 174:1023, 1971
6. Fernstrom JD, Wurtman RJ: Brain serotonin content: physiological regulation by plasma neutral amino acids. Science 178:414, 1972
7. Hartmann E, et al: L-tryptophan, l-leucine and placebo:effects on subjective alertness. Sleep Res 5:57, 1976

8. Yogman MW, Zeisel SH: Diet and sleep patterns in newborns. N Engl J Med 309:1147, 1983

9. Brewerton TD, Reus VI: Lithium carbonate and L-tryptophan in the treatment of bipolar and schizoaffective disorders. Am J Psych 140:757, 1983

10. Growdon JH, et al: Lecithin can suppress tardive dyskinesia. N Engl J Med 298:1029, 1978

11. Jackson IV, et al: Treatment of tardive dyskinesia with lecithin. Am J Psych 136:1458, 1979

12. Cohen BM, et al: Lecithin in the treatment of mania: double-blind, placebo-controlled trials. Am J Psych 139:1162, 1982

13. Nadi NS, et al: Muscarinic cholinergic receptors on skin fibroblasts in familial affective disorder. N Engl J Med 311:225, 1984

14. Snyder SH: Cholinergic mechanisms in affective disorders. N Engl J Med 311:254, 1984

15. Fovall P, et al: Choline bitartrate treatment of Alzheimer-type dementia. Commun Psychopharmacol 4:141, 1980

16. Renvoize EB, Jerram T: Choline in Alzheimer's disease. N Engl J Med 301:330, 1979

17. Wurtman RJ, et al: Brain catechol synthesis: control by brain tyrosine concentration. Science 185:183, 1974

18. Gelenberg AJ, Wurtman RJ: L-tyrosine in depression. Lancet 2:863, 1980

19. Gelenberg AJ, et al: Tyrosine for the treatment of depression. Am J Psych 137:622, 1980

20. Growdon JH, et al: Effects of oral L-tyrosine administration on CSF tyrosine and homovanillic acid levels in patients with Parkinson's disease. Life Sci 30:827, 1982

21. Yamaguchi T, et al: Effects of tyrosine administration on serum biopterin in normal controls and patients with Parkinson's disease. Science 219:75, 1983

22. Goodwin JS, et al: Association between nutritional status and cognitive functioning in a healthy elderly population. JAMA 249:2917, 1983

23. Raskind M: Nutrition and cognitive function in the elderly. JAMA 249: 2939, 1983

24. Schorah CJ, et al: Clinical effects of vitamin C in elderly inpatients with low blood-vitamin-C levels. Lancet 1:403, 1979

25. Manzoor M, Runcie J: Folate-responsive neuropathy: report of 10 cases. Br Med J 1:1176, 1976

26. Botez MI, et al: Neurologic disorders responsive to folic acid therapy. Canad Med Assoc J 115:217, 1976

27. National Institutes of Health Consensus Development Panel: NIH consensus development conference statement: defined diets and childhood hyperactivity. Am J Clin Nutr 37:161, 1983. Also discussed in Clin Peds 21:627, 1982.

28. Feingold BF: Why is your child hyperactive? Random House, New York, 1975

29. Rose TL: The functional relationship between artificial food colors and hyperactivity. J Applied Behavior Analysis 11:439, 1978

30. Rapp D: Does diet affect hyperactivity? J Learning Disab 11:56, 1978

31. Crook WG: Can what a child eats make him dull, stupid or hyperactive? J Learning Disab 13:53, 1980

32. O'Shea JA, Porter SF: Double-blind study of children with hyperkinetic syndrome treated with multi-allergen extract sublingually. J Learning Disab 14:189, 1980
33. Conners CK, et al: Food additives and hyperkinesis: A controlled double-blind experiment. Pediatrics 58:155, 1976
34. Levine MD, Liden CB: Food for inefficient thought. Pediatrics 58:145, 1976
35. Harley JP, et al: Hyperkinesis and food additives: Testing the Feingold hypothesis. Pediatrics 61:819, 1978
36. Williams JI, et al: Relative effects of drugs and diet on hyperactive behaviors: An experimental study. Pediatrics 61:811, 1978
37. Weiss B, et al: Behavioral responses to artificial food colors. Science 207:1487, 1980
38. Swanson JM, Kinsbourne M: Food dyes impair performance of hyperactive children on a laboratory learning test. Science 207:1485, 1980
39. Levy F, et al: Hyperkinesis and diet: A double-blind crossover trial with a tartrazine challenge. Med J Aust 1:61, 1978
40. Augustine GJ, Levitan H: Neurotransmitter release from a vertebrate neuromuscular synapse affected by a food dye. Science 207:1489, 1980
41. Prinz RJ, et al: Dietary correlates of hyperactive behavior in children. J Consulting Clin Psych 48:760, 1980
42. Haslam RHA, et al: Effects of megavitamin therapy on children with attention deficit disorder. Pediatrics 74:103, 1984
43. Coleman M: Serotonin in whole blood of hyperactive children. J Paediatr 78:985, 1971
44. Coleman M, et al: A preliminary study of the effect of pyridoxine administration in a subgroup of hyperkinetic children: a double-blind crossover comparison with methylphenidate. Biol Psych 14:741, 1979
45. Haslam RHA, Dalby JT: Blood serotonin levels in the attention deficit disorder. N Engl J Med 309:1328, 1983
46. Stein TP, Sammaritano AM: Nitrogen metabolism in normal and hyperkinetic boys. Am J Clin Nutr 39:520, 1984
47. News story: Too early to close book on Feingold's diet-behavior hypothesis. Pediatric News 17:13, 1983

CHAPTER 5

A Review of "Life Extension"—The Role of Nutrients in Extending Lifespan

The topic of "Life Extension" has recently been in the limelight due to the publication of a book by Durk Pearson and Sandy Shaw entitled "Life Extension: A Practical Scientific Approach". This 858-page hardcover has reportedly sold more than one million copies, and the authors are said to have made more than 300 TV appearances.

The basic message of this book, for those who haven't read it, is that major lethal disorders, such as heart disease and cancer, can be prevented or significantly delayed by taking megadoses of approximately 25 "nutrient supplements" daily. The authors believe that the average lifespan of individuals who follow this regimen may be increased by several decades, and that the quality of that increased lifespan will also be improved.

Those are certainly honorable goals. I have reviewed the Life Extension book, however, and found it to be extremely inaccurate; some of the recommendations in the book are potentially life-threatening. The purpose of this chapter is to evaluate the Pearson and Shaw (PS) volume. An evaluation of the PS book is a perfect way to end the first section of this book, which has dealt with the question of "whom should you believe?". This chapter will serve as an excellent review of the concepts presented in Chapters 1 and 2 and Appendix A, concepts which are highlighted throughout the rest of the book.

The PS book is a bit unique in the nutrition field because it purports to be scientific, unlike the other books and regimens reviewed in previous chapters, which make no such claim. The authors' intent is to provide for physicians and scientists "A practical scientific approach" (as the book's subtitle proclaims) to extending lifespan by altering nutrient intake and taking prescription drugs. I, with training both as a physician and scientist, and presumably a member of the intended audience, find this book sorely deficient in terms of achieving its stated scientific goals. The PS book disregards the most basic concepts which guide the acquisition and presentation of scientific data.

SCIENCE OR MISINFORMATION?

In the absence of definitive data (and as PS note, such data on the validity of life extension practices are unavailable and will be hard to obtain in humans) much of the discussion depends on interpretation and extrapolation of very shaky, and often contradictory, animal and laboratory data. The true scientist operates according to the null hypothesis, i.e., he assumes that a regimen is worthless and dangerous until proven otherwise. This concept is widely accepted among bona fide scientists, and implies that the burden of proof is upon the proponent of a regimen to show that it is both efficacious (i.e., accomplishes what it promises to accomplish) and safe (i.e., the side effects are minimal, or are acceptable in view of the benefits of the regimen). This is the essence of the scientific method as it applies to the rational selection of various drugs and treatments, and is the method by which the Food and Drug Administration (FDA) decides whether to approve drugs (1-1b).

Pearson and Shaw, on the other hand, assume that a regimen is both safe and effective until proven otherwise. It should be noted that this approach is very similar to that espoused by many (unscientific) alternative health care providers as discussed in Chapters 1 and 2 and Appendix A. The reader is encouraged to read those sections at this time if he hasn't already.

As mentioned previously, the difference between the two approaches may be a philosophical one, but the reader who chooses to adhere to the Pearson and Shaw conception should realize that it *is not* a scientific conception, as these authors lead you to believe. The scientific method puts the burden of proof on Pearson and Shaw to muster the evidence in support of their regimen; I believe that they haven't even come close to meeting that burden of proof.

SCIENTIFIC SHORTCOMINGS OF THE PS BOOK

Referencing

One of the major scientific shortcomings of the PS volume relates to the presentation of the references. As the reader has noticed in this book, references are found at the end of certain statements. This enables the interested reader to determine for himself if the statement made is supported by the reference quoted.

If it isn't, the reader should be suspicious of the book or paper in which the statement is made. Extensive referencing is not always so important if the topic is not controversial (for instance, in a textbook) and if the author is known in scientific circles (such authors may only offer an abbreviated bibliography which is not specifically cited in the text). For most topics, however, and especially controversial ones, detailed citations in the text are absolutely essential. Otherwise, the frustrated reader may have to look up hundreds of references, as I have had to do while reviewing the PS tome, in order to determine if one of the references supports the statements. This makes it very difficult, if not impossible, to trace the evidence upon which the recommendations are based. Since most readers are unlikely to go to this trouble, they will probably blithely believe the "scientific data" which PS purportedly present.

This concern is not strictly theoretical. A careful reading of the references which *are* offered in the PS book does not support the recommendations made, and some of the quoted references directly contradict the conclusions of the PS volume (see below). For instance, PS state in their book that growth hormone (GH) plays an important role in extending lifespan. It is therefore curious that this function of growth hormone isn't even *mentioned* in an authoritative review article on growth hormone (1c) which they reference in their book. Furthermore, Hydergine, which is touted as a potent GH releaser in the PS book, isn't even mentioned in the growth hormone review article. On the other hand, exercise, which PS discount in their book, is described as a growth hormone releaser in the review article.

In addition, although Pearson and Shaw denigrate (and rightly so) the quality of the popular literature, many of their references are from the popular literature, including some of their own articles and booklets. By interspersing these nonscientific citations among legitimate scientific references, they attempt to lend credibility to these writings. Such references have no place in a scientific book. Finally, lectures at meetings or poster sessions are not acceptable references, for two major reasons. First, the information presented in such meetings is not available for a reviewer to critically evaluate. Secondly, many off-the-cuff statements can be made in a lecture which would never be put in writing, because they would be challenged. If a speaker or presentor of poster session is not sufficiently confident of his work to have it published, it does not merit referencing in a scientific book.

It should also be kept in mind that even if a paper appears in a peer-reviewed scientific journal, this is no guarantee of the validity or reproducibility of the data. The journal editorial board and their reviewers try to cull out obviously poor work as much as possible, but they cannot endorse data which are published. Of course, not all journals are even peer-reviewed, and this makes it even more likely that shoddy work will be published. Thus, the presence of even a scientific reference is no guarantee of the conclusions which are offered.

A final comment with respect to references. A single study, even if performed by reputable scientists, does not guarantee the validity or applicability of the conclusions of that study. As mentioned in Appendix A, reproducibility of scientific findings by other researchers, with different subjects, by different methods, is very important in establishing the validity of scientific data. Thus, one must be cautious in making sweeping recommendations on the basis of a single human experiment.

Bias in Reporting Data

Perhaps an even greater departure from acceptable scientific practice than poor referencing is the one-sided presentation (and often, even misrepresentation) of data. This practice is evident throughout the PS book. For instance, on p. 324, PS state:

> "In the Framingham study, 437 men and 475 women were observed for periods up to 10 years . . . There was no clear relation between serum cholesterol and deaths due to heart disease".

This statement is an outright distortion of the actual conclusions of the Framingham study. At the time of publication of PS's book, the Framingham group had published over 100 articles in the scientific literature. Despite this, only *one* is referenced in the life extension book (2). Even that single study is misquoted ! For example, the quoted article focused on HDL, and not total cholesterol, which is the topic of discussion in the citation above. Furthermore, the Framingham study included 5209 men and women, and the HDL study quoted in the PS book actually included 1025 men and 1445 women (not 437 and 475 as in the quote above). Finally, and most importantly, when one examines a review article written by the Framingham group in 1979 (3), and thus available to PS when they were writing their book, based on 18-year follow-up (not 10), the conclusions were:

> "Prospective data at Framingham and elsewhere have shown conclusively that risk of coronary heart disease in persons younger than age 50 is strikingly related to the serum total cholesterol level. Within so-called normal limits (of serum cholesterol) risk (of heart disease) has been found to mount over a five-fold range".

The conclusion in the life extension book is diametrically opposed to that of the Framingham authors; such inaccurate citation cannot be considered scientific. At best, this represents extremely shoddy review work; at worst, it suggests a deliberate attempt to distort the conclusions of the Framingham study. If this were the only such instance in the book, it might be excusable, but that is not the case. Erroneous citations abound in this volume (see next section of this chapter). The reader interested in an unbiased analysis of the cholesterol question is encouraged to consult Chapter 6 for a more detailed discussion and multiple references.

It is also interesting that while PS deny the relatively solid evidence linking serum cholesterol to heart disease, they affirm the minimal-to-non-existent evidence that "many other nutrients (vitamins A, B_1, C, E, and B_6 and zinc, selenium and other antioxidants) are involved in protecting the vessels against atherosclerosis".

Presentation of Anecdote

Another glaring departure from acceptable scientific practice is the recurrent presentation of anecdote. It appears that PS are aware of the unscientific nature of anecdotal evidence—since they state on p.47:

> "It is important to realize that these individual cases (anecdotal evidence) can never be proof of anything because of individual-to-individual biochemical variation. Usually such treatments are not administered double-blind, and therefore the results are strongly subject to biases. When people expect something to happen (like pain relief with a drug that is really a sugar pill), it often does. But this is not evidence for the efficacy of a treatment. On the basis of individual cases, you can find people claiming therapeutic benefits from almost any imaginable substance."

Despite such an accurate analysis of the scientific worthlessness of anecdote, the PS volume is peppered with anecdotes. These are obviously presented in an attempt to convince the reader to disregard the warning above and instead, accept anecdotal evidence in support of the hypotheses propounded in the book. As if the testimonials in the body of the book weren't enough, 58 additional pages of anecdotal evidence are found in the appendix! On page 302, the authors reaffirm that anecdotal data "prove nothing, but they are interesting leads". I would agree that one legitimate scientific use of anecdote is to stimulate the formulation of an hypothesis, which then leads the scientist to perform double-blind, placebo-controlled trials to test the hypothesis. The problem is that many anecdotes, but almost *no* controlled scientific trials of the authors' major hypotheses, are presented in the book. This leads one to believe that PS are not using anecdotes as leads, but rather as proof of their ideas.

Contradictory and Inconsistent Advice

As alluded to above and delineated in more detail below, the PS book is full of inaccurate statements, contradictions and inconsistencies, and the authors frequently do not seem to believe their own advice. Warnings often seem to be inserted to protect the authors from liability rather than to protect the reader. For instance, the following warning, which appears on the first page (p. 611) of appendix G, entitled "Our Current Personal Experimental Life Extension Formula—Quantitative Data", is reproduced verbatim below:

> "The information contained in this appendix is strictly for use by research scientists. This formula is strictly experimental. It is *not* recommended for anyone other than ourselves. These substances in these doses require further safety testing. Pregnant women and children *must not* use this formula. Persons with liver or kidney damage *must not* use this formula. Extensive frequent clinical laboratory tests monitored by a research-oriented physician are necessary, even if one is in perfect health".

Below this warning follows an extensive listing of their "nutrient" and drug regimen (more than 25 chemicals taken daily).

Even a cursory reading of this warning reveals gross inconsistencies. For example, if the authors truly believe their third sentence—that this formula is strictly for themselves—why publish it in a book that is meant for the lay public? It appears they don't believe that the formula is meant only for themselves, because after making that statement, Pearson and Shaw tell us who they *really* don't want to use this regimen—pregnant women, children, and individuals with liver and kidney problems. This is wise because a pregnant woman who delivers a malformed child might sue. Since it appears that PS intend for the reader to disregard their third sentence, they imply that if he does not fall in one of the groups above, he can take this regimen, as long as he gets frequent laboratory tests (which most readers probably won't be able to do, even if they want to).

Many of the arguments in this book are very illogical. For instance, PS discuss thalidomide (p. 571), the tranquilizer which, when taken by pregnant women, was responsible for many deformed babies in Europe. The drug was never approved for sale in the United States. PS are of the opinion that thalidomide should now be approved for use by men and non-pregnant women. They further state that if thalidomide were available, there wouldn't be 1000 people dying from barbiturates annually. This statement implies that people are dying of barbiturate overdoses because safer sedative and hypnotic (sleep-inducing) drugs are unavailable. This is faulty reasoning because many safer hypnotic agents are available. In addition, most deaths from barbiturates are either intentional overdoses or are due to abuse of "barbs" obtained on the street. Availability of thalidomide would not affect either of these mechanisms of barbiturate overdose. Finally, and most importantly, many women are unaware that they are pregnant in the first month of pregnancy, which is precisely the time that the fetus is most sensitive to the teratogenic effects of thalidomide. Thus, making this drug available to "non-pregnant" women would undoubtedly expose many pregnant women as well, and result in the birth of many deformed babies.

Another illogical argument deals with the doses of various substances that the authors recommend. PS recognize that there is an optimal level of all nutrients in the diet. They incorrectly state, however, that the optimal level is that which is just below the toxic (side-effect-producing) dose. This is really a *maximal* dose, not an optimal dose. This is like adding sugar to a cup of coffee until you can't stand the sweet taste, rather than adding an amount which "tastes right". This approach really makes no sense. What you really want in order to optimize the dose is to find a dose which achieves the intended benefits and causes minimal side effects; that dose may be much below the minimal dose that causes any side effects. By optimizing their way, PS are essentially implying that more is better.

PS are quite arrogant in their approach, and apparently believe that if someone disagrees with their ideas, he must be ignorant. For instance, on p. 557, they note that former National Institute of Aging chief Robert Butler didn't want to spend money on aging research because he believed that there is no evidence that it can be done (that is a reasonable assessment of the data). PS say that since he has been to several gerontology meetings, "one can only conclude that perhaps he didn't understand what he heard". This accusation is curious, in view of the fact that Dr. Butler has had training in both medicine and research while Pearson and Shaw have had neither. Such comments are inappropriate in a scientific book. A true scientist would accept the fact that other scientists may look at the same set of data, but reach different conclusions.

Another example of this arrogance is the inclusion of many quotes like the one on p. 526, by Isaac Newton, "No great discovery is ever made without a bold guess". This is an attempt by the authors to link their "bold guess" with Newton's. The difference is that if Newton was wrong in his "bold guess" (the theory of gravity), no harm would result. If PS are wrong in theirs, much damage could result. In addition, unlike PS, Newton didn't misrepresent the work of others, and there wasn't a substantial body of scientific evidence which was incompatible with his "bold guess".

Inappropriate and Potentially Dangerous Medical Advice

Another curious inconsistency is the authors' frequent reference to their own research. In actuality, the book contains not even a single publication of their own aging research in a scientific journal. This is certainly contradictory to their claims of being scientists in the gerontology field.

On p. 433, PS state that they are "scientists, not physicians. We are not licensed to practice medicine, nor do we have the training to do so". Their recommendations, however, go far beyond the scope of research scientists (which they aren't either). For instance, they recommend that a patient undergoing radiation therapy for cancer should request that his thymus be shielded from the radiation. If your radiologist refuses to cooperate with your demand, they insist (p.342), that you "PROMPTLY HIRE ANOTHER RADIOLOGIST, SINCE IT IS YOUR LIFE AND YOUR MONEY!" Such strongly-worded medical advice is clearly inappropriate in a book meant for the layperson. The radiation therapist may have legitimate reasons for not shielding the thymus, e.g., if doing so will interfere with eradication of the cancer. By giving this advice, PS are essentially stating that they know how to handle radiation therapy better than a radiation therapist (who, by the way, is the specialist who administers radiation therapy, *not* a radiologist).

Even more shocking is their recommendation (p. 350) that Hydergine (a prescription drug which PS believe can help salvage tissue from hypoxia— lack of oxygen) be injected "directly into the carotid artery in the neck, which leads to the brain" in emergencies such as "drowning, smoke or carbon monoxide poisoning, heart attack or stroke or severe brain concussion". There are *no* data to show that this would have any beneficial effects. On the other hand, carotid injection could easily cause death. It is unbelievable that such a recommendation is made in the PS book; in my opinion, actually carrying out such a recommendation would constitute medical malpractice!

These are only a few of many instances wherein PS make medical recommendations. I find these recommendations to be totally unsupportable by reasonable scientific data, and to be potentially dangerous. I highly recommend that no advice in this book be followed without at least obtaining the opinion of your physician.

Extrapolation from Animal Studies

One of my most basic objections to the PS book, alluded to previously, is that PS extrapolate unscientifically from animal studies to human recommendations. This practice is fraught with danger in general, but especially so in aging research. It is known (and PS recognize) that aging mechanisms in rodents (the source of most of the animal research) are quite different from aging mechanisms in humans. For instance, PS quote an ad from Monsanto, a company interested in aging research (p. 117):

> "(Studying) Rats and mice who give up the ghost at 2-3 years can't help; their metabolism of nutrients is radically different [from humans] and pretty much their own".

This difference in aging mechanisms between rats and humans is underscored by the observation that restriction of food intake in rodents can significantly lengthen their life expectancy, whereas similar food restriction in primates and humans (as observed in countries where malnutrition is rampant) results in mental retardation, stunting of growth and if anything, decreased life expectancy. Finally, it has been shown that life expectancy is inversely correlated with basal metabolic rate. Since the basal metabolic rate of rodents is several times greater than that of humans, it is unlikely that maneuvers which extend life expectancy in rodents will be relevant to life expectancy in humans.

The preceding conceptual objections to the Pearson and Shaw treatise may seem rather abstract to the reader, but are actually quite important. To illustrate these points, some examples of false or unfounded statements which are made in the "Life Extension" book are listed below. In reviewing the book, I found more than *one hundred* such erroneous statements. Due to space constraints, only the most egregious of these are listed. The page number where the statement is made is given, followed by the statement and then a brief explanation of why the statement is incorrect.

MISINFORMATION IN THE PEARSON AND SHAW BOOK

p. 107—"Since free radicals are able to cause genetic mutations, they have been implicated in the genesis of atherosclerotic plaques (a type of tumor)"

Comment: There is little evidence to implicate free radicals as causes of atherosclerotic plaques. Atherosclerotic plaques are not tumors in the commonly understood way.

p. 126—"As your brain ages, the ability of your brain to make and respond to some of these messenger chemicals drops off. In some cases, we can increase the amounts of the deficient neurotransmitters, thus bringing function in aging brains to young or near young adult levels".

Comment: Brain function in youth and old age is not simply a matter of the *quantity* of neurotransmitters; their microcellular location in the brain and their appropriate delivery to nerve cells at the right time is also very important. Furthermore, it hasn't been clearly demonstrated which nutrients and foods have an effect on neurotransmitter levels in humans, and how this affects brain function (see Chapter 4). In addition, even if neurotransmitter levels are influenced by diet and nutritional supplements, one can't always assume that more is better. For instance, it is widely hypothesized that schizophrenia is characterized by an excess of dopamine in the brain. Therefore, eating foods which can increase dopamine levels might be harmful for schizophrenics. Indeed, PS recognize this, stating that schizophrenics be careful about taking L-DOPA. How about people who aren't currently schizophrenic but who could be made so by excess dopamine? Is it possible that excesses of certain nutrients can do harm? (The answer is yes).

p. 161—Arthritis is usually an autoimmune disease.

Comment: Actually, the most common form of arthritis—osteoarthritis—is not an autoimmune disease. Rheumatoid arthritis, which is much rarer, is believed to be an autoimmune disease.

p. 162—"Symptoms of smoker's cough can be noticeably alleviated in 24 hours with these nutrients" (vitamins A and C, and selenium).

Comment: This is easily tested in a double-blind, placebo-controlled trial. Has the experiment been done? If not, what is the evidence for this?

p. 209—"PABA is a vitamin".

Comment: According to whom? None of the scientific nutrition books which I examined consider PABA to be a vitamin.

p. 219—"Durk has found it to be a safe and effective treatment for his own personal case of male pattern baldness".

Comment: A study of one individual cannot establish the safety and efficacy of anything.

p. 222—"Exercise: More is not necessarily better".

Comment: The authors should heed their own advice as it applies to nutrients, antioxidants, prescription drugs. More certainly isn't always better, but this book clearly suggests otherwise.

p. 258—"Since smoking is not a disease, the FDA may never approve any treatment, no matter how safe, specifically for the purpose of stopping smoking".

Comment: The FDA recently approved a nicotine-containing gum (Nicorette) specifically for the purpose of helping one stop smoking.

p. 265—"In self experiments, we have found that our experimental antioxidant mixture roughly triples the x-ray dosage required to cause our skin to redden and burn".

Comment: Did they really expose themselves to x-rays before and after taking their antioxidant mixture to establish that it required triple the dosage of x-rays to achieve the radiation burn? If they did, that's rather foolhardy. If they didn't, then how can they make this statement?

p. 275—Shulgin developed a recreational drug which provided "the desired alcohol high without the damaging side effects" of alcohol. It was apparently tested in humans, who "couldn't distinguish between the drug and a few martinis". The FDA killed it.

Comment: The FDA would not rule on such a substance since it has no jurisdiction over alcoholic substances. It would be interesting to know what the substance was, what side effects it did have, and how it was "tested" in humans.

p. 289—"The higher growth hormone levels in teenagers have a great deal to do with this difference" [why teenagers can eat like horses without becoming obese].

Comment: Is it the higher growth hormone levels themselves or the fact that teenagers are using the excess calories to actually grow? In other words, if a nongrowing adult stimulates his growth hormone levels, will he also be able to eat like a horse without getting fat? The answer is NO!

p. 289—"Obese people do not have a normal GH response to L-arg, L-ornithine, L-Dopa, fasting, hypoglycemia, exercise or sleep".

Comment: Is this the cause of the obesity, as these authors imply, or is it the result?

p. 308—"There is little strong evidence that high serum cholesterol levels themselves cause heart disease".

Comment: There is a *tremendous* amount of evidence that high serum cholesterol causes heart disease (see Chapter 6).

p. 315—"excess intake of table sugar can contribute to the development of atherosclerosis".

Comment: There is almost *no* evidence to support this statement.

p. 315—"excess insulin is thought to cause cholesterol and other lipids in the blood to be deposited in arterial walls. Diabetics who are able to control their blood sugar levels adequately by dietary means do not generally develop these complications. It appears, therefore, that the insulin diabetics take . . . is responsible for many of these complications".

Comment: The reason that diet-controlled diabetics do not develop as bad complications as insulin-dependent diabetics is that they have a much milder form of diabetes. This is why their diabetes can be controlled by diet only. Thus, insulin-dependent diabetics are a much sicker group of people, and have usually had diabetes for a longer period of time. Insulin does not cause the complications in diabetics—in fact, the opposite is true. The current consensus of scientific experts is that patients who take several shots of insulin per day (and who therefore control their diabetes better) have fewer diabetic complications (4-12). The comments in the PS book are dangerous because they may convince insulin-dependent diabetics to forsake the very life-sustaining therapy that they need.

p. 372—"Some scientists now think it is insulin that is primarily responsible for these (atherosclerotic) changes".

Comment: It would be very interesting to know who these scientists are.

p. 325—"Measurements of total cholesterol do not give any indication of the amounts of HDL and LDL" .

Comment: False. Most studies have shown a significant correlation between total and LDL cholesterol (see Chapter 6).

p. 327—"In human subjects, 3 gm of niacin per day reduced serum cholesterol by 26% after a year".

Comment: Cholesterol advice seems very inconsistent. First the authors tell us that serum cholesterol is unrelated to heart disease, and then they tell us how to lower serum cholesterol. Why reduce serum cholesterol if it makes no difference?

p. 335—"of the original 100 vitamin-C-treated terminal cancer patients, 13 are still alive today and free of cancer".

Comment: This quote refers to a study of terminal cancer patients who received vitamin C. No reference was given to support this statement that 13 of the patients survived as a result of the vitamin C therapy.

p. 339—kids with cystic fibrosis "exhibit abnormally low serum levels of vitamins A and E—reasonably consequences of inadequately controlled free radicals".

Comment: Due to pancreatic disease, kids with cystic fibrosis do not absorb fats or fat-soluble vitamins (like A and E) well. This accounts for their low levels of vitamins A and E in the blood, and has nothing to do with free radicals (12a).

p. 349—"Take your tax money away from FDA legal and regulatory bureaucrats and give it to their scientists instead".

Comment: Does this mean that PS think that the FDA scientists would agree with their ideas?

p. 349—"Talwin is a good nonnarcotic prescription pain reliever".

Comment: Talwin is definitely a narcotic agent, and because it is commonly abused by drug addicts, its formulation has recently been changed.

p. 350—"If you haven't used these antibiotics (tetracycline, penicillin, erythromycin) have your doctor check you for sensitivity in a skin test".

Comment: I know of no general physician or allergist who recommends routine skin testing prior to prescribing any antibiotic, nor is this recommendation made in any textbook which I examined.

p. 350—"Self-treatment with antibiotics is strictly for major emergencies when no physician is available".

Comment: What kind of emergencies are the authors talking about? How do they plan to decide which antibiotic is appropriate? The right dose? The method of administration? I can't think of any infectious emergencies which are amenable to outpatient management without proper cultures and intravenous antibiotics. In such a situation, all efforts should be made to bring the patient to medical attention ASAP rather than attempting self-treatment with any antibiotics.

p. 350—PS describe a case where a child was hit by lightning; "when ambulance arrived, one of the medics applied CPR 'just for the hell of it'".

Comment: What kind of medic would perform CPR "just for the hell of it"? No medic that should work for any ambulance company (or perhaps the story is not entirely accurate?) Then another case of resuscitation is presented— this one involving ice water. What do these two cases of resuscitation have to do with the hypotheses of the book?

p. 351—"these fluorocarbons carry much more oxygen (dissolved in the liquid) than natural blood".

Comment: This statement is technically true—more oxygen is carried in fluorocarbons than in the *liquid* portion of blood. This is because most (>99%) of the oxygen in blood in carried by the *red blood cells*, not the liquid portion of the blood. When red blood cells are included, blood carries much more oxygen than fluorocarbons. Thus, this statement erroneously implies that fluorocarbons are better than your own blood, which is incorrect.

p. 524—we'd like to "test a possible new emergency procedure for victims of carbon monoxide poisoning and mine fires, for example, which result in hypoxic conditions. Part of the victim's blood could be replaced with fluorocarbon blood substitute. This would make oxygen available to the victim's tissues rapidly and avoid many of the safety hazards of blood transfusions".

Comment: Carbon monoxide victims, if they arrive alive in the hospital, are usually successsfully treated with 100% oxygen, under high pressure (hyperbaric) conditions, if available. I am unaware that blood transfusions are ever used to treat victims of mine fires or carbon monoxide poisoning. Replacing their blood with a fluorocarbon substitute would be unnecessary, foolhardy, and would expose the patient to unnecessary risks.

p. 364—"LDL may play a significant role in the genesis of many types of cancer as these lipoproteins carry in the bloodstream the carcinogenic polynuclear aromatic hydrocarbons".

Comment: I am unaware of any reasonable scientific data which support this statement.

p. 365—"500 mg vitamin C taken three times a day reduced serum cholesterol in atherosclerotic humans in one study by about 35 to 40%".

Comment: No references cited to support this statement. Vitamin C is not recognized as an agent which lowers serum cholesterol. In addition, why lower serum cholesterol if it doesn't have any relationship to heart disease? Isn't it a bit inconsistent for these authors to recommend vitamin C to lower cholesterol while eating, *per week*, 1 to 2 dozen eggs, 1 to 2 pounds of butter, several pounds of meat, and 4 to 5 gallons of regular milk (p. 367)?

p. 372—PS state that reactive hypoglycemia occurs "because insulin has a much longer half-life than the sugar".

Comment: There is no such concept as *the* half-life of sugar—how long sugar stays in the bloodstream is dependent on many other things, one of which is the insulin level.

p. 405—"Experimental animals given vitamin E can survive longer and in better condition when they are subjected to a dangerously low oxygen environment. Therefore, heart patients with insufficient circulation should take vitamin E supplements".

Comment: Even assuming that the first sentence is true (and there is little evidence that it is), the second sentence does not logically follow from the first. The problem in heart patients is not low oxygen in the environment. Their problem is inadequate blood flow ("insufficient circulation") to specific areas of the heart. Those are two very different problems, not to mention the fact that experimental animals are different from humans.

p. 421—"Thymus gland drops in weight after injuries; this may be one reason why serious physical injury is so often followed by serious infection".

Comment: More likely reason for increased incidence of infection after major injury is the presence of broken skin (abrasions, lacerations), laying in bed and getting pneumonia, presence of Foley (urinary) catheters, IVs, and other portals of infection (places for infection to enter the body).

p. 434—"Even if you dislike them (side effects of niacin) you may take 3 gms of niacin per day anyway because you dislike your high serum cholesterol and triglycerides even more, and this dose will result in about a 25% reduction in these lipids".

Comment: Again, inconsistent advice. Why are PS so keen on lowering serum cholesterol if they don't consider it a risk factor?

p. 438—"If you already have a family physician, he or she may be willing to consider new *scientific* information, even if he or she has quite properly rejected unsupported allegations of health faddists. If this is not the case, you may want to look for an open-minded doctor".

Comment: This is a subliminal message which is meant to accomplish two things—separate PS from health faddists, and discredit doctors who are not "open-minded" about these "Life Extension" ideas. It also implies—incorrectly—that they have provided "new scientific information" in their book, and that if the reader's physician disagrees with them, the reader should find "an open-minded doctor".

p. 439—"A doctor who is willing to provide copies of your lab reports (as they are received directly from the lab) would probably be willing to consider prescribing low-toxicity prescription drugs such as Diapid, Hydergine, and Deaner".

Comment: Wrong. As a physician, I would be glad to share lab reports with a patient. I would not, however, consider prescribing these drugs on the basis of the unscientific evidence offered in this book.

p. 457—"Finally, if you find a physician with a personal interest in clinical research or life extension or free radical pathology, or simply new-but-non-FDA-approved uses for old familiar drugs, you will have found the best possible profesional assistance for your personal experiment in life extension".

Comment: Well, this description certainly fits me and many of my colleagues, who are interested in clinical research and who have no qualms about prescribing drugs for non-FDA-approved indications. None of my research-oriented colleagues, however, have considered the data presented in this volume sufficient to start prescribing as PS recommend. If PS truly mean that such an individual would be the "best possible professional assistance", they would have to accept my negative opinion of their book.

p. 476—"Beta carotene gives carrots their yellow color".

Comment: I thought carrots had an orange color.

p. 497—"But there will continue to be people willing to buy health products based on a wide variety of untested hypotheses and claims, many not scientifically justifiable on the basis of experiments reported in the scientific literature".

Comment: Boy, that's for sure! Although PS are talking about food faddists here (which they are knocking), these comments could just as easily apply to their own ideas.

p. 507—"We are both professional futurologists".

Comment: What is a professional futurologist?

p. 511—"We intend to use nearly all of the proceeds from this book and our media appearances to fund these (and other) R & D [research and development] programs".

Comment: Excellent idea. Research in the aging field could definitely use the influx of funds. I hope they make at least some of the funds available in the form of grants to others.

p. 513—"Our fourth major research area is the truly rational formulation of free radical modulating regimens. The experimental formulations given in this book are unquestionably far from optimum".

Comment: I certainly agree with the second statement.

p. 519—"Human WBC's often live a couple of years in the body".

Comment: The lifespan of human white cells is more like two *weeks* (13).

p. 575—of Anturane study, "This is a particularly important study since if the first heart attack is not fatal, it is usually followed by a fatal heart attack within several years".

Comment: In the majority of cases, a first heart attack is *not* followed by another heart attack, much less a fatal one. It is true, however, that a person who's had one heart attack is at greater risk of having a second, especially if he doesn't alter the behaviors that contributed to the first one (smoking, hyper-cholesterolemia, high blood pressure, obesity, poorly controlled diabetes).

p. 594—"As scientists, we have access to many drugs that are unavailable to pharmacists, physicians, and their patients due to FDA regulations".

Comment: I'd be interested to know what drugs they can obtain that pharmacists and physicians can't obtain.

p. 595—"usually excellent Consumers Union".

Comment: I wonder what CU would say about this book.

p. 762—"TB is caused by a poor T-cell immune system response".

Comment: TB is actually caused by a type of bacterium (Mycobacteria).

Many statements about Hydergine, a Sandoz Pharmaceuticals product, are made in the PS book. Since I was unable to verify these statements, and since Pearson and Shaw state (p. 319) that some experiments have been reported to Sandoz, I contacted Dr. William Westlin, Director, Medical Services, Sandoz Pharmaceuticals, and asked him if he was able to verify any of the specific statements which I questioned. He responded by stating:

"With regard to the book written for popular audiences called *Life Extension*, may I stress that its contents do *not* have the medical endorsement of Sandoz Pharmaceuticals concerning any of our therapeutic agents. We had no knowledge of this manuscript prior to its publication" (14).

I corresponded further with Dr. Krassner, Associate Medical Director, Medical Services Department, at Sandoz. Dr. Krassner responded as follows to my requests of any documentation that he might have in support of specific statements in the PS book (I have first quoted from the PS book, and then Dr. Krassner's response [15]):

p. 164—"In one study men in their 50s and 60s taking 16 I.U. of Diapid [also a Sandoz product] nasal spray per day had significant improvements in memory and learning and decreased reaction time (the men were faster). In several cases of accident-induced amnesia, people recovered their memory in only hours to days after using Diapid".

Dr. Krassner: "We have no data or statistics which indicate significant improvements in memory and learning following the use of 16 IU of Diapid nasal spray. We are also unaware of any cases of memory recovery with the use of Diapid in cases of accident-induced amnesia"

p. 272—"Hydergine is currently the fifth best-selling prescription drug in the free world outside the United States. In France, where alcoholic drinks such as wine are consumed in large quantities, Hydergine is the number one prescription drug"

Dr. Krassner: "Hydergine is not the 5th best selling drug in the world, outside the U.S. Although very popular, it is not the best selling drug in France"

p. 275—"Experiments have been done in cats in which their brains did not receive adequate oxygen to function normally. Irreversible brain damage occurred in 15 minutes. But in cats whose brains were equally deprived of oxygen but who also received Hydergine . . . there was no brain damage for forty-five minutes. Because of this protective property, Hydergine is administered in many countries in Europe just before an operation so that if anything goes wrong, doctors will have more time to correct the situation before brain damage occurs".

Dr. Krassner: "Physicians in Europe do not routinely use Hydergine preoperatively [before surgery] or for resuscitation . . . While animal studies (cats) in European hands have shown a decrease in brain damage resulting from oxygen deprivation following Hydergine administration, I am unaware of any country in which Hydergine is routinely administered in neurological cases preoperatively"

p. 304—"Hydergine is effective in helping about 60% of the asthma sufferers who try it".

Dr. Krassner: "While Hydergine apparently elevates cAMP levels (see my review enclosed), I am unaware of any studies indicating that Hydergine is effective in helping 'about 60% of asthma sufferers who used it'".

p. 319—"Although the patents on Hydergine have expired, the Sandoz Corporation still spends about 40 percent of their research budget on this truly remarkable drug".

Dr. Krassner: "Sandoz does not spend 40% R&D budget on Hydergine. It spends 2-3% of its annual budget on Hydergine studies—most of which is for new dosage forms and delivery systems".

p. 350—"Hydergine . . . is very effective in preventing brain damage from hypoxia (insufficient oxygen) in emergencies such as drowning, smoke or carbon monoxide poisoning . . . Hydergine . . . can be injected intravenously or, better yet, directly into the carotid artery in the neck"

Dr. Krassner: "We have no evidence that Hydergine in humans can improve the outcome of resuscitation nor has it been used as a carotid injection".

p. 471—"Parlodel [also a Sandoz drug] stimulates release of growth hormone (GH) when there is too little GH, but normalizes GH levels when too high"

Dr. Krassner: "I have been unable to find any literature to support this Parlodel GH level statement"

My purpose in detailing the above is certainly not to denigrate these Sandoz products. Parlodel (bromocriptine), for instance, has revolutionized the treatment of several hormonal and tumor conditions, as explained in a recent review (16). Rather, my purpose is to demonstrate that the PS book is replete with inaccuracies. Furthermore, these are potent drugs, and can have significant side effects (e.g., psychotic reactions [17]). Thus, they are not to be taken lightly, especially in the absence of convincing evidence of their efficacy. Such evidence appears to be sorely lacking in the PS book.

These are just some selected false, inaccurate or poorly documented claims in the Pearson and Shaw book. Several, like the one which states that insulin causes diabetic complications, are dangerous. One must be skeptical of the whole book if so many erroneous statements could be found. I would therefore recommend that none of the hypotheses or recommendations in this book be accepted without checking with a reliable medical information source.

MERITS OF THE PEARSON AND SHAW BOOK

This review may seem as one-sided and unobjective as the "Life Extension" book itself, and the reader may wonder if I believe that there is *nothing* of value in the PS book. On the contrary, I believe that the authors present several interesting and reasonable hypotheses, most of which have previously been presented in the scientific literature and which should be tested in clinical trials. As a matter of fact, some of the ideas *are* being tested in clinical trials—for instance, the value of carotene in the prevention of cancer. Individuals who would rather not await the definitive data may choose to take some of the supplements described in the PS book. Many of the controversial recommendations which are made in the book, however, are not scientifically supportable in humans at the current time.

Another factor to consider is that even if some of these substances actually have the beneficial effects which are attributed to them, one often cannot be confident of the quality or even identity of materials which are widely obtainable as "nutritional supplements". This is because nutritional supplements are not subject to inspections or quality controls by any (federal or other) agencies.

Consequently, the consumer may not be getting what he thinks he's getting. For instance, most bottles of vitamin C which proclaim "all-natural" sources of vitamin C actually contain synthetic vitamin C. The cost of obtaining vitamin C from natural sources would be prohibitive. Another example is the recent finding that some samples of bone meal had significant amounts of lead in them. When one realizes that bone removes lead from the rest of the body, this makes sense. The buyer of that bone meal, however, undoubtedly did not bargain for a supplement of poisonous lead.

The reader may wonder about the scientific status of the topics raised in the PS book. PS declare that lifespan can be prolonged and its quality enhanced by taking an alphabet-soup of "nutritional supplements". What is the actual unbiased scientific evidence in support of this concept? Are there any interventions that can reasonably be expected to increase lifespan? We are fortunate that a review article on this very topic appeared very recently in the New England Journal of Medicine (18). The reader interested in life extension ought to read this well-documented (194 references!) up-to-date unbiased article. This article should be understandable by non-medical readers, and is probably available in most hospital libraries.

This article concludes that there are several interventions which have been shown to increase lifespan in animal experiments, but none in humans. Many of these interventions also decrease body weight in experimental animals, and this may be the common denominator between these approaches. Food restriction, however, is not a realistic modality for prolonging human lifespan, as was noted earlier in this chapter. The article ends with a hopeful note—that application of new techniques in molecular biology, immunology, nutrition, endocrinology, exercise physiology, and the neurosciences may lead to the development of effective regimens to increase the quantity and quality of human life.

Another topic which receives much attention in the PS tome is free radicals. Free radicals are very reactive chemicals which are produced in all living things. PS believe that the production of free radicals is responsible for most conditions which ail humans, including aging, and that supplements (called antioxidants) which deactivate free radicals can delay the aging process and prevent the development of these degenerative diseases. The hypothesis that free radicals are responsible for human disease and aging is not novel; in fact, it was first proposed in the 1950s. Despite the passage of three decades and much research, this concept remains conjectural and controversial today. Despite this, PS present the free radical theory as if it was well-accepted dogma. Readers who want a more balanced view of the potential role of free radicals and antioxidants in health and disease are encouraged to consult some recent review articles on this subject (19-24). The controversial nature of free radicals can be noted by reviewing a recent article and the correspondence which it spawned (25,26).

It is interesting to note that one review on free radicals (20) doesn't even *mention* their role in aging, while the other reviews only mention aging in passing. Instead, the focus is on the role of free radicals in cell damage after heart attacks and during organ transplantation. It should also be noted that several recent papers state that free radicals are useful in certain human diseases. For instance, it is widely believed that the body's infection-fighting cells (white blood cells) kill bacteria by generating free radicals (27), and drugs which generate free radicals may be useful in treatment of malaria strains which are resistant to current antimalaria drugs (28,29).

Finally, there are only a few human studies of the administration of antioxidants, and none of these studies have dealt with the aging issue. It is also unclear what side effects, if any, antioxidants may have. Therefore, it is difficult for me to draw any conclusions on this topic at the present time. In the absence of such data, however, ingestion of antioxidant supplements cannot be recommended.

Many other subjects are discussed in the PS book. Some have been dealt with above, but others are a bit far afield from the nutrition orientation of this book and thus cannot be dealt with herein.

THE BOTTOM LINE: EVALUATING THE PS BOOK

In summary, of greatest concern is that the PS book purports to be scientific, but in reality, disregards many scientific concepts. These unscientific practices include presentation of a one-sided literature review, misrepresentation of the scientific work of others, extrapolating animal data to human recommendations, poor referencing, and relying on anecdote instead of controlled clinical trials. These practices make it improbable that the regimens recommended are either efficacious or safe.

REFERENCES

1. Medical News: FDA prepares to meet regulatory challenges of the 21st century. JAMA 254:2189, 1985
1a. Medical News: Reviewing new, very complicated drugs. JAMA 254:2215, 1985
1b. McMahon FG: How safe should drugs be? JAMA 249:481, 1983
1c. Catt KJ: Growth hormone. Lancet 1:933, 1970
2. Gordon T, et al: High density lipoprotein as a protective factor against coronary heart disease. The Framingham Study. Am J Med 62:707, 1977
3. Kannel W, et al: Cholesterol in the prediction of atherosclerotic disease. New perspectives based on the Framingham Study. Ann Int Med 90:85, 1979
4. Cahill GF, et al: "Control" and diabetes. N Engl J Med 294:1004, 1976

5. Karlsson K, Kjellmer I: The outcome of diabetic pregnancies in relation to the mother's blood sugar level. Am J Obstet Gynecol 112:213, 1972

6. Lavaux JP, Pirart J: The course of diabetic retinopathy: A statistical study on its development, progression and regression in 4400 diabetics. Diabetologia 11:358, 1975

7. Job D, et al: Effect of multiple daily insulin injections on the course of diabetic retinopathy. Diabetes 25:463, 1976

8. Greene DA, et al: Effects of insulin and dietary myoinositol on impaired peripheral motor nerve conduction velocity in acute streptozotocin diabetes. J Clin Invest 55:1326, 1975

9. Rasch R: The effect of diabetic control on kidney weight, glomerular volume and glomerular basement membrane thickness. Diabetologia 13:426, 1977

10. Mauer SM, et al: Studies of the rate of regression of the glomerular lesions in diabetic rats treated with pancreatic islet cell transplantation. Diabetes 24:280, 1975

11. Fox CJ, et al: Blood glucose control and glomerular capillary basement membrane thickening in experimental diabetes. Br Med J 2:605, 1977

12. Yetiv JZ: Recent advances in diabetes research and therapy. In: Recent Advances in Clinical Therapeutics, Yetiv JZ, Bianchine JR (eds.), Academic Press, New York, 1981

12a. Rudolph AM: Pediatrics. 17th edition, Appleton Century Crofts, 1982, pp. 1438

13. Humbert JR (ed.): Neutrophil physiology and pathology. Seminars Hemat 12:1, 1975

14. Personal communication, William Westlin, M.D., September 24, 1984

15. Personal communication, Michael B. Krassner, M.D., Ph.D., February 15, 1985

16. Vance ML, et al: Bromocriptine. Ann Intern Med 100:78, 1984

17. Turner TH, et al: Psychotic reactions during treatment of pituitary tumors with dopamine agonists. Br Med J 289:1101, 1984

18. Schneider EL, Reed JD: Life extension. N Engl J Med 312:1159, 1985

19. Dormandy T: An approach to free radicals. Lancet 2:1010, 1983

20. Kathryn Simmons (medical news): Defense against free radicals has therapeutic implications. JAMA 251:2187, 1984

21. Halliwell B, Gutteridge JMC: Lipid peroxidation, oxygen radicals, cell damage, and antioxidant therapy. Lancet 1:1396, 1984

22. Letters to the editor: Oxygen radicals and cell damage. Lancet 2:577, 1984, and 2:1095, 1984

23. McCord JM: Oxygen-derived free radicals in postischemic tissue injury. N Engl J Med 312:159, 1985

24. Editorial: Metal chelation therapy, oxygen radicals, and human disease. Lancet 1:143, 1985

25. Fink R, et al: Increased free-radical activity in alcoholics. Lancet 2:291, 1985

26. Letters to the editor: Free radicals and alcoholics. Lancet 2:774 and 955, 1985

27. Fantone JC, Ward PA: Role of oxygen-derived free radicals and metabolites in leucocyte-dependent inflammatory reactions. Am J Pathol 107:397, 1982

28. Allison AC, Eugui EM: A radical interpretation of immunity to malaria parasites. Lancet 2:1431, 1982

29. Clark IA, et al: Free oxygen radicals in malaria. Lancet 1:359, 1983

SECTION TWO

NUTRIENTS—THE GOOD, THE BAD AND THE UGLY

CHAPTER 6

Cholesterol and Fats in Health and Disease

Perhaps no other nutritional topic has received more attention in the scientific and lay press than the role of cholesterol and lipids (fats) in causing disease. After considerable research, much of it only reported in the last two years, there finally appears to be a consensus among experts in the field. Indeed, a consensus conference statement, entitled "Lowering Blood Cholesterol To Prevent Heart Disease", was recently issued under the auspices of the National Institutes of Health (1). The panel of experts concluded that "it has been established beyond a reasonable doubt that lowering definitely elevated cholesterol levels . . . will reduce the risk of heart attacks due to coronary heart disease". This chapter will review the evidence that led to the above conclusion, and discuss the consensus statement in more detail. The interested reader is also referred to several excellent editorial and review articles for further detail (2-9).

Although agreement has now been reached, the consensus message has only slowly been filtering to the medical community and lay public. It is sad to realize that many physicians are still not treating levels of hypercholesterolemia (high cholesterol in the blood) which clearly increase the risk of heart disease (10). For instance, of 1600 physicians surveyed, 25% said they initiate drug therapy only when cholesterol levels are >400, and another 28% reported that they never use drugs for hypercholesterolemia under any circumstances! Many patients are unaware of their cholesterol level or its importance; in contrast, many know their blood pressure. This situation is now improving, however, and at least 4 major articles which discussed the cholesterol issue appeared in the lay press in 1984 (11).

Americans have actually been living healthier for about the last decade. The incidence of stroke (12), and coronary heart disease—CHD—(13-15), have recently decreased, and many attribute this to improvement in the national diet (16). Progress has also been made in other areas, including decreased smoking (17), increased exercising (18), and improved control of hypertension (19). It is interesting to note, however, that CHD mortality began decreasing in the mid-1960s, before major changes in these habits became widespread, and before public recognition of the nutrition-heart disease link. Thus, many attribute at least part of the decrease in CHD to advances in coronary care and prehospital care (paramedics), and general improvements in medical care.

Despite this encouraging decline in mortality, CHD remains the leading cause of death in the U.S. Therefore, efforts to disseminate information which may further decrease CHD mortality must be intensified.

LIPOPROTEINS

The 2 major lipids, cholesterol (CHOL) and triglyceride (TG), circulate in the blood as lipid-protein complexes known as lipoproteins. As can be noted from Table 6-1, lipoproteins are composed of different amounts of protein (called apoprotein), CHOL, and TG. Each lipoprotein contributes both CHOL and TG to the serum pool of these substances. Thus, a high serum CHOL may be due to a high level of VLDL, LDL or HDL, or any combination of the three. Since it's not only the *amount* of cholesterol but also the *distribution* among lipoproteins that affects the risk of heart disease, this is more than an academic issue. For instance, let's consider 3 individuals who have an identical total CHOL (TC) in their blood (see Figure 6-1). The one who has the most of his TC carried in the HDL subfraction (Subject C), will have the lowest risk of CHD. The difference among these individuals is further clarified by examination of the LDL/HDL ratio. The higher this ratio, the greater the CHD risk.

This example is not hypothetical, because there are individuals with elevated TC levels which are due to increased HDL, a condition known as hyper-alphalipoproteinemia. It should be noted, however, that by far the most common cause of hypercholesterolemia is an elevated LDL level.

The various lipoproteins are synthesized in different locations in the body and appear to have different functions. For instance, it appears that LDL carries cholesterol from the liver to the periphery of the body, while HDL does the opposite, bringing cholesterol from the tissues back to the liver for safe disposal. This is why HDL is often referred to as a "scavenger", and why it is thought to be beneficial. In this regard, it has been shown that LDL, when added to a preparation of smooth muscle and endothelial cells like those found in coronary arteries, is cytotoxic to the cells (kills them) (20). The addition of HDL inhibited this LDL-induced cytotoxicity. The interested reader should consult 3 recent review articles on lipoprotein metabolism for further details (21,22a).

PATHOGENESIS OF ATHEROSCLEROSIS

Although much has been said of lipids and vascular disease, atherosclerosis is not solely due to lipids. In addition to the lipid hypothesis (23), the injury (24)

Table 6-1

| Lipoprotein | Synonyms | Apoproteins | | Composition | | |
		Major	Minor	%protein	%CHOL	%TG
Chylomicrons		C-I C-II C-III	A-I A-II B	2	7	84
VLDL (Very Low Density Lipoprotein)	Prebeta	B C-I C-II C-III E	E	8	20	51
LDL (Low Density Lipoprotein)	Beta	B	C-I C-II C-III	21	45	11
HDL (High Density Lipoprotein)	Alpha	A-I A-II	C-I C-II C-III D	50	22	4

Composition of the major lipoproteins
Modified from refs. 21–22a.
CHOL = cholesterol   TG = triglycerides

and transformation (25) hypotheses have been proposed. The injury hypothesis states that arterial injury is the primary event; arterial injury, which may be due to hypertension or other causes, is followed by lipid deposition. The transformation hypothesis holds that the first event in atherogenesis (development of atherosclerosis) is the transformation and undesirable multiplication of arterial smooth muscle cells. This latter event has been shown to occur *in vitro*—addition of LDL to muscle cells in culture stimulated them to multiply (26).

It is quite likely that all three mechanisms play a role in atherogenesis, and the order in which they do so may be of academic interest only. This combination of factors may explain why two individuals with similar lipid profiles have markedly different rates of atherosclerosis. It does appear reasonable, however, that if one of these three factors is treated, the overall process of atherogenesis may be slowed down, or hopefully, even reversed. This concept is the major impetus behind the treatment of hypercholesterolemia.

HYPERLIPIDEMIA AS A RISK FACTOR FOR ATHEROSCLEROSIS

Hyperlipidemia (HLP) means the elevation of either CHOL or TG, or both. This chapter will focus on hypercholesterolemia because it is felt to be a much

Figure 6-1

	Subject A	Subject B	Subject C
C	265	265	265
HDL	35	50	65
TG	250	250	250
LDL	180	165	150
LDL/HDL Ratio	$^{180}/_{35} = 5.1$	$^{165}/_{50} = 3.3$	$^{150}/_{65} = 2.3$
CHD risk	High	Medium	Low

Comparison of lipoprotein levels in three individuals with identical total cholesterol levels
See text for explanation.

more common and stronger risk factor for CHD than hypertriglyceridemia. The latter will be briefly discussed at the end of this chapter. The question as to what constitutes a "normal" or elevated CHOL level has received much attention recently, and was addressed in detail at the recent consensus conference. Before discussing this, a short section on lipid measurement is in order.

Lipid Measurement

It is currently recommended (1) that total cholesterol, triglycerides, and HDL be measured at least once in all adults. Some recommend measurement of HDL only if the TC is above 250. Measurement of lipoproteins other than HDL is not routinely performed in most laboratories, and is primarily a research technique. LDL, which is often reported, is not actually measured. Instead, it is calculated from the other values [LDL = TC-HDL-(TG/5)]. Some labs also calculate and report the ratio of LDL/HDL, because this ratio is believed to be a better predictor of CHD risk than TC, LDL, or HDL alone.

These lipids should always be measured after a 12-14 hour (overnight) fast. If elevated, the lipid should be measured again and the two values averaged to obtain a reliable baseline. This rationale also applies to a low HDL measurement.

If the TC value is markedly elevated (>300), measuring lipids in first-degree relatives would be prudent.

Concept of "Normal" Lipid Levels

As mentioned above, the term "normal" is hard to define. The usual statistical definition of normal includes all values within two standard deviations of the mean. For TC, this would be an upper value of about 270 in the United States. Table 6-2 lists the mean and 90th percentile for TC, TG, LDL and HDL, for men and women of various ages (27). Many laboratories consider a TC value of up to 300 to be normal (28). However, "normal" in the statistical sense isn't always good; e.g., it is "normal" for 50,000 Americans to die on the highways annually. Thus, we should really strive to define not what level of TC is statistically normal, but which level is *optimal*. Stated another way, At what TC level is CHD and total mortality lowest?

Hypercholesterolemia as a Risk Factor

Today, the question is not *whether* hypercholesterolemia increases the risk of CHD, but rather, *at what level* does cholesterol become a significant risk factor?

Table 6-2

Age	Men (Percentile)							
	50th	90th	50th	90th	50th	10th	50th	90th
	Total cholesterol		LDL-Cholesterol		HDL-Cholesterol		Triglycerides	
20–29	172	215	108	147	45	32	90	182
30–39	194	234	128	171	44	32	109	232
40–49	206	254	138	180	44	32	123	250
50–59	211	261	144	188	45	31	122	242
60–69	210	258					116	222
70–79	205	249					112	212

Age	Women (Percentile)							
	50th	90th	50th	90th	50th	10th	50th	90th
	Total cholesterol		LDL-Cholesterol		HDL-Cholesterol		Triglycerides	
20–29	164	207	100	138	52	38	65	114
30–39	176	219	113	151	54	39	71	130
40–49	195	241	124	168	56	39	84	163
50–59	222	275	144	196	58	40	111	194
60–69	228	280					108	203
70–79	228	280					110	200

50th and critical percentiles of total cholesterol, triglycerides, LDL and HDL, in men (upper panel) and women (lower panel)
Modified from ref. 27.

Figure 6-2

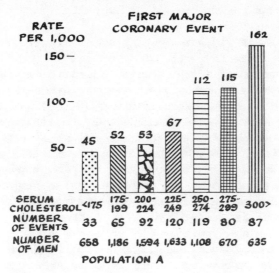

Relationship of serum cholesterol to rate of major coronary events over a 10-year follow-up period

Heart disease incidence increased 4-fold as serum cholesterol climbs from <175 to >300. From refs. 39, 40.

Such a level does not exist. Most epidemiologic studies have shown that risk of heart disease increases continuously as TC climbs from 180 upwards (29-38). Figure 6-2, taken from the Cooperative Pooling Study, demonstrates the relationship between TC and CHD (39,40). Other studies, such as the Framingham study, have reported similar results. Although one might argue that most of these studies are old, even the most recent data document a 3 to 4-fold increase in coronary heart disease as CHOL increases from 180 to above 270 (41).

Despite the consistency of their data, epidemiologic studies cannot prove cause and effect. Other types of studies, however, also support the hypothesis that increased serum CHOL increases the risk of CHD. For instance, atherosclerosis can be induced in animals, including primates, by feeding them a high CHOL diet (42). Removal of the high CHOL diet causes a regression of the atherosclerosis.

Finally, and of greatest importance, are the interventional trials in which serum CHOL level in a large group of people was decreased by diet and/or drugs. These individuals, who were chosen because of their high risk of developing CHD, were then followed up for several years to determine if the intervention had decreased their chance of developing heart disease.

Two major types of intervention have been studied: diet and drugs. In the former, serum CHOL levels were decreased by modifying the diet (lowering fat, especially saturated fat, and cholesterol content of the diet). In drug studies, the experimental group usually received the active drug while the control group received a placebo ("sugar" pill).

Several long-term trials have shown beneficial results for *dietary* intervention (43-47). These studies, however, have been attacked on various grounds (48), not the least of which is the fact that although they did show a significant decrease in CHD mortality, *overall* mortality was unaffected in most of these studies. Furthermore, there are at least two major studies (49,50) which showed little change in CHD mortality despite dietary intervention. In fact, an unassailable diet study cannot be reasonably conducted, because a double-blind dietary trial is not achieveable, not to mention problems with patient compliance. In addition, some have argued that a 10-15% decrease in serum cholesterol in middle-aged men, sustained for a period of 5-10 years is "too little, too late", and that longer term and more marked decreases in cholesterol levels are needed if CHD and total mortality is to fall significantly. In view of these difficulties, it is almost surprising that *any* study has shown that dietary intervention is of benefit.

In view of the unlikelihood that a definitive diet study will ever be performed, we must consider the current best available evidence to make our decisions and recommendations. It is my opinion (and the consensus of many experts in the field), that the evidence favoring the diet-CHD link is overwhelming, and that dietary modification will further decrease the morbidity and mortality of CHD in the United States.

Although this book deals primarily with diet, a brief discussion of drug intervention, especially the Lipid Research Clinics (LRC) Trial (51), may be in order. The LRC study was a multicenter randomized double-blind trial in which the cholesterol-lowering drug cholestyramine was tested for its effect in decreasing CHD. Middle-aged men with a TC>265 were enrolled in the trial and followed for 7-10 years. All participants followed a moderate cholesterol-lowering diet.

The group taking cholestyramine achieved a TC 8.5% lower than that in the placebo group, and experienced a 19% reduction in nonfatal heart attacks and a 24% decrease in CHD death. In addition, incidence rates of new positive exercise tests, angina (chest pain), and need for bypass surgery were 25%, 20% and 21% lower, respectively, in the cholestyramine group.

As might be anticipated, not all subjects in the cholestyramine group took the medication as instructed. The more medication a patient took, the lower his TC (Table 6-3). Those who took the full amount of medication (6 packets per day) experienced a 28% decrease in LDL, which led to a 50% fall in CHD incidence! In addition, placebo patients who achieved a fall in serum TC with dietary control also had a decrease in CHD.

It was thus concluded that it was the fall in TC, and not the means used to achieve it, that decreased CHD mortality. This indirectly, but persuasively, sug-

Table 6-3

| Mean daily packet count | % change in LDL | |
	Cholestyramine	Placebo
0–1	−6.6	−4.8
1–2	−8.7	−3.6
2–3	−13.1	−6.9
3–4	−16.5	−6.3
4–5	−20.9	−6.0
>5	−28.3	−8.4

Relationship of cholestyramine intake to decrease in LDL.
The more medication taken, the greater the fall in LDL. Modified from ref. 51.

gests that if a TC fall of 10% is induced by any means, including diet, a 25% fall in CHD incidence can be expected.

Although the LRC was a drug study of middle-aged men with high TC levels, the conclusions of the study have been extrapolated to women, and to men in other age groups and with lower TC levels. It has been argued that the results should also be applied to other means by which TC can be decreased—such as diet. Although it may not be scientifically accurate to conclude from the LRC data that lowering TC by diet is as beneficial as lowering it with cholestyramine, this assumption seems reasonable in view of other supporting evidence, and in view of the fact that it is very unlikely that a moderate cholesterol-lowering diet presents any danger to the general population.

HIGH DENSITY LIPOPROTEIN (HDL)— THE "GOOD" CHOLESTEROL

When cholesterol is discussed, one usually thinks of total cholesterol or LDL, both of which contribute to CHD, and which should be lowered. High density lipoprotein (HDL), however, is inversely correlated with CHD. This means that a high level of HDL is predictive of a low risk of developing CHD, and vice versa.

Table 6-4

HDL Level (mg/dl)	Rate of coronary events per 1000 patients over 4 year follow-up	
	Men	Women
< 25	176.5	0.0*
25–34	100.0	164.2
35–44	104.5	54.5
45–54	51.0	49.2
55–64	59.7	39.7
65–74	25.0	13.9
> 75	0	20.1
all levels	77.1	43.6

Relationship of HDL level to incidence of heart disease.
As HDL level increases, incidence of CHD decreases. Modified from ref. 58.
*there were only four women in this category (HDL<25) and none died during the 4 years.

What isn't known yet is what will happen if a person starting with a low HDL increases his HDL level. It is widely assumed and hoped that such a person will decrease his CHD risk.

Although Barr (52) initially suggested in 1951 that HDL protects against CHD, not much attention was paid to HDL until the mid-1970s when Miller and Miller (53) resurrected and expanded upon this hypothesis. Since then, much research has focused on HDL, including several recent reviews and editorials (54-56).

That high HDL is associated with lower CHD mortality has been shown in several studies. In the Cooperative Lipoprotein Phenotyping Study (57), HDL levels in persons with CHD were significantly lower than in healthy controls. The famous Framingham study provides even stronger evidence for the HDL relationship (58). Between 1969 and 1971, lipoprotein levels were measured in 2815 men and women, who were then followed for 4 years. A low HDL was associated with an increased risk of CHD in both men and women (Table 6-4). Indeed, persons with an HDL<35 had a CHD incidence 8 times greater than those with HDL>65. This inverse correlation with HDL has been reaffirmed in a more recent analysis of the Framingham cohort (59).

It should be realized that all the evidence in favor of HDL, though very consistent, is epidemiologic in nature. No study has yet demonstrated that an intervention which raises HDL lowers CHD risk. It may be that low HDL is simply a *marker* for high CHD risk, rather than a *cause* of CHD. If this is true, low HDL may well predict high CHD risk, but raising the HDL may not alter the risk of CHD.

Having said that, let's now briefly survey the factors that are related to high HDL, because despite the foregoing discussion, it is more likely than not that raising HDL will decrease the risk of CHD. Thus, raising HDL is a reasonable recommendation as long as the method used to achieve it is essentially risk-free or has other benefits.

Femaleness is one factor that is associated with increased HDL. Mean HDL levels are 45 for men, and 55 for women. This difference has been proposed as an explanation for the lower incidence of CHD in women. Being Black is also associated with a high HDL (57). Neither of these factors, however, are amenable to change.

Interestingly, estrogen tends to raise HDL, while progestins tend to lower it (60). Since most contraceptive pills currently marketed contain varying amounts of both types of compounds, a specific brand of birth control pill may raise, lower or have no effect on HDL level. The specific type of progestin used also affects lipoprotein level (60). Furthermore, one must consider the total picture: although it is true that estrogen raises the HDL level, it also raises LDL and TG. Thus, the beneficial effects of raising HDL may be offset by the negative effects of raising LDL.

Although race and gender cannot be altered, several factors which can be changed affect HDL levels. One of the best publicized of these is exercise. Marathon runners and other athletic individuals have higher HDL levels than controls (61,62). Most of the 40 million runners in the United States, however, are recreational runners, not marathoners. Fortunately, recreational runners also have a significant elevation in HDL, though not as much as marathoners (63). When middle-aged men exercised 3 times per week (walking, jogging, swimming, skiing or cycling), 30 minutes each time, HDL increased 11% and TG decreased 17% (63).

A more recent study evaluated the effects of exercise on lipoproteins in both sexes. Men and women had different responses to exercise (64). Men had a 5.1% increase in HDL and a 6% decrease in LDL while women showed essentially no change in HDL and a 4.3% decrease in LDL.

Aerobic sports such as swimming (65) and running (66,67) increase HDL. Competitive bodybuilding (many repetitions, less weight) also seems to elevate HDL, especially when compared to powerlifting (heavy weights, fewer repetitions) (68). Recreational weight training also seems to increase HDL (69), though the HDL rise in this study was not statistically significant.

One might ask the interesting question as to whether people *less* active than normal sedentary individuals would have lower HDL levels. A recent letter to the editor suggests this to be the case (70). Bedridden patients with recent spinal cord injuries had the lowest HDL (27 mg%), with progressively increasing HDL levels in patients with older spinal cord injuries (who were more active), normal sedentary individuals, joggers and marathoners.

Perhaps related to exercise is the effect of weight loss on HDL. A negative association has been noted between obesity and HDL level (71-73). For instance, HDL increased 16% and triglycerides decreased 37% after a weight loss of 36 pounds in grossly obese subjects who initially weighed almost double their ideal body weight (74). Increase in HDL correlated significantly with weight loss (the greater the weight loss, the greater the increase in HDL). There is a suggestion that weight loss may increase HDL more in men than women (75), but this is as yet unclear. Another well-publicized factor which raises HDL is *moderate* alcohol intake (76). The effect of alcohol on HDL, however, seems to vary with the exercise level of the subject (77). HDL was measured in 16 marathon runners, 15 joggers and 13 sedentary men before and after alcohol abstinence. At baseline, the marathoners had the highest HDL (58.3 mg%), while the joggers (49.4 mg%) and inactive men (49.8 mg%) had similar HDLs. A 3-week period of abstinence resulted in a significant decrease in HDL in the inactive men, but not in the joggers or runners. Resumption of alcohol intake increased HDL back to its original level in the inactive men, but had no effect on HDL in the joggers or runners.

One might conclude from this study that drinking is equal to jogging (but not as good as marathon running) in elevating HDL. Thus, there might not be much incentive for the beer drinker watching the joggers run in front of his house to go out and join his brethren.

This may not be an accurate interpretation of these data, especially in view of a more recent study (78), discussed below. It may also be worth noting that there may have been other differences among the 3 groups of men that may have accounted for their differential HDL responses to alcohol intake. For instance, the runners were significantly older and ate more carbohydrate and potassium than the other two groups.

Most important of all, however, is that alcohol and jogging seem to elevate two different subgroups of HDL. Of the two subgroups, HDL_2 is associated with reduced CHD, while HDL_3 apppears to be unrelated to CHD (79,80). The higher HDL levels in women are due to higher HDL_2 levels (81), as are the higher HDL levels in runners (82,83). Both of these factors (female gender and exercise) are known to be associated with decreased CHD risk, as would be expected from the HDL_2 elevation. Unfortunately, alcohol elevates HDL_3, not HDL_2 (78), so that alcohol-mediated HDL elevation would not be expected to improve CHD risk. Thus, although the abstaining joggers and drinking inactive men discussed in the previous study (77) had similar HDL levels, the HDL subgroup distribution of the joggers appears to be better from a cardiovascular point of view than that of the drinkers.

Finally, it has not been demonstrated that HDL elevation, regardless of the way used to achieve it, can actually decrease CHD risk. Thus, it would be unwise to recommend a means of elevating HDL which is *known* to have deleterious effects (alcohol). On the other hand, exercise is known to have other beneficial effects, in addition to possible salutary effects on HDL. These include attainment of ideal body weight, decreased prevalence of smoking among exercisers, improved diet, and a psychological sense of well-being (it might be argued that the last one is also seen with alcohol intake). Some of these concepts were discussed in an accompanying editorial (84).

It is interesting to note that HDL increases after cessation of smoking (85). It was suggested by these authors, however, that coincidental changes in diet and activity level may have been partially responsible for the HDL increase. The fact, however, that 3 subjects who resumed smoking after 6 weeks of abstinence had subsequent falls of HDL to baseline further supports a cause and effect relationship.

The last HDL reports to be discussed deal with the effects of drugs on HDL levels. Some drugs which are used to treat high levels of TG (nicotinic acid and clofibrate) increase HDL (86), as do some drugs used in the treatment of epilepsy (87). Of more significance is that cimetidine produced a modest but statistically significant rise in HDL in 10 normal subjects (88). This is important because cimetidine (Tagamet) is one of the most frequently prescribed drugs. More recently, it was reported that a patient with familial Type III hyperlipoproteinemia had a more than doubling in the initially very low HDL level (23 mg%) associated with cimetidine therapy (89). There are undoubtedly other drugs which affect HDL levels which are as yet unidentified.

IS REGRESSION OF ATHEROSCLEROSIS POSSIBLE?

The title of this section represents one of the questions that individuals with CHD often ask their physicians. This topic has received much attention in both the scientific and lay press (90-93). If regression is possible, it provides further evidence for the diet-heart hypothesis. Perhaps of even greater importance is that the potential for regression also provides incentive for patients to alter risk factors, even after they have experienced a heart attack or some other CHD event.

After an extensive review of the literature, it appears very clear to me that regression of atherosclerosis is *possible*. Perhaps more relevant are questions such as, What factors are most important in inducing regression? and, How frequently does regression occur? Although we don't have all the answers to these questions, we can venture an educated guess. A case report published in 1976 (94) demonstrates the degree of regression possible. A 49 year-old woman with high blood pressure (despite treatment with 3 medications), hyper-cholesterolemia (TC = 340), and a strong family history of heart disease, had severe angina pectoris. A special x-ray (arteriogram) showed a 90% blockage of blood flow to the right kidney due to atherosclerosis, and this was thought to be responsible for her refractory high blood pressure.

Her high CHOL was treated with diet and a CHOL-lowering drug (cho-lestyramine). The patient's CHOL fell from 340 to about 160, and the ar-teriogram was repeated after 3 ½ years. Incidentally, her blood pressure had normalized in the meantime despite the fact that she had been taken off her blood pressure medications. The repeat kidney arteriogram showed significant regres-sion of the blockage in the right kidney artery, and this was probably the reason that her blood pressure had normalized.

Although this case is encouraging, it is anecdotal, and as explained in the appendix, it is hard to interpret anecdotal "evidence". However, studies in ani-mals, including primates, have also shown significant regression when choles-terol-free diets were fed (95,96). A few studies involving human patients have also documented regression and have shown it to occur in approximately 30% of hypercholesterolemic patients who zealously adhere to a low-cholesterol diet and drug therapy (97,98).

In one of these studies, for example (97), arteriograms of the femoral (leg) arteries were performed in 25 patients at initial evaluation and again 13 months later. During the 13 months, hyperlipidemia and hypertension were treated with diet and drugs. Regression was observed in 9 (36%) of the patients, no change observed in 3, and progression in 13. Of most interest is the fact that patients who were successful in controlling their BP and CHOL were more likely to have regression of their atherosclerosis than those who weren't successful.

In some patients, diet and drugs cannot control serum CHOL, and only heroic measures may be effective. When such measures are successful, they may also demonstrate regression. For instance, two recent papers (99,100) describe a *6-year-old* girl with a *CHOL >1000* and severe heart disease. She underwent two heart bypass surgeries without success, and then had a simultaneous heart-liver transplant. This girl had a rare condition known as homozygous familial hyper-cholesterolemia wherein liver LDL receptors are absent or dysfunctional. Since these receptors are needed to remove cholesterol from the bloodstream, their absence leads to a very high blood CHOL.

After the heart-liver transplant, the child's CHOL fell to 268! Cholesterol deposits under her skin (tendinocutaneous xanthomas) regressed dramatically during the 10 weeks of follow-up. This case provides further evidence that regression is possible, although it sometimes requires heroic measures.

Chelation Therapy for Regression?

In view of the popularity of "chelation therapy", it may be worthwhile to scientifically evaluate the alleged ability of this "treatment" to promote regression of atherosclerosis. This topic has been recently reviewed by several authors (101-105), all of whom concluded that there is no scientific validity to this practice, and that there are significant risks of harm.

It was originally proposed in 1955 that repeated administration of a calcium-binding (chelating) agent such as EDTA could remove calcium from atherosclerotic deposits ("plaques") and therefore promote the regression of these lesions (106). This would presumably open up the blood vessel and increase the blood flow to the organ involved. Many uncontrolled and inadequately described studies reported in the 1950s and 1960s suggested that patients receiving this therapy improved. These studies have been reviewed in detail (105). This reviewer (105) was unable to find a single study which contained the research methodologies and elements required to objectively assess treatment efficacy. Thus, a study which scientifically demonstrates that chelation therapy is effective has yet to be done, more than 30 years after this hypothesis was advanced. It is noteworthy that the companies which manufacture EDTA have so little faith in its potential use in atherosclerosis that they have not funded or performed any clinical studies to test it.

Another reason for the widespread disinterest among physicians in the potential efficacy of chelation therapy is that no scientifically valid rationale has been proposed for why chelation therapy *should* work. As has been pointed out by Dr. Peter Frommer, Deputy Director of the National Heart, Lung and Blood Institute,

"In the majority of patients with arteriosclerosis, calcium deposits are an insignificant part of the total lesion. It's predominantly a fibrous overgrowth which would be left behind even if the calcium were removed and would be more than enough to cause trouble. And besides, when calcium in the blood is chelated, why would it be replenished from these inaccessible bits of calcium rather than from the accessible relatively large stores of calcium in bone?" (104)

Thus, there is no scientific rationale in support of chelation therapy, and there are no scientific studies (not even poorly controlled ones) which show this "remedy" to be of value. Furthermore, the safety of chelation therapy is questionable. Chelation therapy can lead to low blood calcium levels, potentially resulting in uncontrolled muscle contractions (tetany), heart rhythm abnormalities, convulsions, respiratory arrest and kidney failure. Thus, chelation therapy cannot be considered medically acceptable in the treatment of atherosclerosis (107,108). Multiple scientific bodies (American Heart Association, American College of Physicians, American Academy of Family Physicians, American Society for Clinical Pharmacology and Therapeutics, American College of Cardiology, and American Osteopathic Association) have reviewed the data and found no scientific evidence to support the claims of benefit in patients with atherosclerosis (101).

Some would consider the administration of EDTA for atherosclerosis to be medical malpractice. In fact, a recent lawsuit awarded $550,000 to a patient who developed kidney disease severe enough to necessitate dialysis after a series of EDTA infusions (109, also described in 105).

Thus, it is quite clear that EDTA has not been proven efficacious, and has serious, potentially fatal, side effects. As discussed in the first chapters and Appendix A of this book, the onus of proving the efficacy of chelation therapy rests with its proponents. It is not the obligation of science to pursue and disprove all improbable pseudo-medical practices which have a cult following. Thus, anyone who receives chelation therapy is experimenting, traveling uncharted territory. Unfortunately, since the person is not enrolled in a trial, any potentially useful information is lost.

Pritikin Diet for Regression?

One diet popularly recommended with the promise of inducing regression is the Pritikin diet. In a provocatively entitled ("Bypass surgery? Consider an alternative: Pritikin") newspaper advertisement which appeared in the Los Angeles Times in 1983, the late Pritikin boldly stated, "Many patients recommended for bypass surgery could control their heart disease just as effectively with drugs and a diet and exercise program". In the ad, he quotes a study carried out at his Longevity Center: "In 1976, 64 patients recommended for bypass surgery went to Pritikin instead. Today, 80 percent still have not required surgery" (110).

This ad suggests that all 64 patients were doing just fine at followup. In fact, as noted in the ad, 12 patients (19% of the 64 patients) did require bypass surgery during the five-year followup. Three (5%) had died from cardiac disease, 19 (30%) still had angina or had developed it anew, and 4 (6%) had heart attacks during the followup period. Since there was no control group (e.g., patients who had undergone bypass but not the Pritikin program), it is impossible to state whether these results are better, worse, or about equal to those that would have been achieved with bypass surgery. Using historical controls, especially from studies a decade old, is fraught with danger because several important advances have been made in the last decade. For instance, certain drugs have only been commonly used in the last 10 years (beta blockers and more recently, calcium channel blockers) and mortality after bypass surgery has decreased significantly in the last decade. For instance, the Coronary Artery Surgery Study (CASS) had 780 patients very similar to those in the Pritikin group (111). Half of the CASS group had bypass surgery, while the other half received medical therapy. The five-year mortality for the two groups was 5% and 8%, respectively. These numbers are very similar to those in the Pritikin study.

It is also impossible to tell which component of the Pritikin program— diet, exercise, maintenance of ideal body weight, cessation of smoking, improved control of blood pressure—may have been responsible for any beneficial effects of the program. This is not necessarily a drawback, however, because the components of the Pritikin program noted above are widely viewed as safe and effective.

Two diets are recommended by Pritikin—the "regression" and "maintenance" diets. For $8000, the Pritikin Longevity centers offer a 26-day inpatient diet-and-exercise program, utilizing the regression diet. Presumably in recognition of the fact that it is very difficult to adhere to the regression diet in a setting outside the inpatient longevity centers, patients are encouraged to follow the "maintenance" diet once they go home. Both diets are composed of 80% carbohydrates, 10-15% protein, and 5-10% fat (112). The major difference between the diets is that the "less restrictive" maintenance diet allows a cholesterol intake of up to 100 mg/day, while the upper limit of the regression diet is 25 mg/day.

In the Pritikin book (112) and in literature provided by the longevity center in Santa Monica, California, Pritikin mixes very sensible advice with some incredibly optimistic promises and downright false statements. The sensible advice includes cessation of smoking, weight control, and abstinence from alcohol. The optimistic statements include "essential hypertension can be controlled or eliminated with appropriate nutrition, salt restriction and weight reduction". Although these non-drug means of hypertension control are very important (see Chapter 10), there remain many individuals who require antihypertensive medications despite adhering to the above. The false statements include, "You may be surprised to learn that the best food sources for proteins are grains, roots, vegetables, and fruits in an unrefined, minimally processed form", (I was indeed very surprised to read this!), and "Almost any amount of sugar is too much". These and other false statements are discussed in a Consumer Reports evaluation of the Pritikin Program (113).

The real question about the Pritikin program, however, is whether it delivers the primary benefit which it promises—namely, a decrease in the risk of heart disease. In addition to the paper quoted above (110), Pritikin has published several others which support the utility of his diet (114-120). For instance, an analysis of 893 patients observed at the Longevity Center showed:

(a) a 26% decrease in mean serum cholesterol (from 235 to 175), (b) smoking was discontinued by 85% of the smokers, (c) obese patients lost an average of 13 pounds, (d) of 218 hypertensives requiring blood pressure medication at the beginning of the 28 day stay, 186 (85%) left normotensive and drug-free, (e) half of the insulin-dependent diabetics left insulin-free with controlled blood sugar after the 4-week intervention program

The publication of papers, however, especially those lacking control groups and performed under the auspices of a for-profit organization, hardly inspires confidence in the validity of the results. A Canadian group of investigators compared the American Heart Association (AHA) diet with the Pritikin maintenance diet in patients with peripheral vascular disease (blockage of arteries in the legs) (121,122). These papers suggest that the Pritikin maintenance program is no better than the less restrictive American Heart Association diet consisting of 50-55% carbohydrate, 15-20% protein and 25-30% fat (123).

This conclusion does not carry very much weight, however, considering the small sample sizes in these two studies. The number of patients in each experimental group was so small (about 20 patients each) that the statistical power of these studies was very limited. In fact, there were trends suggesting greater reduction in serum cholesterol in the Pritikin diet group (which makes sense) but these did not attain statistical significance—either because the trends were not real (i.e., they were due to chance) or because the sample sizes were too small.

In addition, the conclusion that a diet which restricts fat to 5-10% of total calories is no better than one which restricts fat to 25-30% is rather curious, because this conclusion contradicts the current AHA recommendations and those of the recent consensus conference (1). These recommendations are that if moderate fat restriction (25-30% fat) does not decrease serum lipids sufficiently, a more marked fat restriction should be followed. These results also contradict Barndt's study (97). He found that regression of atherosclerosis was more likely in patients who adhered more faithfully to diet and hypolipidemic drugs.

What is one to make of all of this? I believe that there is truth to both points of view. The AHA recommendations are good for the population at large, are relatively easy to live with, and carry little risk of any nutrient deficiencies. The AHA diet is also good as a first step in treating individuals with hyperlipidemia. Hyperlipidemic individuals who do not respond adequately to the 25-30% fat AHA diet should be encouraged to further restrict fat and cholesterol, in essence heading toward the Pritikin maintenance diet. Whether they actually reach the goal of 5-10% fat established by the Pritikin maintenance diet will be determined by the individual. It is only a rare person who will be able to adhere to such an ascetic diet, but if he can, he may avoid the need for hypolipidemic drugs. It is my opinion that most patients who remain hyperlipidemic despite faithful adherence to a 25% fat diet (with less than 10% saturated fat) are likely to require pharmacologic therapy. If a person is willing to do so, however, a further reduction in fat intake to 10% of total calories may obviate the need for hypolipidemic agents.

The bottom line, then, is that the *concept* of both the Pritikin and the AHA diets (low fat, high carbohydrate, especially of the complex variety) is a good one. The difference is really only a matter of degree, with the Pritikin diet being more restrictive. For those who can stick to it, all the power to them. Most people, however, won't be able to adhere to a 5-10% fat diet; these individuals will still benefit by reducing their fat intake as much as they can, along the lines of the Pritikin diet.

Physicians interested in receiving the packet of Pritikin information referred to above should write Pritikin Longevity Center, 1910 Ocean Front Walk, Santa Monica, CA 90405 [phone #—1(800)421-0981].

FISH OIL FOR HEART DISEASE?

This book has dealt with many popular regimens which have been demonstrated to lack scientific foundation. The reader may consequently be suspicious that I am not being as objective as I promised to be. Unfortunately, regimens that have not been adequately subjected to scientific scrutiny are unlikely to be of value, and this may explain why most of the popular regimens previously discussed are no better than placebo.

The popular idea of using fish oil to ameliorate heart disease appears *not* to belong in this category of undocumented regimens. Although still experimental, there does appear to be solid scientific evidence in support of this practice. I have seen two advertisements for fish oil in the popular literature (124,125) and both are surprisingly factual and accurate, and thus very unusual compared to most advertisements of popular regimens. Both ads quote studies from the medical literature, which enhances their credibility. In fact, the second ad lists 15 references from the scientific literature!

In order to understand the potential use of fish oil, we must first learn something about prostaglandins (PGs). Although many PGs have been discovered, the two that have attracted the most attention, and which are of interest to us, are prostacyclin (PGI_2) and thromboxane (TXA_2). These two PGs, although made from the same precursor (biological "raw material"), have opposite biological effects. Prostacyclin is a vasodilator (dilates arteries) while thromboxane is a vasoconstrictor (constricts arteries). In addition, prostacyclin decreases the tendency of platelets to aggregate (and thus lead to blood clots), while thromboxane enhances this tendency. Thus, it has been proposed that the degree of vasoconstriction and platelet aggregation is determined by the ratio of thromboxane to prostacyclin production.

Since vasoconstriction increases blood pressure, and since platelets and blood clots are thought to play a role in heart disease, TXA_2 has often been thought of as a "bad" prostaglandin while PGI_2 is considered "good". This is obviously overly simplistic—if we had no thromboxane to close blood vessels and enhance blood clotting, we might bleed to death from the most trivial injury! In our atherosclerosis-prone and high blood pressure-prone population, however, lowering the amount of thromboxane and increasing that of prostacyclin may be of benefit. As a matter of fact, the widely recommended one-aspirin-per-day is thought to decrease risk of strokes and heart disease by decreasing thromboxane production and platelet aggregation.

Both PGI_2 and TXA_2 are made from aracidonic acid. Arachidonic acid is found in animal fat in the diet, and is also made in the human body. PGI_3 and TXA_3 are prostaglandins analogous to PGI_2 and TXA_2, except that they are made from eicosapentaenoic acid (EPA), which is found largely in fish and other foods of marine origin (126). EPA is not made in the human body. Thus, when marine foods are eaten, especially if they replace animal fat, less PGI_2 and TXA_2 is made and more PGI_3 and TXA_3 is made.

One last piece of information relevant to this hypothesis is that while PGI_2 and PGI_3 have similar vasodilator and antiplatelet properties, the biological effects of TXA_2 and TXA_3 are different—TXA_2 causes vasoconstriction and platelet aggregation, while TXA_3 does not. Thus, if someone eats lots of marine foods, they will have less TXA_2 and more TXA_3 than a "normal" person. This individual would consequently have less tendency to vasoconstriction and platelet aggregation.

What evidence supports this hypothesis? There are several types of evidence. The first is epidemiologic: Greenland Eskimos, whose high-fat diet consists almost exclusively of Arctic marine foodstuffs have low serum cholesterol, and a very low incidence of heart disease (127,128). Eskimos in Denmark, on the other hand, who eat a Western diet, have higher cholesterol levels and more heart disease than their more primitive brethren in Alaska and Greenland (129). Marine-eating Eskimos have also been noted to have a low prevalence of hypertension (130) and their platelets have a decreased tendency to aggregate (131). It has been proposed, therefore, that the type of fat that the Greenland Eskimos eat decreases their risk of CHD. The relationship of Eskimo diet to disease has been recently well reviewed (132). A more recent epidemiologic study (132a) also shows that eating fish may be related to decreased incidence of CHD. CHD mortality over a 20-year follow-up period was more than 50% lower in men who consumed at least one ounce of fish per day compared to those who did not eat fish.

Although these data suggest a relationship between diet and a low incidence of heart disease, interpretation of epidemiologic data, as has been pointed out previously, is limited. Several interventional studies, however, support and extend these epidemiologic data.

Sinclair, a scientist with interest in Eskimo diets, obtained a deep-frozen seal and himself ate a strict Eskimo diet for 100 days (133,134). His LDL/HDL ratio fell from 1.3 to 1.0. TXA_2 and PGI_2 production decreased while small amounts of the 3-series thromboxane and prostacyclin (TXA_3 and PGI_3) appeared in his semen. His bleeding time was markedly prolonged (>50 minutes, compared to a normal value of 10 minutes). Platelet aggregation was decreased and spontaneous bleeding was observed.

The effect of an EPA-rich diet on platelet aggregation and bleeding time was studied in 10 healthy men whose usual diet was partly replaced by fish for 11 weeks (135). The diet, which contained 2-3 g of EPA/day decreased platelet aggregation and increased bleeding time. The hypolipidemic effect of a fish-rich diet is impressive. In one study, 20 markedly hyperlipidemic were given high-fish diets, which were compared to the traditional low-fat diet containing large amounts of vegetable oil (135a). For instance, a subgroup of these patients (who had type V hyperlipidemia) had a decrease in their TG from a baseline of 1353 mg% to 281 mg%! CHOL in this group decreased from 373 to 207. Other studies of increasing dietary fish intake have confirmed these findings (136-139).

Although these studies are interesting, some people may not want, or may be unable, to increase their intake of seafood to such an extent. Thus, an attempt was made to ascertain whether cod liver oil, taken as a supplement to a normal Western diet, could duplicate the beneficial results achieved by increased fish intake. A daily cod liver oil supplement containing 10 g of EPA was given to 8 healthy volunteers for 25 days (140). Triglycerides, HDL and LDL were unaltered, but bleeding time increased and platelet count and aggregation decreased. Upright blood pressure was reduced during cod liver oil supplementation. Other studies have confirmed these effects of cod liver oil supplements (141-144).

The studies quoted above have all been short-term studies of healthy volunteers. Whether long-term fish oil supplementation would show similar effects remains to be determined. Perhaps of greater importance is whether these dietary manipulations would have the same beneficial effects in subjects with heart disease. There are a few studies which suggest this to be the case. Hay et al (145) gave EPA-rich oil to 13 patients with heart disease; beneficial effects on the platelets were noted. The Japanese have also published suggestive data (146).

On the other hand, one must also consider the adverse effects of the caloric excess (about 300 calories/day) induced by the oil supplement. If the diet was otherwise unchanged, the caloric excess would amount to a weight gain of more than 25 pounds in a year. To maintain caloric balance, the dietary intake must be decreased 300 calories/day.

It is difficult at the present time to recommend the intake of fish oil supplements, in view of the fact that most studies have been short-term and have used healthy volunteers. The impressive falls in TG and CHOL in one study quoted above (135a) argue persuasively at least for consideration of fish oil therapy, because the current hypolipidemic drugs are far from ideal. It should be noted, however, that neither the beneficial nor the deleterious long-term effects of such supplementation in heart disease patients are known. Rather than taking a supplement, it would be preferable to obtain extra EPA by increasing fish (and other seafood) intake and decreasing red meat intake. This approach would also decrease saturated fat and cholesterol intake, and would therefore enhance the serum-cholesterol-lowering effects of the diet. The interested reader is encouraged to review the editorial (146a) and correspondence (146b) relating to the study quoted above (135a).

A recent communication raises another potential option (147). These authors noted that linolenic acid (found in linseed and other vegetable oils) can be converted to EPA in the human body. EPA in the blood and platelets of subjects who changed their diet by replacing butter with linolenic-acid-rich-margarine increased, and platelet aggregation decreased. Thus, it appears that dietary intake of linolenic acid may be another way of increasing (indirectly) EPA in the body.

THE LOW-CHOLESTEROL DIET AND CANCER

It has been demonstrated in previous sections of this chapter that a diet low in cholesterol and saturated fat results in low serum cholesterol, which is associated with a lower cardiovascular mortality. Some have argued, however, that one does not "get something for nothing", and that the low cholesterol diet is associated with an *increase* in non-cardiovascular mortality, especially from cancer. Since reduction of cardiovascular mortality is not of much benefit if it is offset by increased non-cardiovascular mortality, this hypothesis bears careful scrutiny.

Since diet has been shown to have a significant effect on heart disease, diabetes, and other chronic diseases, it seems reasonable that it could also have an effect on carcinogenesis (development of cancer). A conference co-sponsored by the National Heart Lung and Blood Institute and the National Cancer Institute was held in mid-1981 to review data from 17 studies and determine whether low serum cholesterol levels or the low cholesterol diet may lead to increased non-cardiovascular mortality (148).

Of some comfort is the fact that no relationship between serum cholesterol and cancer mortality was noted consistently in all 17 studies. Eight of the studies found an inverse association between serum cholesterol and cancer mortality among men, but none of the 17 studies found such an association in women. In four studies—Framingham, Hawaii, Stockholm and Hiroshima-Nagasaki—an inverse association was found between serum CHOL and colon cancer. No other specific sites of cancer showed a significant relationship in more than one or two studies.

It must be noted that in these studies, cholesterol levels in all subjects were "naturally occurring". None of the population groups studied was on any sort of cholesterol-lowering diet or medication.

It is important to note that in the studies that did show increased cancer risk, this was observed only at a serum CHOL level *below* 180. In no study was a decrease in serum CHOL from 250 to 190 associated with an increase in non-cardiovascular mortality. Serum CHOL had to be below 180 before cancer mortality was increased (in some studies). This finding has been recently confirmed (149).

These data suggest that some individuals, especially men, with naturally low serum cholesterol may be at an increased risk of dying from cancer. This does not necessarily imply a cause-and-effect relationship. For instance, the tendency toward low cholesterol may be carried on the same gene that carries a tendency to cancer. If this hypothesis is correct, low cholesterol may merely be a "marker" for increased cancer risk.

Of greater importance, perhaps, is that these studies say nothing about the risk of dying from cancer in an individual who starts out with a naturally high cholesterol and who then lowers it by diet or medications. This may be a totally different circumstance from the person with a naturally low serum cholesterol, and the studies reviewed above did not really deal with this type of individual.

Finally, this whole discussion may be moot, even if it's shown that reducing serum CHOL from a high initial level to below 180 does increase non-cardiovascular mortality. The reason that this is moot is that it is exceedingly difficult to lower even a "moderately" elevated serum cholesterol of 250 to below 180. Only a small percentage of hypercholesterolemic individuals would be able to achieve such a reduction. Thus, this concern would not constitute a realistic problem for most hypercholesterolemic individuals.

There are several possible reasons for the association of low serum cholesterol with excess non-cardiovascular risk (150):

1) The influence of "competing risks", i.e., if all patients are followed to death, if their risk of dying from one disease (e.g., cardiovascular) is low, their risk of death from other causes is likely to increase. Expressed in another way, people who would have died from heart disease may have had cancer also. If the risk of heart disease is decreased, they are given the opportunity to die from their cancer. However, since only a small percentage (10-15%) of the patients in the study groups usually die during a study period, such an explanation appears unlikely. In addition, elevated HDL levels, which are also associated with low cardiovascular risk, were not associated with increased non-cardiovascular mortality (151).

2) Excess non-cardiovascular mortality is due to a third factor, which accounts for both the low cholesterol and the increased incidence of cancer. The gene linkage explanation given above (low cholesterol is only a "marker") is an example of this third factor.

3) Cancer causes low cholesterol levels. This is the old "chicken and egg" argument. If there is an association between two conditions, it may be spurious, as discussed in 1 and 2 above, or it may reflect a cause-and-effect relationship. If

the latter applies, which factor causes which is not always clear. Although it has been suggested that low cholesterol causes cancer, the converse could be equally true. For instance, an undiagnosed cancer could alter body chemistry in such a way as to depress serum cholesterol long before the cancer is diagnosed. If one were to measure cholesterol levels in 1000 people, 50 of whom had undiagnosed cancer, those people would have low serum CHOL levels, if this hypothesis is correct. When these individuals were later diagnosed as having cancer, and their cholesterol levels are compared to the 950 without cancer, the cancer patients would have lower levels.

This hypothesis assumes that cancer was "incubating" when the low serum CHOL was measured. If the hypothesis is correct, cancer is more likely to be diagnosed in the few years after the cholesterol levels are measured than later on. Some studies (e.g, 149) have tried to deal with this issue by eliminating all cancers diagnosed within 2-5 years after the cholesterol levels are measured. In most studies, the relationship between low serum CHOL and cancer became weaker, but did not disappear, after this adjustment. Thus, this issue remains unclear.

4) Of course, it is possible that low CHOL *causes* cancer. Although some potential mechanisms for this have been proposed, they are rather sketchy at the present time. For instance, it has been suggested that low serum cholesterol might have an adverse effect on cell plasma membrane fluidity, which could depress the cell's ability to combat carcinogenesis. It is also known that low serum cholesterol is associated with low serum retinol (a form of vitamin A). There is much data that suggests that retinol has anticancer properties (see Chapter 8). Thus, it may be that the low serum retinol associated with low serum cholesterol is responsible for the increased cancer risk (152,153). If this is the case, this is really an example of a third factor, as explained in #2 above. Finally, it has been suggested that polyunsaturated fats, which are known to lower serum cholesterol, may contribute to carcinogenesis because of their potential free-radical-enhancing activities. The latter is extremely controversial at the present time, and lack of adequate data does not allow a reasonable scientific opinion on this topic.

In view of the above discussion, it seems reasonable to attempt to lower one's serum CHOL no lower than about 180. The major benefits, in terms of cardiovascular disease, will be achieved at this level, without incurring the potential risk of lower levels. In addition, eating a diet high in retinol and carotene would be reasonable. Furthermore, not exceeding a polyunsaturated fat intake of 10% of total calories would be prudent, and is consistent with the AHA and recent consensus recommendations. Finally, it should be emphasized that avoidance of tobacco is much more important, in terms of decreasing cancer risk, than is alteration of serum CHOL.

COFFEE AND HYPERCHOLESTEROLEMIA

Concern that coffee may increase serum CHOL and consequently increase the risk of heart disease has waxed and waned over the years until the recent publication of a Norwegian study (154), which rekindled interest in this issue. Two other studies, both performed in the United States and published in 1985, have also supported an *association* between coffee intake and increased cholesterol levels (155,156). The latter study (156) found an association only when coffee intake exceeded 2-3 cups per day. Several other studies, however, have found no correlation between coffee and cholesterol (157-160).

Interestingly, most of the investigators who have found a correlation between coffee and cholesterol do not believe this to be a cause-and-effect relationship (154-156). Several explanations for the relationship have been offerred:

1) Modest (161) proposed that stress could produce an artifactual relationship between coffee and cholesterol—stress may increase serum CHOL (162,163) and coincidentally also increase coffee drinking.

2) Roeckel (164) suggested that cream added to coffee might raise serum CHOL and actually be responsible for the coffee-cholesterol relationship.

3) Ockene (165) speculated that the diet of heavy coffee drinkers may differ in other ways, which account for the relationship.

4) Coffee drinkers are more likely to be smokers, and smoking increases the risk of CHD.

The role of caffeine content of the coffee is unclear. At least one study (155) suggests that the coffee-cholesterol association, if one exists, is not due to the caffeine in coffee; tea, which also contains caffeine, does not appear to elevate serum CHOL. In addition, another study (156) found that the relationship between coffee and cholesterol was *strengthened* after correction for the potential confounding factors noted above.

It should be readily obvious that this issue is extremely complex, especially when it is investigated by epidemiologic means, such as the studies above. It is impossible to intelligently comment on the possibility of a causal relationship until some interventional data become available. In the meantime, it may be prudent to limit coffee intake for other reasons. At the present time, however, the proscription of coffee cannot be recommended on the basis of scientific studies.

HYPERTRIGLYCERIDEMIA

Although this chapter has focused primarily on hypercholesterolemia, a brief discussion of hypertriglyceridemia is in order. Table 6-2 lists the mean and 90th percentile values for TG in American men and women of various ages. As was true of CHOL levels, the statistical distribution of TG levels says nothing about whether high TG levels are related to CHD. It used to be thought that TG levels in the 200-500 range increased the risk of CHD, but current thinking is that they don't. In September, 1983, a Consensus Development Conference reviewing the treatment of hypertriglyceridemia was held at the National Institutes of Health. The following discussion summarizes their conclusions (166).

It is known that fasting TG levels above 500-1000 carry a significant risk of pancreatitis, which is a life-threatening, hard-to-treat condition. Therefore, it is recommended that TG levels >500 be treated, with diet first, but with drugs if necessary.

About 5% of the population has TG levels between 250 and 500, and these levels require individual assessment and treatment. Although TG levels in this range *are* associated with an increased risk of cardiovascular disease, this does not appear to be an independent association. This is because TG is directly correlated with obesity and inversely correlated with HDL. This means that obese people with low HDLs tend to have high TGs. This suggests that TG is not *etiologic* in CHD, but rather, is a *marker* for other characteristics which predispose to heart disease. Thus, the current evidence suggests that two patients with similar body weight and HDL and other risk factors will have a similar risk of heart disease even if one has a TG level of 400 compared to 150 for the other.

Hypertriglyceridemia is frequently secondary to other factors, and can be easily treated by dealing with those factors. These include obesity, excessive alcohol intake, drug (thiazide diuretics, estrogen, some beta blockers) ingestion, diabetes mellitus (especially if poorly controlled), hypothyroidism, uremia, nephrotic syndrome, and liver disease. If the TG level remains elevated despite treatment of the underlying disorder, drug therapy should be considered.

In the absence of hypercholesterolemia, other risk factors, or family history of premature CHD, there is no evidence for increased cardiovascular risk in patients with TG between 250 and 500. In view of known and potential side effects of drug therapy, it is certainly not indicated in this clinical circumstance. The more common situation, however, is that other risk factors are present, and in this situation, the decision of whether to treat is more difficult to make. It would seem reasonable in this situation to attempt to normalize TG levels by nonpharmacologic means. Fortunately, non-drug therapy for hypertriglyceridemia is much more effective than non-drug therapy for hypercholesterolemia.

Changes in lifestyle—weight control and increased exercise, and alcohol and dietary fat restriction—are the cornerstone of nonpharmacologic therapy of hypertriglyceridemia. Attainment of ideal body weight will dramatically decrease, and often normalize, TG levels. Some individuals are also very sensitive to alcohol, and abstaining may further reduce TG level. Caloric restriction in the hyperlipidemic patient should be achieved primarily by decreasing intake of saturated fat and alcohol (actually, this is a good way to decrease caloric intake in anyone). Weight loss can be further enhanced by increased physical activity, which can also independently reduce TG levels. Exercise also simultaneously increases HDL levels, which may be salutary.

The vast majority of patients with borderline hypertriglyceridemia (TG between 250 and 500) will normalize their TG level if they comply with nonpharmacologic therapy. The assistance of a trained dietitian may enhance compliance with this dietary prescription. Up to a year should be allowed for the patient to comply with dietary therapy before drug therapy is contemplated. In fact, many physicians do not believe that the benefits of drugs in borderline hypertriglyceridemia outweigh their known and potential risks. Consequently, many do not recommend drug treatment in this condition even if nonpharmacologic therapy is unsuccessful.

If drug therapy is necessary, three drugs are currently recognized as useful: clofibrate, gemfibrozil and nicotinic acid. Clofibrate has fallen out of favor since the demonstration of *increased* mortality in the clofibrate-treated group in the World Health Organization Clofibrate Trial. In addition, clofibrate may raise CHOL levels in some patients. Although there is limited clinical experience with gemfibrozil, it is chemically similar to clofibrate and its side effects resemble those of clofibrate. The major advantage of nicotinic acid is that it tends to lower both TG and CHOL. Some patients are, however, unable to tolerate the flushing and itching side effects of the drug. Taking aspirin one-half hour before the nicotinic acid may prevent these side effects. Some of the longer-acting preparations of nicotinic acid may also decrease the incidence or severity of these side effects. More severe side effects of nicotinic acid include hyperuricemia, hyperglycemia, and hepatic dysfunction. Gastrointestinal complaints are frequent with all three of these drugs.

SUMMARY AND RECOMMENDATIONS

It is my hope that the preceding discussion has convinced the reader that treating hypercholesterolemia is very likely to decrease the risk of CHD. The objective of this final section is to briefly summarize the information presented in this chapter and explain how the cholesterol-lowering diet may be implemented. Much of this recommendation section draws upon and/or is consistent with the NIH Consensus Conference Statement published in 1985 (1). This statement was briefly discussed in the beginning of this chapter, and should be read by the interested reader.

First of all, the recommendation is made that the public at large, and not only known hypercholesterolemic patients, adopt the cholesterol-lowering diet. In others words, this is a national plan, not a selective one for specific individuals.

Although there are those who disagree with this national diet plan, most experts endorse it. The selective approach would require extensive resources to identify the individuals who are at high risk of developing CHD. Perhaps of greater importance is the fact that most CHD events occur in individuals with "average" CHOL levels. Thus, targeting society's resources at only the upper 5-10% of the population will neglect the health of the majority, who also stand to gain by switching to a cholesterol-lowering diet. Finally, since there is *no* evidence that lowering serum CHOL to the 180-200 level has *any* harmful effects, it seems clear that adoption of such a goal nationally is wise.

The first step in dietary control is reduction of dietary fat to <30% of total calories (compared to the current national average of about 40%) and cholesterol to <250-300 mg per day (compared to national average of about 450 mg). No more than one-third of the fat consumed (10% of total calories) should be as saturated fat (compared to about 20% national average currently). The dietary fat reduction from 40 to 30% of total calories should be primarily at the expense of saturated fat, such as animal and dairy fats. Dairy products should not be eliminated since they are the primary dietary source of calcium; instead, low-fat or non-fat dairy products should be eaten. The fat calories should be replaced primarily by complex carbohydrates such as breads, cereals, legumes, fruits and vegetables. These foods are low in fat, high in complex carbohydrates, high in nutrients (e.g., vitamins), low in salt, and high in potassium and fiber.

Most individuals on this diet will experience a 10-20% decrease in their serum CHOL. An occasional patient, however, does not respond to this diet, and a stricter diet or the prescription of hypocholesterolemic drugs or both may be indicated. It is important not to expect patients to change their diets overnight, and patience and encouragement on the part of the health care team will enhance compliance. If despite adherence to the diet serum CHOL remains high, a further restriction of dietary fat to 20-25% of total calories may be useful. Although such a diet may seem radical by comparison with the American diet, this type of diet is ingested in many of the Mediterranean countries with pleasure. It should also be kept in mind that many vegetarians in the United States voluntarily eat a diet containing even less dietary fat. Again, the major factor is a slow change with adequate assistance from the health team(e.g., dietitian).

The low-fat diet is recommended for all individuals in the United States, but especially for those in the upper half of the cholesterol distribution. This translates to a serum CHOL of about 200-210 for most middle-aged American adults. All members of the family, except for children under 2 years of age, should be encouraged to eat this type of diet. This will enhance compliance for the hypercholesterolemic individual, as well as treat other family members who may otherwise be destined to develop hypercholesterolemia.

REFERENCES

1. NIH Consensus Development Conference Statement: Lowering blood cholesterol to prevent heart disease. JAMA 253:2080, 1985
2. American Heart Association Special Report: Recommendations for treatment of hyper-lipidemia in adults. Circulation 69:1065A, 1984
3. Kannel WB, Gordon T: The search for an optimum serum cholesterol. Lancet 2:374, 1982
4. Stamler J: Public health aspects of optimal serum lipid-lipoprotein levels. Prev Med 8:733, 1979
5. Editorial: Is reduction of blood cholesterol effective? Lancet 1:317, 1984
6. Murchison LE: Hyperlipidaemia. Br Med J 290:535, 1985
7. Stamler J: Lifestyles, major risk factors, proof and public policy. Circulation 58:3, 1978
8. Rahimtoola SH: Cholesterol and coronary heart disease: A perspective. JAMA 253:2094, 1985
8a. Truswell AS: Reducing the risk of coronary heart disease. Br Med J 291:34, 1985
8b. Borhani NO: Prevention of coronary heart disease in practice. Implications of the results of recent clinical trials. JAMA 254:257, 1985
9. Harlan WR, Stross JK: An educational view of a national initiative to lower plasma lipid levels. JAMA 253:2087, 1985
10. National Heart Lung and Blood Institute: National Cholesterol Education Program. Modern Medicine,,March, 1985, pp.72
11. Cholesterol:And now the bad news. Time, 3/26/84, pp.56
Giving cholesterol a bad name. Newsweek, 1/23/84, pp.75
Killer cholesterol — grim new size-up. US News & WR, 12/24/84, pp.8
America's nutrition revolution. Understanding the link between diet and disease has changed our eating habits. Newsweek, 11/19/84, pp. 111
12. Garaway WM, et al: The declining incidence of stroke. N Engl J Med 300:449, 1979
13. Walker WJ: Changing United States lifestyle and declining vascular mortality: cause or coincidence? N Engl J Med 297:163, 1977
14. Walker WJ: Changing U.S. lifestyle and declining vascular mortality — a retro-spective. N Engl J Med 308:649, 1983
15. Goldman L, Cook EF: The decline in ischemic heart disease mortality rates. An analysis of the comparative effects of medical interventions and changes in lifestyle. Ann Int Med 101:825, 1984
16. Jones JL: Are health concerns changing the American diet? DHEW pub. # (NFS) 159, Government Printing Office, Washington, D.C., 1977, pp.27
17. MRFIT Trial Research Group: Multiple risk factor intervention trial:risk factor changes and mortality results. JAMA 248:1465, 1982
18. The Surgeon General's Report on Health Promotion and Disease Prevention. Public. # 79-55071A, Washington, D.C., 1979
19. Folsom AR, et al: Improvement in hypertension detection and control from 1973-4 to 1980-81. The Minnesota Heart Survey experience. JAMA 250:916, 1983

20. Hesler JR, et al: LDL-induced cytotoxicity and its inhibition by HDL in human vascular smooth muscle and endothelial cells in culture. Atherosclerosis 32:213, 1979
21. Brown MS, et al: Regulation of plasma cholesterol by lipoprotein receptors. Science 212:628, 1981
22. Goldstein JI, et al: Defective lipoprotein receptors and atherosclerosis. Lessons from an animal counterpart of familial hypercholesterolemia. N Engl J Med 309:288, 1983
22a. Schaefer EJ, Levy RI: Pathogenesis and management of lipoprotein disorders. N Engl J Med 312:1300, 1985
23. Gofman JW, et al: Blood lipids and human atherosclerosis. Circulation 2:161, 1950
24. Ross R, et al: Pathogenesis of atherosclerosis. N Engl J Med 295:369, 420, 1976
25. Benditt EP: The origin of atherosclerosis. Sci Am 236:74, 1977
26. Glueck CJ: Classification and diagnosis of hyperlipoproteinemia. In: "Hyperlipidemia: Diagnosis and therapy", Rifkind BM, Levy RI (eds.), Grune & Stratton, New York, 1977, pp.17
27. Rifkind BM, Segal P: Lipid Research Clinics program for reference values for hyperlipidemia and hypolipidemia. JAMA 250:1869, 1983
28. McManus BM, et al: "Normal" blood cholesterol levels. N Engl J Med 312:51, 1985
29. Kleinbaum DG, et al: Multivariate analysis of risk of coronary heart disease in Evans County, Georgia. Arch Intern Med 128:943, 1971
30. Carlson LA, Bottiger LE: Ischemic heart disease in relation to fasting values of plasma triglycerides and cholesterol. Stockholm Prospective Study. Lancet 1:865, 1972
31. Friedman GD, et al: Kaiser Permanente epidemiologic study of myocardial infarction. Study design and resultd for standard risk factors. Am J Epidemiol 99:101, 1974
32. Goldbourt U, et al: Clinical myocardial infarction over a five-year period. A multivariate analysis of incidence, the Israel Ischemic Heart Disease Study. J Chron Dis 28:217, 1975
33. Gordon T, et al: Predicting coronary heart disease in middle-aged and older persons. The Framingham Study. JAMA 238:497, 1977
34. Kannel WB, et al: Cholesterol in the prediction of atherosclerotic disease. New perspectives based on the Framingham study. Ann Int Med 90:85, 1979
35. Robertson TL, et al: Epidemiologic studies of coronary heart disease and stroke in Japanese men living in Japan, Hawaii, and California. Incidence of myocardial infarction and death from coronary heart disease. Am J Cardiol 39:239, 1977
36. Pooling Project Research Group: Relationship of blood pressure, serum cholesterol, smoking habit, relative weight, and ECG abnormalities to incidence of major coronary events: final report of the pooling project. J Chron Dis 31:202, 1978
37. Keys A: Seven countries:a multivariate analysis of death and coronary heart disease. Harvard University Press, Cambridge, MA, 1980
38. Shekelle RB, et al: Diet, serum cholesterol and death from coronary heart disease. The Western Electric study. N Engl J Med 304:65, 1981
39. Inter-Society Commission for Heart Disease Resources. Atherosclerosis Study Group and Epidemiology Study Group: Primary prevention of the atherosclerotic diseases. Circulation 42:A55, 1970
40. Blackburn H, et al: Revised data for 1970 Inter-Society for Heart Disease Resources Report (letter to the editor). Am Heart J 94:549, 1977

41. Kannel WB, Gordon T: The search for an optimum serum cholesterol. Lancet 2:374, 1982
42. Wissler RW: Development of the atherosclerotic plaque, in "The myocardium:Failure and infarction (Braunwald E, ed.). HP Publishing Co., New York, 1974, pp. 155-66
43. Dayton S, et al: A controlled clinical trial of a diet high in unsaturated fat in preventing complications of atherosclerosis. Circulation 40 (suppl 2):1, 1969
44. Research Committee to the Medical Research Council: Controlled trial of a soya bean oil in myocardial infarction. Lancet 2:693, 1968
45. Leren P: The Oslo Diet Heart Study: Eleven-year report. Circulation 42:935, 1970
46. Miettinen M, et al: Effect of cholesterol-lowering diet on mortality from coronary heart disease and other causes. A twelve year clinical trial. Lancet 2:835, 1972
47. Hjermann I, et al: The effect of diet and smoking interventions on the incidence of coronary heart disease. Lancet 2:1303, 1981
48. Olson R: Cholesterol and the heart: Will we mislead the public? Mod Med 51:15, 1983
49. Research Committee to the Medical Research Council: Low-fat diet in myocardial infarction — a controlled trial. Lancet 2:501, 1965
50. MRFIT Research Group: Multiple Risk Factor Intervention Trial. Risk factor changes and mortality results. JAMA 248:1465, 1982
51. LRC Program: The lipid Research Clinics Coronary Primary Prevention Trial Results. I. Reduction in incidence of coronary heart disease. II. The relationship of reduction in incidence of coronary heart disease to cholesterol lowering. JAMA 251:351, 365, 1984
52. Barr DP, et al: Protein-lipid relationship in human plasma. II. In atherosclerosis and related considerations. Am J Med 11:480, 1951
53. Miller GJ, Miller NE: Plasma high-density lipoprotein concentration and development of ischemic heart disease. Lancet 1:16, 1975
54. Lees RS, Lees AM: High density lipoproteins and the risk of atherosclerosis. N Engl J Med 306:1546, 1982
55. Havel RJ: High density lipoproteins, cholesterol transport and coronary heart disease. Circulation 60:1, 1979
56. Grundy SM: High density lipoproteins and atherosclerosis. Med Times 107:87, 1979
57. Castelli WP, et al: HDL cholesterol and other lipids in coronary heart disease. The Cooperative Lipoprotein Phenotyping Study. Circulation 55:767, 1977
58. Gordon T, et al: High density lipoprotein as a protective factor against coronary heart disease. The Framingham Study. Am J Med 62:707, 1977
59. Gordon T, et al: Lipoproteins, cardiovascular disease and death. The Framingham Study. Ann Int Med 141:1128, 1981
60. Wahl P, et al: Effect of estrogen/progestin potency on lipid/lipoprotein cholesterol. N Engl J Med 308:862, 1983
61. Wood PD, et al: The distribution of plasma lipoproteins in middle-aged runners. Metabolism 25:1249, 1976
62. Lehtonen A, Viikari J: Serum triglycerides and cholesterol and serum high density lipoprotein cholesterol in highly physically active men. Acta Med Scand 204:111, 1978
63. Huttunen JK, et al: Effect of moderate physical exercise on serum lipoproteins. A

controlled clinical trial with special reference to serum high density lipoproteins. Circulation 60:1220, 1979

64. Brownell KD, et al: Changes in plasma lipid and lipoprotein levels in men and women after a program of moderate exercise. Circulation 65:477, 1982

65. Smith M ,et al: Exercise intensity, dietary intake, and high density lipoprotein cholesterol in young female competitive swimming. Am J Clin Nutr 36:251, 1982

66. Quig DW, et al: Effects of short-term aerobic conditioning and high cholesterol feeding on plasma total and lipoprotein cholesterol levels in sedentary young men. Am J Clin Nutr 38:825, 1983

67. Herbert PN, et al: High density lipoprotein metabolism in runners and sedentary men. JAMA 252:1034, 1984

68. Hurley BF, et al: High density lipoprotein cholesterol in bodybuilders v powerlifters. JAMA 252:507, 1984

69. Goldberg L, et al: Changes in lipid and lipoprotein levels after weight training. JAMA 252:504, 1984

70. La Porte RE, et al: HDL cholesterol across a spectrum of physical activity from quadriplegia to marathon running (letter). Lancet 1:1212, 1983

71. Avogaro P, et al: HDL cholesterol, apolipoprotein A and B, age index and body weight. Atherosclerosis 31:85, 1978

72. Goldbourt U, Medalie JH: High density lipoprotein cholesterol and incidence of coronary heart disease — the Israeli ischemic heart disease study. Am J Epidemiol 109:296, 1979

73. Follick MJ, et al: Contrasting short- and long-term effects of weight loss on lipoprotein levels. Arch Intern Med 144:1571, 1984

74. Streja DA, et al: Changes in plasma high density lipoprotein cholesterol concentration after weight reduction in grossly obese patients. Br Med J 281:770, 1980

75. Brownell KD, Stunkard AJ: Differential changes in plasma high density lipoprotein cholesterol levels in obese men and women during weight reduction. Arch Intern Med 141:1142, 1981

76. Hulley SB, Gordon S: Alcohol and high density lipoprotein cholesterol. Circulation 64 (suppl 3):57, 1981

77. Hartung GH, et al:Effect of alcohol intake on high density lipoprotein cholesterol levels in runners and inactive men. JAMA 249:747, 1983

78. Haskell WL, et al: The effect of cessation and resumption of moderate alcohol intake on serum high density lipoprotein subfractions. A controlled study. N Engl J Med 310:805, 1984

79. Miller NE, et al: Relation of angiographically defined coronary artery disease to plasma lipoprotein subfractions and apolipoproteins. Br Med J 282:1741, 1981

80. Ballantyne FC, et al: High density and low density lipoprotein subfractions in survivors of myocardial infarction and in control subjects. Metabolism 31:433, 1982

81. Krauss RM: Regulation of high density lipoprotein levels. Med Clin North Am 66:403, 1982

82. Nye ER, et al: Changes in high density lipoprotein subfractions and other lipoproteins induced by exercise. Clin Chim Acta 113:51, 1981

83. Wood PD, et al: Increased exercise level and plasma lipoprotein concentrations:a one-

year, randomized controlled study in sedentary middle-aged men. Metabolism 32:31, 1983

84. Lieber CS: To drink (moderately) or not to drink? N Engl J Med 310:846, 1984

85. Stubbe I, et al: High density lipoprotein concentrations increase after stopping smoking. Br Med J 284:1511, 1982

86. Thompson GR: Dietary and pharmacological control of lipoprotein metabolism. In: Lipoproteins, atherosclerosis and coronary heart disease. Miller NE, Lewis B (eds.) Elsevier, Amsterdam, Holland, 1981, pp.129

87. Nikkila EA, et al: Increase in serum high density lipoprotein in phenytoin users. Br Med J 283:99, 1978

88. Bolton CH, et al: Effects of cimetidine on serum and lipoprotein lipids in normal subjects (abstract). Br J Clin Pharmacol 15:152P, 1983

89. Miller NE, Lewis B: Cimetidine and HDL cholesterol. Lancet 1:529, 1983

90. Gresham GA: Is atheroma a reversible lesion? Atherosclerosis 23:379, 1976

91. Brooks SH, et al: Determinants of atherosclerosis progression and regression. Arch Surg 113:75, 1978

92. Malinow MR: Atherosclerosis: Progression, regression and resolution. Am Heart J 108:1523, 1984

93. Blankenhorn DH, Sanmarco ME: Angiography for study of lipid-lowering therapy. Circulation 59:212, 1979

94. Basta LL, et al: Regression of atherosclerotic stenosing lesions of the renal arteries and spontaneous cure of systemic hypertension through control of hyperlipidemia. Am J Med 61:420, 1976

95. Armstrong ML, et al: Regression of coronary atheromatosis in rhesus monkeys. Circ Res 27:59, 1970

96. Malinow MR: Experimental models of atherosclerosis regression. Atherosclerosis 48:105, 1983

97. Barndt R, et al: Regression and progression of early femoral athersclerosis in treated hyperlipoproteinemic patients. Ann Int Med 86:139, 1977

98. Kuo PT, et al: Use of combined diet and colestipol in long-term (7-7.5 years) treatment of patients with Type II hyperlipoproteinemia. Circulation 59:199, 1979

99. Starzl TE, et al: Heart-liver transplantation in a patient with familial hypercholesterolemia. Lancet 1:1382, 1984

100. Bilheimer DW, et al: Liver transplantation to provide low-density-lipoprotein receptors and lower plasma cholesterol in a child with homozygous familial hypercholesterolemia. N Engl J Med 311:1658, 1984

101. Diagnostic and therapeutic technology assessment. Chelation therapy. JAMA 250:672, 1983

101a. Shaw D: Chelation therapy (letter). NZ Med J 96:144, 1983

102. Cashion WR: What about chelation? Tex Med 80:6-7, 1984

102a. Gotto AM: Chelation therapy in 1984. Tex Med 80:36, 1984

103. Pentel P, et al: Chelation therapy for the treatment of atherosclerosis. An appraisal. Minn Med 67:101, 1984

104. Soffer A: Chelation clinics. An abuse of the physician's freedom of choice. Chest 86:157, 1984

105. Rathmann KL, Golightly LK: Chelation therapy of atherosclerosis. Drug Intell Clin Pharm 18:1000, 1984
106. Clarke NE, et al: The in vivo dissolution of metastatic calcium — An approach of atherosclerosis. Am J Med Sci 229:142, 1955 107. Department of Health and Human Services: EDTA chelation therapy for atherosclerosis. HRST Assessment Report Series, vol. 1, #18, 1981
108. Anon: EDTA chelation therapy for arteriosclerotic heart disease. Medical Letter 23:49, 1981
109. DePalma v. Levin. U.S. District Court , EDNY, No. 78 Civ 227, 2 November, 1981
110. Barnard RJ, et al: Effects of an intensive exercise and nutrition program on patients with coronary artery disease: Five-year follow-up. J Cardiac Rehab 3:183, 1983
111. CASS Principal Investigators: Myocardial infarction and mortality in the Coronary Artery Surgery Study (CASS) randomized trial. N Engl J Med 310:750, 1984
112. Pritikin N, McGrady P: The pritikin program for diet and exercise. New York, Grosset & Dunlap, 1979
113. Anon: The Pritikin program: Claims vs. facts. Consumer Reports, October 1982, pp. 513
114. Barnard RJ, et al: Effects of an intensive, short-term exercise and nutrition program on patients with coronary heart disease. J Cardiac Rehab 1:99, 1981
115. Barnard RJ, et al: Response of non-insulin-dependent diabetic patients to an intensive program of diet and exercise. Diabetes Care 5:370, 1982
116. Hall JA, Barnard RJ: The effects of an intensive 26-day program of diet and exercise on patients with peripheral vascular disease. J Cardiac Rehab 2:569, 1982
117. Weber F, et al: Effects of a high-complex-carbohydrate low-fat diet and daily exercise on individuals 70 years of age and older. J Gerontology 38:155, 1983
118. Barnard RJ, et al: Long-term use of a high-complex-carbohydrate, high-fiber, low-fat, diet and exercise in the treatment of NIDDM patients. Diabetes Care 6:268, 1983
119. Barnard RJ, et al: Effects of a high-complex carbohydrate diet and daily walking on blood pressure and medication status of hypertensive patients. J Cardiac Rehab 3:839, 1983
120. Pritikin N: Guest editorial. Optimal dietary recommendations: A public health responsibility. Prev Med 11:733, 1982
121. Hutchinson K, et al: Effects of dietary manipulation on vascular status of patients with peripheral vascular disease. JAMA 249:3326, 1983
122. Brown GD, et al: Effects of two "lipid-lowering" diets on plasma lipid levels of patients with peripheral vascular disease. J Am Diet Assoc 84:546, 1984
123. Subcommittee of Diet and Hyperlipidemia, Council on Arteriosclerosis: A maximal approach to the dietary treatment of hyperlipidemias. Diet C. The low cholesterol, high polyunsaturated fat diet. New York, AHA, 1973
124. MaxEPA advertisement: Low heart disease rate linked to Eskimo secret. In Household magazine, distributed locally, San Diego, CA, 1983
125. Steve Blechman, for Dale Alexander Cod Liver Oil: EPA-rich cod-liver oil. A potential breakthrough in the prevention and treatment of cardiovascular disease. Brochure picked up in health food store, 1983

126. Dyerberg J, et al: Eicosapentaenoic acid and prevention of thrombosis and athero-sclerosis. Lancet 2:117, 1978

127. Nutrition Canada. The Eskimo survey report. Ottawa: Department of National Health and Welfare, 1975

128. Arthaud B: Cause of death in 339 Alaskan natives as determined by autopsy. AMA Arch Pathol 90:433, 1970

129. Bang H, et al:Plasma lipid and lipoprotein pattern in Greenlandic West-Coast Eskimos. Lancet 1:1143, 1971

130. Dahl LK: Salt intake and salt need. N Engl J Med 258:1152, 1958

131. Dyerberg J, Bang H: Haemostatic function and platelet polyunsaturated fatty acids in Eskimos. Lancet 2:433, 1979

132. Editorial: Eskimo diets and diseases. Lancet 1:1139, 1983

132a. Kromhout D, et al: The inverse relation between fish consumption and 20-year mortality from coronary heart disease. N Engl J Med 312:1205, 1985

133. Sinclair HM: Advantages and disadvantages of an Eskimo diet. In: Drugs Affecting Lipid Metabolism. Fumagalli R, et al (eds.), Elsevier/North Holland, Amsterdam, 1980, pp.363-70

134. Sinclair HM: The relative importance of essential fatty acids of the linoleic and linoleic families: studies with an Eskimo diet. Prog Lipid Res 20:897, 1981

135. Thorngren M, Gustafson A: Effects of 11-week increase in dietary eicosapentaenoic acid on bleeding time, lipids and patelet aggregation. Lancet 2:1190, 1981

135a. Phillipson BE, et al: Reduction of plasma lipids, lipoproteins, and apoproteins by dietary fish oils in patients with hypertriglyceridemia. N Eng J Med 312:1210, 1985

136. Von Lossonczy TO, et al: The effect of a fish diet on serum lipids in healthy human subjects. Am J Clin Nutr 31:1340, 1978

137. Bronsgeest-Schoute HC, et al: The effect of various intakes of w3 fatty acids on the blood lipid composition in healthy human subjects. Am J Clin Nutr 34:1752, 1981

138. Siess W, et al: Platelet membrane fatty acids, platelet aggregation and thromboxane formation during a macketel diet. Lancet 1:441, 1980

139. Woodcock BE, et al: Beneficial effect of fish oil on blood viscosity in peripheral vascular disease. Br Med J 288:592, 1984

140. Lorenz R, et al: Platelet function, thromboxane formation and blood pressure control during supplementation of the Western diet with cod liver oil. Circulation 67:504, 1983

141. Sanders TAB, et al: Effects on blood lipids and haemostasis of a supplement of cod liver oil, rich in eicosapentaenoic and docosahexaenoic acids in healthy young men. Clin Sci 61:317, 1981

142. Sanders TAB, Roshanai, F: The influence of different types of w3 polyunsaturated fatty acids on blood lipids and platelet function in healthy volunteers. Clin Sci 64:91, 1983

143. Brox JH, et al: The effect of cod liver oil and corn oil on platelets and vessel wall in man. Thrombosis Haemostas 46:604, 1981

144. Goodnight SH, et al: The effect of dietary w3 fatty acids on platelet composition and function in man: a prospective controlled study. Blood 58:880, 1981

145. Hay CRM, et al: Effects of fish oil on platelet kinetics in patients with ischemic heart disease. Lancet 1:1269, 1982

146. Terano T, et al:Effect of oral administration of highly purified eicosapentaenoic acid

on platelet function, blood viscosity and red cell deformablility in human subjects. Atherosclerosis 0:000, 1983 or 84

146a. Glomset JA, et al: Fish, fatty acids, and human health. N Engl J Med 312:1253, 1985

146b. Letters to the editor: Fish, consumption and mortality from coronary hear disease, N Engl J Med 313:820, 1985

147. Renaud S, Nordoy A: "Small is beautiful": linolenic acid and eicosapentaenoic acid in man. Lancet 1:1169, 1983

148. National Institutes of Health: Summary of workshop on cholesterol and non-cardiovascular disease mortality. May 11–12, 1981 Bethesda, MD. Also published in Prev Med 11:360, 1982

149. Salmond CE, et al: Are low cholesterol levels associated with excess mortality? Br Med J 290:422, 1985

150. Hlatky MA, Hulley SB: Plasma cholesterol. Can it be too low? Arch Intern Med 141:1132, 1981

151. Gordon T. et al: Lipoprotein, cardiovascular disease, and death. The Framingham study. Arch Intern Med 141:1128, 1981

152. Kark JD, et al: Serum retinol and the inverse relationship between serum cholesterol and cancer. Br Med J 284:152, 1982

153. Merenah CB, et al: Hypercholesterolemia and non-cardiovascular disease: metabolic studies on subjects with low plasma cholesterol concentration. Br Med J 286:1603, 1983

154. Thelle DS, et al: The Tromso Heart Study: does coffee raise serum cholesterol? N Engl J Med 308:1454, 1983

155. Klatsky AL, et al: Coffee, tea and cholesterol. Am J Cardiol 55:577, 1985

156. Williams Pt, et al: Coffee intake and elevated cholesterol and apolipoprotein B levels in men. JAMA 253:1407, 1985

157. Dawber TR, et al: Coffee and cardiovascular disease: Observations from the Framingham study. N Engl J Med 291:871, 1974

158. Korvar MG, et al: Coffee and cholesterol. N Engl J Med 309:1249, 1983

159. Shekelle RB, et al: Coffee and cholesterol. N Eng J Med 309:1249, 1983

160. Hofman A, et al: Coffee and cholesterol. N Engl J Med 309, 1249, 1983

161. Modest G: Coffee and cholesterol. N Eng J Med 309:1248, 1983

162. Dreyfuss F, Czaczkes JW: Blood cholesterol and uric acid of healthy medical students under the stress of an examination. Arch Intern Med 103:708, 1959

163. Friedman M, et al: Changes in the serum cholesterol and blood clotting time in men subjected to cyclic variations of occupational stress. Circulation 17:852, 1958

164. Roeckel IE: Coffee and cholesterol. N Engl J Med 309:1248, 1983

165. Ockene IS et al: Coffee and cholesterol. N Engl J Med 309:1248, 1983

166. NIH: National Institutes of Health Consensus Development Conference Statement: Hypertriglyceridemia. NIH, Bethesda, MD, 1984

CHAPTER 7

Sugar, Hypoglycemia and Diets for Diabetics

Sugar has certainly been a popular topic (and scapegoat), especially in the lay press, but also in the scientific literature. Although it has been blamed, often irrationally, for every ill to which man is subject, there is little evidence to support most of these incriminations. This is not to say that sugar is good for you, but by blaming sugar for ills for which it isn't responsible, one only avoids dealing with the items or factors which *are* responsible. This chapter will review the role of sugar and other carbohydrates in the metabolism of the human body, and then review some very interesting recent data which question age-old concepts in the dietary treatment of diabetes. Finally, the role of hypoglycemia in disease (and non-disease) will be examined.

A REVIEW OF CARBOHYDRATE METABOLISM

Types of Carbohydrate

Sugar is a member of a group of substances known as carbohydrates so-called because they are composed of *carbo*n and water—*hydrate*. There are four major subtypes of CHO (the abbreviation for carbohydrate): monosaccharides, disaccharides, oligosaccharides and polysaccharides (Figure 7-1). These types of CHO are composed of one or a combination of several different 6-carbon compounds; the most common 6-carbon compound in all carbohydrates is glucose. The other 6-carbon compounds are fructose, galactose and mannose. These four 6-carbon compounds—glucose, fructose, galactose, and mannose—comprise the first class of CHO, the monosaccharides. These four compounds all have the same number of carbon, hydrogen and oxygen atoms; they differ from one another in the arrangement of these atoms. This difference leads to variations in their biologic properties.

Figure 7-1

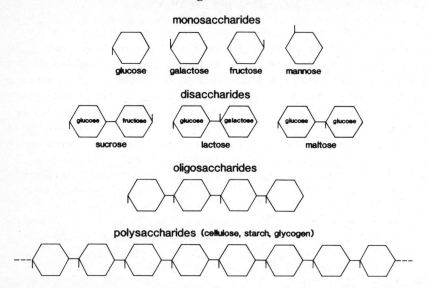

Four major subtypes of carbohydrates
See text for explanation.

Disaccharides, the second class of CHO, are sugars composed of two mono-saccharides which are bound together. Different combinations of monosac-charides yield different disaccharides. For instance, if glucose is attached to fructose, sucrose—table sugar—is formed. If glucose and galactose are com-bined, lactose (milk sugar) results. Maltose, another disaccharide, is derived from the combination of 2 glucose molecules.

Oligosaccharides (*oligo* means "a few") are composed of a few monosac-charides joined together. They are not an important source of dietary carbohy-drate and will not be further discussed.

The fourth and calorically most important class of carbohydrate are the polysaccharides. As the name suggests, these compounds are composed of many repeating monosaccharide (usually glucose) subunits. As is diagrammatically shown in Figure 7-1, both cellulose, and starch and glycogen, are made from many repeating glucose subunits. The difference between these two types of polysaccharides is that cellulose contains some bonds that cannot be broken by human intestinal enzymes, whereas all the bonds in starch and glycogen can be broken (digested) by human enzymes. The difference between starch and glycogen is that starch is made by plants whereas glycogen is made by animals. Both are made for the purpose of storing energy for the future.

Carbohydrate Metabolism

Glucose is the common carbohydrate "currency" of the human body. It is the main circulating carbohydrate in the blood (often called "blood sugar"). All other carbohydrates are converted to glucose before further metabolism. For example, all disaccharides, oligosaccharides and polysaccharides (at least the digestible variety), are digested to glucose in the intestines. After absorption into the bloodstream, the glucose may be taken to organs (e.g., the brain) where it will be metabolized ("burned") for energy. Glucose may also be converted to glycogen or fat, to store energy for the future. Consider an analogy of a monetary system wherein all currency must be converted to $1 bills. Thus, when a $100 bill (a polysaccharide)is "eaten", it will be broken down to $1 bills (glucose), some of which will be "burned" for energy, while others will go to the liver to be stored as $10 bills (glycogen) and yet others will be stored as $50 bills (fat). Incidentally, this concept applies to protein metabolism as well as to carbohydrate metabolism. When protein is eaten, it is broken down (digested) to single amino acids; these amino acids are then rebuilt into human proteins.

Carbohydrate digestion starts in the mouth, where the salivary glands secrete the enzyme amylase. Salivary amylase initiates the breakdown of starch in the mouth. More amylase is made by the pancreas and is delivered to the small intestine, where carbohydrate digestion continues and absorption of the monosaccharides (like glucose) occurs. As the reader will recall from Chapter 1, starch blockers were alleged to interfere with carbohydrate digestion by "blocking" the action of amylase. Unfortunately for starch blocker manufacturers, all clinical studies to date have shown starch blockers to be ineffective. There are diseases, however, wherein amylase (and other enzymes) are made in insufficient quantities, and these diseases result in malabsorption of various nutrients. Cystic fibrosis is one such disease, while lactose intolerance is a milder disease that is characterized by a partial or total inability to digest lactose due to the absence of the necessary enzyme (lactase).

Insulin Secretion and Regulation of Blood Sugar

Although many body chemicals are important in the regulation of carbohydrate metabolism, insulin is often considered the most important. This hormone has many functions which have been the object of extensive research for more than half a century. Simplistically speaking, the major function of insulin is to facilitate the uptake of blood glucose into various cells of the body, especially muscle, liver and adipose (fat) tissues. In so doing, insulin controls the amount of sugar that is left in the bloodstream. Insulin is not necessary for the absorption of glucose from the intestine or its uptake in the brain.

If insulin is deficient, glucose will still be absorbed in the intestine and used in the brain, but the other tissues will not be able to utilize the excess glucose as they would if insulin were available. Consequently, the excess glucose will remain in the bloodstream, resulting in a condition called hyperglycemia (high blood sugar). Whereas normal *fasting* blood sugar is 80-100 mg% (it is normally higher after eating), a diabetic in poor control often has a blood glucose of 300-400 mg%, and levels over 1000 mg% are not unheard of! When blood sugar rises above 180-200 mg%, glucose can start "spilling" into the urine. This accounts for the name of the disease diabetes mellitus, which means "sweet urine".

Blood sugar level is regulated as follows: within minutes of eating, the gastrointestinal tract has already evaluated the amount of food eaten and signals the pancreas to secrete the proper amount of insulin. The pancreas carefully monitors food intake and blood sugar continuously, and insulin (and other hormone) secretion is modified accordingly. Blood sugar is carefully maintained in a narrow range regardless of how much carbohydrate has been ingested. Very rarely, the pancreas may secrete a bit too much insulin in response to food, and blood sugar decreases below normal levels. Low blood sugar is known as hypoglycemia, but the exact level at which true hypoglycemia can be diagnosed depends on the age and sex of the patient. Hypoglycemia is discussed in detail later in this chapter.

With this introduction on carbohydrate metabolism in mind, let us now consider the evidence against sugar.

THE CASE AGAINST SUGAR

Although both the mono- and disaccharides discussed above are considered sugars, most people are referring to the disaccharide sucrose when they discuss "sugar". Sucrose differs from blood sugar (glucose) in an important way. The latter is essential for life, and its absence from the bloodstream can result in coma and death. It is not necessary to eat either glucose or sucrose in order to maintain a normal level of blood sugar, because blood glucose can be derived from all types of carbohydrate. In fact, glucose can also be made from protein (this is what happens during fasting). Indeed, Eskimos ingest almost no carbohydrate and seem no worse off for it.

The situation for Americans, however, is quite different from that of Eskimos, in that we supposedly ingest excessive amounts of sugar. At this point, a clear distinction should be drawn between sugars (mono- and disaccharides) and carbohydrate in general, although this distinction is becoming somewhat blurred in light of new research. As will be discussed in this chapter and in Chapter 11, carbohydrates, especially the high-fiber, complex carbohydrates, are now widely recommended. Increased carbohydrate intake is advised both for healthy individuals, and, with some rare exceptions, for patients with diabetes, heart disease, diverticulosis, etc.

For many years, carbohydrates were the object of bad press, having often been labeled as "fattening". As the reader undoubtedly recognizes, fat is more than twice as "fattening" as carbohydrate. In addition, fats have other negative health effects, as discussed in Chapter 6. As this has become better appreciated, complex carbohydrates have gained favor, usually as a replacement for fat-derived calories, with recommendations for protein calories remaining essentially unchanged.

The reader may wonder, "If both simple sugars and complex carbohydrates are broken down to glucose, why is one type of carbohydrate (sugar) worse than the other (polysaccharide)?" For healthy (i.e., non-diabetic) individuals, this comes down to two major reasons: (1) empty calories, and (2) cavities. A food containing empty calories is often referred to as having "low nutritional density". The concept of nutritional density is an attempt to evaluate the amounts of nutrients—vitamins, minerals, protein— available per number of calories in a certain food. For instance, while an orange and a piece of caramel both may contain 100 calories, and both may be carbohydrate calories, the orange would contain vitamin C, other vitamins, and fiber, while the piece of caramel would not. If you ate a lot of foods with low nutritional density, you would either achieve your quota of calories without attaining your recommended daily intake of various nutrients, or you might achieve your adequate nutrient intake, but at the expense of ingesting too many calories (and therefore gaining weight). The latter is especially likely since although sweets have many calories, they tend not to be filling, and thus excess calories are likely to be ingested. The gustatory advantages of sweets (their good taste) also increase the likelihood that excess calories will be eaten. If a person is very active and burns many calories, some calories can be obtained from foods with low nutritional density without undue concern.

The second negative aspect of excessive sugar consumption is that of dental cavities (caries). Although it is fairly widely accepted that sugar is a major factor in the development of dental caries (see ref. 1 for a recent review), even this concept appears to be controversial, as evidenced by a series of letters to the editor of the Lancet (2). It seems that it is not the absolute amount of sugar eaten that is most important, but rather the timing, the type, and pH of the substance. Sugary foods eaten between meals, in a sticky form (e.g., caramel, peanut brittle), and in an acid medium, are thought to be most cariogenic (cavity-forming). Of course, dental hygiene and preventive care, and other aspects of diet (e.g., fluoride), are also important in preventing dental decay. Some experts have suggested that not only simple sugars, but also complex carbohydrates, can be cariogenic. From a brief review of the literature, it is reasonable to conclude that reduction of sugar intake will result in a decreased incidence of cavities.

Are there other bad effects of sugar besides low nutritional density (and maybe consequent obesity) and dental caries? Although sugar has been blamed, primarily in the popular literature, for many of man's ills, there's little scientific evidence to support this view. However, since decreasing sugar intake is unlikely to be harmful, and may confer benefits, it seems reasonable to attempt to reduce one's sugar intake, but probably not with the quasi-religious zeal that some would recommend. This is especially true in view of some recent data which suggest that simple carbohydrates, like sugar, may not be that different from complex carbohydrates after all.

DIETS FOR DIABETICS

It has been estimated that there are more than 10 million diabetics in the United States. Prior to the discovery of insulin, a diagnosis of diabetes mellitus (DM) usually implied very strict dietary control of the disease, or certain death. Upon its discovery in 1921, insulin was hailed as "the cure" for DM, and it was anticipated that the lifespan of diabetics would become normal. Many suggested that diabetics would no longer have to watch their diet.

We now know that, unfortunately, this is not the case. Life expectancy for those who develop diabetes before the age of 20 (so-called juvenile-onset or more accurately, Type I diabetes—see ref. 3 for new nomenclature) is reduced by approximately one-third (4). Life expectancy becomes progressively longer as the age of onset of DM increases, but the *likelihood* of developing the disease also increases with age (5). For instance, 17% of people over 65 years of age, and 26% of 85-year-olds, are diabetic (6).

It has also become obvious that despite the discovery of insulin, diet remains the cornerstone of management of this disease. For instance, more than 50% of adult-onset (Type II) diabetics can totally eliminate the need to take insulin or oral medication if they achieve normal ("ideal") body weight (7). Even if ideal body weight is already achieved and the type II diabetic still requires antidiabetic medication (an unusual situation), appropriate diet can still be extremely important. Diet is also important for type I diabetics. For example, Anderson and Ward (8) showed that 11 of 20 lean insulin-requiring (type I) diabetic men were able to discontinue insulin injections after beginning a high-carbohydrate, high-fiber (HCF) diet. Despite discontinuation of insulin, blood glucose levels decreased; an added benefit was that mean serum cholesterol values dropped from 206 to 147 mg% on this diet. Other studies have confirmed these findings. Thus, it is estimated that 2-3 million diabetics could control their disease by diet alone!

Since diet can play such a major role in diabetic control, it is important to define exactly what kind of diet is beneficial. Ideas on this issue have changed significantly over the past few decades, and some fascinating recent research calls into question our current ideas (see also Chapter 11). It must be emphasized that diabetic dietary management cannot be learned by reading a book. It is *imperative* that the diabetic who is interested in implementing the diets and concepts described in this chapter discuss them with his physician and dietitian.

It used to be argued that since DM is a disease of improper carbohydrate (CHO) metabolism, diabetics should restrict their CHO intake, to "lighten the load" on the body's metabolic machinery. This approach was widely accepted despite the lack of scientific evidence to support this practice. Over the past two decades, it has been recognized that not only is dietary CHO restriction not necessary in managing DM, but rather, that *increased* carbohydrate intake may actually be beneficial (7,9,10—see reference 10 for a recent review of the utility of high-CHO high-fiber diets in DM). This dietary approach is now fairly well accepted and has led both the American Diabetes Association and the British Diabetic Association (10-12) to recommend high-carbohydrate diets (50-60% of ingested calories versus the national average of 40%). This increase in CHO intake should be made up mostly (if not exclusively) of complex carbohydrates, and at the expense of dietary fat. The attitude toward most of the simple CHO has not changed, although as will be discussed below, some complex CHO may behave metabolically like simple CHO (and vice versa).

In addition to improving glucose tolerance, high CHO diets, by definition, reduce fat intake. It is currently believed that reducing fat (especially saturated fat) intake is healthy. Thus, especially in diabetics, who are already predisposed to atherosclerosis, increasing CHO intake and consequently decreasing fat intake, is indicated. It should be noted that high CHO diets can increase serum triglycerides in some individuals. Some physicians believe that elevated triglyceride levels (>300 mg%) increase the risk of atherosclerosis, although this is controversial (see Chapter 6). If an individual, however, already has borderline elevated serum triglycerides, it would be wise to recheck them after switching to a high CHO diet. It appears that if the high-CHO diet also contains a lot of fiber (as it often does), triglycerides are less likely to increase (8).

Dietary recommendations are useless, however, if patients, for reasons of cost, convenience, or palatability, will not follow them. This is one of the advantages of the high CHO diet. It can be prepared inexpensively and palatably, and consists of foods already widely available—cereals, fruits, vegetables, grains and legumes. Diets for the diabetic are extremely hard to follow if the rest of the family is eating a "regular" diet. In view of the advantages of the HCF diet, even for nondiabetics, many organizations are now recommending this type of diet for the general population (see Chapters 11, 12 and 13). Thus the diabetic and his family can eat the same diet, with benefit for all, and this will enhance compliance with the dietary prescription.

COMPLEX AND SIMPLE CARBOHYDRATES—DOGMA DISPROVED?

As if the upheaval in carbohydrate recommendations for diabetics wasn't enough, data have been published in the last few years which impugn the basis for differentiating complex from simple carbohydrates. The original hypothesis was that complex CHO are healthier for diabetics because they are more slowly digested to glucose than simple sugars. Due to this presumed slow digestion, glucose is more slowly absorbed from the gut, which enables the diabetic to handle it more easily. Simple sugars, on the other hand, were thought to be absorbed quickly, causing a rapid rise in blood sugar, which the diabetic system would be unable to handle.

It appears that this classical concept, though plausible, is in for some revision. The new thinking has been recently summarized (13,14). The problem, says diabetologist Jesse Roth, M.D., is that, "I believed it [the dogma described above]. Everyone believed it. But no one ever tested it" (13).

Since the new findings are more pleasant to consider than the original dogma, they have received considerable coverage both in the scientific and the popular press (15-17). Because it had been shown that ice cream caused modest increases in blood sugar in diabetics (18), many of the articles written suggested that ice cream was acceptable as part of the diabetic diet, and this led some experts to call for restraint, in the fear that open season on ice cream had been announced for diabetics (19,20).

The reason for such concern is perhaps substantiated by the opening statement of reference 14: "Would you believe that mashed potatoes may be worse than a dish of ice cream in terms of glucose control for diabetics?" The answer, in fact, obtained in short-term feeding experiments, seems to be "yes". The fact that various carbohydrates evoke different "glycemic responses" was first noted by Otto and colleagues in Germany in 1973 (21). The term glycemic response refers to the increase in blood sugar after a standard amount (often 50 g) of a carbohydrate is eaten. The notion that various carbohydrates have different glycemic responses was popularized by Crapo (22) and Jenkins (23) and their colleagues.

Glycemic response is quantified by the glycemic index (GI). The GI is defined as:

$$\frac{\text{blood glucose area of the test food}}{\text{blood glucose area of a standard food}} \times 100$$

This is graphically illustrated in Figure 7-2. The GI enables comparisons to

Figure 7-2

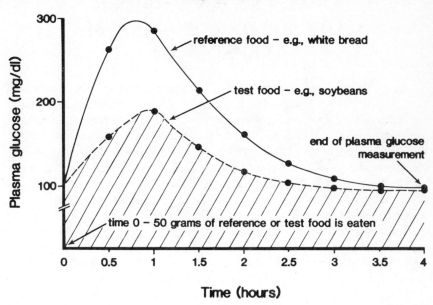

Graphic explanation of how the glycemic index is calculated

be made between different foods and between the same foods in different sub-jects and laboratories. Most studies have used 50 grams of white bread as the standard food. Table 7-1 is modified from the review article by Jenkins and colleagues (14), and summarizes GI data from various references (22-26).

A glycemic index under 100 means that the food causes less of a blood glucose rise than white bread. It is currently assumed that foods which cause less glycemia (blood sugar rise) are "better" for diabetics, and possibly for healthy individuals as well. Thus, lower GI's are presumed to be better than higher GI's. Several interesting observations can be made from Table 7-1. For instance, wholemeal wheat bread has the same GI as white bread, while ice cream has a much lower GI (=52) than a Russet baked potato (=135!). The degree of agreement between laboratories in the GI's of the same foods suggests that these findings are real. Among the monosaccharides, fructose has a much lower GI (=30) than glucose (=138), and the disaccharide sucrose (table sugar) is inter-mediate (=86). The lowest GI's in the table belong to legumes, such as baked beans, kidney beans, soybeans (having the lowest GI in the table—20), chick peas and lentils. Fruits, despite their sweetness, had surprisingly low GI's (e.g., cherries = 32 and peach = 40), except for raisins, which had a GI of 93.

Caution has been sounded, however, about overinterpretation of the glycemic index data (27). It has been noted that in the measurement of GIs, test foods have

Table 7-1

Food	Mean GI (range)	Food	Mean GI (range)
Breads:		**Legumes:**	
White	100	Baked beans	
Wholemeal		(canned)	60
(wheat)	99	Kidney beans	54
Wholegrain (rye)	58	Soybeans (dried)	22
		Soybeans (canned)	20
Cereal products:		Chick peas	49
Buckwheat	74	Green peas (dried)	56
Millet	103	Red lentils	43
Rice (brown)	96		
Rice (white)	83 (58–104)*	**Sugars:**	
Spaghetti (white)	66 (59–72)	Fructose	30
Spaghetti		Glucose	138
(wholewheat)	61	Honey	126
Corn	87	Maltose	152
		Sucrose	86
Breakfast cereals:			
All Bran	73	**Vegetables:**	
Cornflakes	119	Peas, frozen	74
Porridge oats	85 (71–96)	Potato (instant)	116
Shredded wheat	97	Potato (boiled)	81 (67–101)
		Potato (Russett,	
Fruit:		baked)	135
Apple	53	Potato (sweet)	70
Banana	79 (66–90)	Yam	74
Cherries	32		
Grapefruit	36	**Dairy products:**	
Grapes	62	Ice cream	52
Orange	66	Milk, skim	46
Peach	40	Milk, whole	49
Pear	47	Yogurt	52
Plum	34		
Raisins	93		

Glycemic indices of various foods

*Ranges are derived from several different studies. Most of above numbers were obtained in normal volunteers: some were also derived from diabetics. Modified from ref. 14.

index data (27). It has been noted that in the measurement of GIs, test foods have been given singly, which may not be relevant to ingestion of a mixed meal. In other words, the glycemic index of a mixed meal may not be at all similar to the GIs of the individual foods in the meal. Furthermore, the effect of ingesting a food once (as while measuring the GI) may be very different from the effects of chronic ingestion. Finally, other nutritional aspects of foodstuffs must be evaluated in addition to the GI. For instance, while ice cream may not have an adverse glycemic index, it is very high in calories and saturated fat, both of which are bad the diabetic (and nondiabetic, for that matter).

Several recent papers (28-30) have confirmed and extended the initial findings of Crapo and Jenkins and their colleagues. Bantle and his colleagues (28) measured the effects of 5 carbohydrates as components of a mixed meal, rather than singly. They confirmed that in normal subjects as well as in type I and II diabetics, fructose caused the smallest increments in plasma glucose level, and that sucrose, potato, wheat, and glucose produced similar increments in plasma glucose. Slama and his colleagues (29) also studied mixed meals, comparing the effects of rice versus sucrose in type I and II diabetics. There was no difference in plasma glucose curves. Finally, although it had been shown that fructose had a low GI in single-meal experiments (31), none of these carbohydrates had been studied chronically until Crapo and Kolterman showed that in *normal* subjects, the low glycemic index of fructose was maintained during a two-week feeding period (30). It will be interesting to see if similar results will be obtained with chronic feeding studies (although 2 weeks is hardly chronic) of other carbohydrates in *diabetics*.

These few studies suggest that single-meal experiments may be correlated with longer-term effects of these foods. Obviously, more experiments will have to be performed before this can be said with certainty. This is especially true in view of the fact that small groups of subjects have been studied. These and other comments were raised in some editorials and letters to the editor (32-34).

Why various carbohydrates induce such different glycemic responses is unclear at the present time. Says Jenkins, "We never cease to be amazed. We are unable to predict and we are still trying to explain what we find. We thought we would find most of the foods not too dissimilar. We expected some differences, but not massive differences" (13).

To complicate matters, it appears that the form (cooked or raw) and texture and consistency (coarse or fine) of a substance influences the GI (35). For instance, a rice slurry has a higher GI than rice grains. It is postulated that the temperature and method of preparation of a food may also affect the glycemic index. It has been suggested that differences in the polyphenol content (36) or type of bond (37) in various carbohydrates may account for the differences in GI. One disturbing consequence of these findings is that the time-honored concept of diabetic exchange diets, which considers similar portions of various complex carbohydrates to be interchangeable, may be due for an overhaul. For instance, a one-ounce portion of mashed potatoes has always been considered equivalent to a one-ounce serving of rice or cereal, and these have been routinely exchanged in the diabetic diet. The studies above suggest that this is inappropriate. It may also explain the pleas of diabetic patients telling their physicians that they have not been "cheating" on their diet. If their diabetic control is poor, perhaps that is because they have been overdosing on potatoes rather than cakes or candy bars!

As noted previously, these findings are preliminary, and any diabetic who is considering implementing changes in his diet on the basis of this information is advised to consult his physician and dietitian. It may be easier for diabetics who monitor their blood sugar regularly to adopt some changes along these lines, because they will be able to evaluate the glycemic effect of these foods for themselves. Those who use an insulin pump probably already have a good idea of the glycemic index of foods that they commonly eat, and probably are already used to adjusting their pre-meal insulin bolus according to the foods they plan to consume.

SUMMARY OF CURRENT DIETARY RECOMMENDATIONS FOR DIABETICS

To summarize, the following diet resembles that currently recommended by both the American and British Diabetic Associations (10,11). Such a dietary prescription is aimed simultaneously at improving day-to-day diabetic control, decreasing the need for hypoglycemic drugs (whether oral drugs or insulin) and reducing the risk of longterm diabetic complications:

1) Energy intake should equal energy expenditure; if overweight, reduce calorie intake and/or increase exercise until ideal body weight is achieved.

2) Exclude from the diet, as much as possible, simple carbohydrates, except in the treatment of hypoglycemic reactions. As more information is obtained, this recommendation may change to selectively allow some sugars such as fructose.

3) Obtain 50-60% of calories (some recommend even more) from complex carbohydrates, especially legumes and other fiber-rich carbohydrates, realizing that recent research suggests that not all complex carbohydrates are beneficial to blood glucose (e.g., potato). High carbohydrate intake will reduce fat intake to 20-30% of total calories, keeping protein intake at 15% of total calories. Several studies (discussed in Chapter 11) have shown that diabetic control is improved with a high-carbohydrate, high-fiber diet.

4) The decrease in fat intake should come primarily from the saturated fat component.

5) Keep in mind that the exchange system, though still useful, may have to be somewhat modified in view of the research discussed above.

6) Discourage high salt intake.

7) Moderate use of artificial sweeteners facilitates compliance with the dietary prescription. This topic is discussed in a later section of this chapter.

HYPOGLYCEMIA

Hypoglycemia, as noted earlier in this chapter, means low blood sugar. There are two major types of hypoglycemia—postprandial (occurring after eating) and fasting (occurring more than 5 hours after last caloric intake). When the lay press refers to hypoglycemia, it invariably refers to the first type, also known as reactive hypoglycemia (RH). The second type, fasting hypoglycemia, is rare but important because it often suggests a serious underlying medical disorder (38), and should be promptly evaluated by a physician. Therefore, fasting hypoglycemia will not be further discussed herein.

Although much has been written about RH in the lay literature, few physicians and other health professionals, and even fewer patients, are even remotely aware of the scientific literature dealing with the topic. Several recent review articles should be consulted by the interested reader for further detail (39-41).

The accurate definition of RH has several components:

1) The patient must have episodes of a *documented low blood sugar* which are accompanied by

2) Symptoms and signs which include sweating, shaking, palpitations (heart

pounding in the chest), piloerection (goose pimples), lightheadedness, confusion, and mental obtundation (slowness).

3) Symptoms usually occur 2-3 hours after eating, more commonly (but not necessarily) after eating simple carbohydrates.

4) Symptoms are usually short-lived (they last less than an hour or two), and go away by themselves even if nothing is done.

5) Symptoms improve with food ingestion.

6) Symptoms *do not* occur when blood sugar is normal—because the individual cannot have reactive hypoglycemia without the *hypoglycemia*.

7) The person is otherwise healthy (not diabetic, no bowel surgery, etc.)

This list of diagnostic criteria specifically excludes symptoms like lethargy and chronic fatigue or depression, since, contrary to popular belief, these are not due to RH. RH is an episodic, not a chronic, phenomenon. Symptoms are very rarely noted less than an hour after eating, because blood sugar has not had a chance to fall. We have yet to define what constitutes a "low blood sugar". This used to be arbitrarily defined (and still is by some) as a blood glucose <50-55 mg%. However, Fariss (42) tested blood sugar in 4928 healthy young men (army inductees)two hours after giving them 100 grams of glucose, as simulation of a meal. He found that one-quarter (24.4%) of the men had a plasma glucose under 60 mg% 2 hours after the glucose load. Had he also measured plasma glucose level 3 hours after the sugar load, he would have found more individuals with low blood sugar. Since these were healthy individuals without symptoms of RH, the obvious conclusion is that many normal people have blood sugar levels in a range that is often arbitrarily considered "hypoglycemic".

The question then arises as to how low plasma glucose must fall to be considered truly abnormal. One could consider the widely accepted statistical definition of abnormality—values which are below two standard deviations below the mean. Merrimee and Tyson (43) measured plasma glucose every 12 hours in 12 men and 12 women who fasted for 72 hours. Although plasma glucose values obtained during fasting may not be entirely relevant to the diagnosis of RH, the findings in this study were interesting. When all the subjects' lowest glucose values during the fast were averaged, the men had an average low of 66.4 mg% and the women 47.8 mg%. At no time while fasting did any male subject have a plasma glucose <50 mg%, whereas over half the female subjects had such values. A value of 55 mg% for men and 35 mg% for women denoted 2 standard deviations below the mean in these normal subjects.

In view of the limitation of this study (fasting rather than postprandial measurements), Lev-Ran and Anderson (40) compared glucose tolerance tests (GTT's) in 650 people with normal carbohydrate metabolism with GTT's in 118 individuals with suspected RH. The lowest glucose values (nadirs) after the sugar load in the normal subjects averaged 64.8 mg%. Five percent of these normal subjects had nadirs below 43 mg% and 2.5% (the statistically "abnormal" group) had values below 39 mg%! None of these subjects experienced any untoward symptoms during the tests. The subjects in the bottom 2.5% tended to be women under age 30.

Individuals with suspected RH underwent identical GTT's. Many of these patients were well read in the lay literature and cited publications in support of their belief that they had RH. Despite this, only 16 of the 118 individuals had symptoms typical of hypoglycemia that *coincided* with nadirs of plasma glucose. Nadirs in these 16 patients ranged from 33 to 48 mg%. The remaining 102 subjects included some who had no complaints during the GTT and others with multiple complaints that didn't correlate with low plasma glucose. Their mean nadir was 61.3 mg%. This mean and range of nadirs in the suspected hypoglycemia group were not different from those in the normal group.

Sixteen of the 118 suspected hypoglycemia patients underwent placebo GTT in addition to the regular GTT. The placebo was a sugarless diet drink which was indistinguishable from the drink used in the actual GTT. Since it contained no sugar, the placebo drink should not have caused any symptoms even in a person with real RH. Two of these 16 patients had symptoms which coincided with blood glucose nadirs during the real GTT, but no problems during the placebo test. These two patients, therefore, had real RH. On follow-up of one and two years, both were relieved of their symptoms on a diet free of concentrated simple carbohydrates. The other 14 who underwent the placebo as well as the real GTT did not have RH—they had symptoms regardless of whether placebo or sugar-containing GTT drinks had been administered. Not surprisingly, all these patients had tried various diets without lasting benefit.

Overall, of the 118 patients who believed they had true RH, the authors were able to document the condition in only 5 individuals. This suggests that most individuals who have been diagnosed as having RH do not.

Lest the medical reader become complacent about our understanding of RH, Lev-Ran and Anderson described a rather unusual patient. This gentleman suffered from arthritis of the hip, which was worse after a meal rich in sugar. During GTT, he recorded hip pain when his plasma glucose reached a nadir of 44 mg%. A low carbohydrate diet reduced his hip pain significantly during the 18 months that he was followed up.

As mentioned previously, women normally have significantly lower plasma glucose levels than men. It therefore appears that gender must be considered in evaluating a patient for the diagnosis of RH. Age and weight may also influence plasma glucose level following GTT (44). In this study (44), younger and heavier women had a greater tendency toward low blood sugar than older and lighter women. Incidence of low blood sugar (<59 mg%) was 31% in the younger overweight women compared to 2% in the older nonoverweight group. This does not, however, mean that 31% of younger overweight women in this study had

RH. Many of these women did not have symptoms accompanying their low blood sugar.

Two factors which are thought to influence the level of plasma glucose at which symptoms are noted are the previous blood sugar level and the rapidity of its fall. For instance, a diabetic who has a postprandial plasma glucose level of 250 mg% may experience hypoglycemic symptoms if the level drops rapidly to 60 mg%, whereas an equally rapid drop from 80 to even 50 mg% may not evoke symptoms.

In view of the foregoing discussion, it should be obvious that a diagnosis of RH is not easily made. It is a tribute to the impressive chemical machinery of the human body that true RH is as rare as it is. The fact, however, that the disease is uncommon and that the diagnosis made with difficulty is not a reason for over-diagnosing it.

The reader may wonder, "If RH is not the cause of the symptoms which are commonly attributed to it, what *is* responsible for those symptoms?" Although the answer to this question isn't clear, one recent study has shed light on this question (41). In this study, 192 patients underwent GTT for evaluation of suspected RH. Eighty-six of these patients also took the Minnesota Multiphasic Personality Inventory (MMPI), a psychologic test. The MMPI scores of the suspected RH patients were significantly different ($p < 0.01$) from those of controls. The psychologic pattern found in the suspected RH patients indicated physical expression of emotional problems (the psychologic term is conversion reaction).

This is not to imply that these individuals are crazy or are imagining the symptoms which they describe. Rather, this study simply suggests that the human brain is very powerful and inadequately understood by physicians, and that certain psychologic or situational problems may manifest themselves through somatic complaints. Many of the complaints which have been attributed to RH, including lethargy, headache, anxiety, depression and insomnia, are ubiquitous and do not really require specific explanation. Using a medical-sounding label to account for these symptoms legitimizes their presence, and in a sense, "takes the load" off the patient. However, attaching the hypoglycemia label precludes facing the real reason for the depression, lethargy, headache, or whatever, and that is why misdiagnosing these complaints as hypoglycemia is unfortunate.

These concepts were the subject of an editorial and an opinion paper in the New England Journal of Medicine (45,46). These authors described the way their patients learned about hypoglycemia—from friends, relatives, TV, and magazine articles. They noted that the diagnosis of hypoglycemia has its advantages—it is socially acceptable (indeed, almost "chic"), the patient feels better just by identifying the "problem", and such identification suggests simple dietary modifications which will "cure" the problem. Health professionals also deserve part of the blame for either inappropriately suggesting the diagnosis without adequate evaluation or facilitating its erroneous application. This gets them "off the hook", seemingly absolving them from the responsibility to properly investigate either the organic, or more likely, the psychosocial factors responsible for the symptoms.

Frequently, depression is responsible for symptoms which are erroneously diagnosed as RH. Health professionals who diagnose RH in these circumstances may rationalize, "What's the harm in perpetuating a little myth? After all, we aren't giving unnecessary medications or recommending surgery". As pointed out above, such misdiagnosis *is* harmful, by precluding proper evaluation of the real reasons for the "hypoglycemic" symptoms. Some patients will not accept the doctor's opinion of "non-hypoglycemia", but with time and patience, most should be able to, thereby opening the door for evaluation of the real underlying problem.

Although it almost seems unnecessary, in view of the rarity of real RH, a brief discussion of treatment may be in order. Various recommendations have been made, ranging from strict diets totally eliminating carbohydrate to more liberal ones which suggest stepwise elimination of specific foods known to evoke the response, regardless of the nutritional composition of the presumed offending substance. The former diet is almost impossible to follow (unless you're an Eskimo), and the latter is difficult to implement (i.e., figuring out exactly what item in a 5-course dinner was responsible for the symptoms). In addition, diets which are highly restricted in carbohydrates are of necessity liberal in fat, which certainly is not healthy.

The current recommended dietary treatment of RH is to decrease and almost totally eliminate the intake of simple carbohydrates (or perhaps, those foods with high glycemic indexes?) while increasing intake of foods with low glycemic indexes, primarily certain complex carbohydrates. Such a diet was accompanied by symptomatic improvement in every one of 8 RH patients (47). Thus, this approach has both theoretical and experimental support. Although this study didn't mention it, frequent small feedings (e.g., 6 per day) are also recommended in the treatment of RH. However, due to the rarity of actual RH, it is likely that most health professionals will not have the opportunity to test these recommendations.

ASPARTAME—THE NEW ARTIFICIAL SWEETENER

"Of the three artificial sweeteners that have whet the palates of millions of Americans over the years, the one souring ingredient common to them all has been controversy." So began a recent article dealing with artificial sweeteners

(48). It is not my purpose here to re-review reams of arguments on artificial sweeteners. The interested reader is referred to the above article, and a review evaluating the safety of saccharin (49). This review article concluded: "In humans, available evidence indicates that the use of artificial sweeteners, including saccharin, is not associated with an increased risk of bladder cancer. Until there is firm evidence of its carcinogenicity in humans, saccharin should continue to be available as a food additive, and reports of adverse health effects associated with its use should be monitored".

The purpose here is to evaluate aspartame, which is the new kid on the block. Aspartame (NutraSweet) is an artificial sweetener recently approved by the FDA (50). It was approved in 1981 as a sugar substitute for dining table use, in hot beverages and cold cereals, in powdered prepared beverages, gelatins, puddings, and in chewing gum. In July, 1983, it was further approved for use in soft drinks. It has since been the target of debate, which will be briefly reviewed below.

Unlike saccharin, which is truly an artificial product (i.e., it is not normally found in nature), aspartame is a dipeptide. This means that it is composed of two naturally-occurring amino acids, L-aspartic acid and L-phenylalanine. Amino acids are the building blocks of all proteins which we eat, and indeed, aspartame is digested in the human body to these two amino acids. Although natural doesn't necessarily mean good, we are comforted to know that amounts of these amino acids which can be derived from reasonable daily intakes of aspartame are very small compared to normal protein sources of these amino acids.

Concerns which have been raised about aspartame include possible excess intake of the two amino acids. An excess of phenylalanine could be potentially harmful to individuals with phenylketonuria (PKU), and indeed, all foods which contain aspartame have a warning to this effect on the label. Some studies of aspartame in rats (e.g.,51,52) have shown increases in brain and plasma levels of various amino acids; this is not surprising since the dose used in these rat studies is the human equivalent of approximately 70 12-ounce cans of soda consumed at a single sitting! In more realistic (though still very high) dose tests in humans, aspartame had little effect on plasma amino acid and methanol concentrations in both adults (53) and infants (54,55).

Despite this, alarms continue to be sounded from various individuals, asking for a reconsideration of the approval of this sweetener. As has been pointed out, *any* substance can be harmful if the dose administered is sufficiently large. At this time, there is no data to suggest that aspartame is at all harmful if taken in reasonable amounts. It has been used in soft drinks in Canada for several years without any documented harmful effects. The Council on Scientific Affairs has concluded that "consumption of aspartame by normal humans is safe and is not associated with serious adverse health effects". Considering the potential disadvantages of the other two major sweeteners—sugars and saccharin—most individuals would probably choose aspartame. The interested reader may wish to contact the manufacturer, G.D. Searle & Co., Searle Consumer Products, Division of Searle Pharmaceuticals Inc., Box 5110, Chicago, Illinois, 60680, for further information.

The Community Nutrition Institute, a consumer advocacy group, and other consumer groups contended that the FDA approved aspartame without proper testing. The groups asked FDA to hold public hearings on the topic, but the agency refused, saying all safety issues had been adequatly addressed. The issue went to court and in a September 24, 1985 ruling, the federal appeals court upheld the FDA's position, stating that the consumer groups "failed to raise any material issues of fact requiring FDA to hold a hearing." The judges added, "The court will not substitute its judgement on highly technical matters for that of the agency charged with supervision of the industry."(57)

REFERENCES

1. Sheiham A: Sugars and dental decay. Lancet 1:282, 1983
2. Letters to editor: Sugar and dental decay. Lancet 1:598, 827, 873, 1983
3. Yetiv JZ: Recent advances in diabetes research and therapy. In: Recent Advances in Clinical Therapeutics, vol. 1. Yetiv JZ, Bianchine JR (eds.), Grune & Stratton, New York, 1981. pp. 141-73.
4. Rosenbloom AL: Long-term complications of Type I (insulin-dependent) diabetes mellitus. Ped Annals 12:665, 1983
5. Horwitz DL: Diabetes and aging. Am J Clin Nutr 36:803, 1982
6. Bennett PH: Report of work group on epidemiology. National Commission on Diabetes. Vol III, Part I. Washington, D.C. U.S. Dept. of Health, Education and Welfare, NIH publication #76-1021, pp. 65, 1976
7. Flood TM: Diet and diabetes mellitus. Hosp Pract 14:61, 1979
8. Anderson JW, Ward K: High-carbohydrate high-fiber diets for insulin-treated men with diabetes mellitus. Am J Clin Nutr 32:2312, 1979
9. Carbohydrate restriction in diabetes deemphasized. Ped News, Jan. 1983, pp. 56
10. Editorial: High carbohydrate high fibre diets for diabetes mellitus. Lancet 1:741, 1983
11. Committee of the American Diabetes Association on Food and Nutrition: Principles of nutrition and dietary recommendations for individuals with diabetes mellitus. Diabetes 28:1027, 1979
12. Nuttall FO: Dietary recommendations for individuals with diabetes mellitus. Am J Clin Nutr 33:1311, 1979
13. Kolata G: Dietary dogma disproved. Nutritionists find that some complex carbohydrates act like simple sugars and vice versa. Science 220:487, 1983
14. Jenkins DJA, et al: The glycaemic response to carbohydrate foods. Lancet 2:388, 1984
15. Byrne M: Potatoes equal to ice cream? Diabetic diet dogma shaken. Med Tribune 5/25/83, p.3
16. Jacobson AS: Nutrition and the unexpected. Med Tribune, ibid, p. 30
17. Editorial: Untitled. Ped News, 5/83, p.32

18. Nathan DM, et al: Ice cream in the diet of insulin-dependent diabetic patients. JAMA 251:2825, 1984

19. Horwitz N: Experts:'Wait and see' on new diabetic diet data. Med Trib 9/14/83, p.1

20. Letters to the editor: Utility of studies measuring glucose and insulin responses to various carbohydrate-containing foods. Am J Clin Nutr 39:163, 1984

21. Otto H, et al: Kohlenhydrataustauch nach Biologischen aquivalenten. In: Otto H, Spaether, eds. Diatetik bei Diabetes Mellitus. Berne:Verlag Hans Huber, 1973, pp.41-50

22. Crapo PA, et al: Postprandial plasma glucose and insulin responses to different complex carbohydrates. Diabetes 26:1178, 1977

23. Jenkins DJA, et al: Glycemic index of foods: a physiological basis for carbohydrate exchange. Am J Clin Nutr 34:362, 1981

24. Schauberger G, et al (Otto's group): Exchange of carbohydrates according to their effect on blood glucose. Diabetes 26:415, 1978

25. Jenkins DJA, et al: The glycemic index of foods tested in diabetic patients: a new basis of carbohydrate exchange favoring the use of legumes. Diabetologia 24:257, 1983

26. Crapo PA, et al: Comparison of serum glucose, insulin and glucagon responses to different types of complex carbohydrate in non-insulin dependent diabetic patients. Am J Clin Nutr 34:184, 1981

27. Mann JI: Blood glucose response to carbohydrate (letter). Lancet 2:811, 1984

28. Bantle JP, et al: Postprandial glucose and insulin responses to meals containing different carbohydrates in normal and diabetic subjects. N Engl J Med 309:7, 1983

29. Slama G, et al: Sucrose taken during mixed meal has no additional hyperglycaemic action over isocaloric amounts of starch in well-controlled diabetics. Lancet 2:122, 1984

30. Crapo PA, Kolterman OG: The metabolic effects of 2-week fructose feeding in normal subjects. Am J Clin Nutr 39:525, 1984

31. Crapo PA, et al: Comparison of the metabolic responses to fructose and sucrose sweetened foods. Am J Clin Nutr 36:256, 1982

32. Letters to editor: Glucose and insulin responses of diabetic patients to different carbohydrates. N Engl J Med 309:1251, 1983

33. Jenkins DJA (editorial): Dietary carbohydrates and their glycemic responses. JAMA 251:2829, 1984

34. Letters to editor: Rice or sucrose in the diabetic diet. Lancet 2:585, 1984

35. Wong S, O'Dea K: Importance of physical form rather than viscosity in determining the rate of starch hydrolysis in legumes. Am J Clin Nutr 37:66, 1983

36. Thompson LU, et al: Relationship between polyphenol intake anf blood glucose response of normal and diabetic individuals. Am J Clin Nutr 39:745, 1984

37. Goddard MS, et al: The effect of amylose content on insulin and glucose responses to ingested rice. Am J Clin Nutr 39:388, 1984

38. Santiago J, et al: Fasting hypoglycemia in adults. Arch Intern Med 142:465, 1982

39. Dargaville R: Hypoglycemia. Aust Fam Phys 11:901, 1982

40. Lev-Ran A, Anderson RW: The diagnosis of postprandial hypoglycemia. Diabetes 30:996, 1981

41. Johnson DD, et al: Reactive hypoglycemia. JAMA 243:1151, 1980

42. Fariss BL: Prevalence of post-glucose load glycosuria and hypoglycemia in a group of healthy young men. Diabetes 23:189, 1974

43. Merrimee TJ, Tyson JE: Stabilization of plasma glucose during fasting. Normal variations in two separate studies. N Engl J Med 291:1275, 1974

44. Jung Y, et al: Reactive hypoglycemia in women: Results of a health survey. Diabetes 20:428, 1971

45. Yager J, Young RT: Non-hypoglycemia is an epidemic condition. N Engl J Med 291:907, 1974

46. Cahill GF, Soeldner JS: A non-editorial on non-hypoglycemia. N Engl J Med 291:906, 1974

47. Sanders LR, et al: Refined carbohydrate as a contributing factor in reactive hypoglycemia. South Med J 75:1072, 1982

48. Lecos C: Sweetness minus calories = controversy. FDA Consumer, Feb, 1985, pp.18

49. Council on Scientific Affairs: Saccharin. Review of safety issues. JAMA 254:2622, 1985

50. Gunby P: FDA approves Aspartame as soft-drink sweetener. JAMA 250:872, 1983

51. Yokogoshi H, et al: Effects of aspartame and glucose administration on brain and plasma levels of large neutral amino acids and brain 5-hydroxyindoles. Am J Clin Nutr 40:1, 1984

52. Wurtman RJ: Neurochemical changes following high-dose aspartame with dietary carbohydrate. N Engl J Med 309:429, 1983

53. Steginik LD, et al: Plasma amino acid concentrations in normal adults fed meals with added monosodium L-glutamate and aspartame. J Nutr 113:1851, 1983

54. Steginik LD, et al: Blood methanol concentrations in one-year-old infants administered graded doses of aspartame. J Nutr 113:1600, 1983

55. Filer LJ: Effect of aspartame loading on plasma and erythrocyte free amino acid concentrations in one-year-old infants. J Nutr 113:1591, 1983

56. Council on Scientific Affairs: Aspartame. Review of safety issues. JAMA 254:400, 1985

57. Updates: Court affirms FDA's OK of aspartame. FDA Consumer, Dec. 1984-Jan. 1985, pp. 2

CHAPTER 8

Multivitamins and Megavitamins—Are They Megahealthy?

Use of nutritional supplements, especially vitamins, is widespread in the United States. The goal of this chapter is to evaluate the scientific evidence on the safety and efficacy of multivitamins and megavitamins for the various purposes for which they are taken (the reader is also referred to a two-part review article for further detail [1]). Minerals are similarly discussed in Chapter 9.

VITAMINS AND THE RDAs—A BRIEF OVERVIEW

The party line of orthodox medicine has always been that if one eats a balanced diet, the Recommended Dietary Allowance (RDA) of various nutrients is very likely to be met. The RDAs are defined by the Food and Nutrition Board, a committee of the National Academy of Sciences, as "the levels of intake of essential nutrients considered . . . on the basis of available scientific knowledge, to be adequate to meet the needs of *practically all* healthy persons" (1a). Contrary to popular belief, therefore, the RDAs are not *minimums*. There is a term which defines the real minimum amount, known as the MDR—Minimum Daily Requirement, the amount of a nutrient which must be taken to prevent true deficiency. The RDA is usually 2 to 6 times the MDR, and thus provides a respectable margin of safety. Nevertheless, it is true that the major objective of the RDAs is to define basic nutritional requirements; RDAs don't really address the potential benefits (if any) of mega-intakes of various vitamins.

The nutritional scientists who formulate the RDAs probably feel that the preponderance of the evidence must show that benefits of megadoses of a certain vitamin outweigh the risks before they can recommend such practice. This is a conservative and appropriate approach for the RDA committee, (an approach

159

Table 8-1

Vitamin	Males	Females
A (RE/IU.*)	1000/3300	800/2640
D (micrograms/IU)**	5/200	5/200
E (αTE/IU)†	10/15	8/12
Thiamine (mg)	1.4	1.0
Riboflavin (mg)	1.6	1.2
Niacin (mg)	18	13
Pyridoxine (mg)	2.2	2.0
Cobalamin (ug)	3.0	3.0
Folacin (ug)	400	400
Vitamin C (mg)	60	60

1980 RDAs

*Vitamin A is measured in retinal equivalents (RE) or international units (IU).

**Vitamin D is measured in micrograms or in international units (IU).

†Vitamin E is measured in alpha tocopherol equivalents (αTE) or in international units (IU).

Numbers given are for adult men and women. RDA's for children, and pregnant or lactating women may vary. No RDAs were established in 1980 for vitamin K, biotin or pantothenic acid.

From the Food and Nutrition Board, National Academy of Sciences, National Research Council Committee on Dietary Allowances, 1980.

discussed recently in several papers [1b-1e]). This approach is analogous to that used by the Food and Drug Administration (FDA) in approving drugs, i.e., that safety and efficacy must be proved beyond reasonable doubt before a drug is approved. A more liberal, though still a reasonable and scientific approach, will be adopted in this chapter.

The current RDAs (Table 8-1) are awaiting revision as this book goes to press (January, 1986). The new RDAs, which were due out in 1985, have been delayed for an unspecified period of time due to lack of agreement between the scientific bodies which are responsible for them. It is anticipated that several changes in these (1980) RDAs will be made, but the identity of these changes is unclear.

Only four fat-soluble (A, D, E and K) and nine water-soluble substances (B_1, B_2, B_3, B_6, B_{12}, folic acid, pantothenic acid, biotin, and C) are currently recognized as vitamins. Every day, one hears of "newly discovered vitamins" like choline, inositol, B_{15} (pangamic acid) and B_{17} (Laetrile). These substances are not recognized by medical experts as vitamins, because they fulfill neither of the criteria of definition as vitamins: (1) no dietary requirement for these compounds has been demonstrated, and (2) no deficiency disease occurs if they are absent from the diet. Laetrile has already been thoroughly discussed in Chapter 1, and some of the other compounds are discussed in other chapters of this book.

In touting these unrecognized vitamins, vitamin enthusiasts often argue that their favorite substance is actually a necessary nutrient for humans, i.e., it is an as-yet-undiscovered vitamin. One major argument which refutes this view is that many individuals have been maintained for extended periods of time by what is known as total parenteral nutrition (TPN). Individuals undergoing TPN receive all their nutrients intravenously, and may take nothing by mouth for months. They receive essential amino acids, fats, and carbohydrates, as well as all the recognized vitamins and other nutritional factors. The fact that these individuals are able to survive for months without conventional food and without the appearance of any deficiency symptoms suggests that all the important vitamins essential to life have been discovered, and can be supplied intravenously.

Table 8-2 is a summary of the salient characteristics of the 13 vitamins, including their common food sources and deficiency diseases. Due to space constraints, a more detailed discussion of vitamin basics cannot be presented here. The lay reader is referred to several popular books for this information (e.g., 2-4). For the medical or paramedical professional, the basic nutrition or physiology text accompanying his course of study would be suitable for reviewing the basics. For readers inclined to delve into the biochemistry of nutrition in more detail, Lehninger's biochemistry textbook is highly recommended (5). In addition, two recent reviews on megavitamin therapy have appeared in the scientific literature and should be consulted for further reference (6,7).

FAT-SOLUBLE VITAMINS

Vitamin A and Carotenoids

Much scientific interest and research has been directed at vitamin A and related compounds, especially at their potential in preventing carcinogenesis (development of cancer). This is attested to by the recent publication of multiple review articles on this topic (8-16).

Metabolism

Prior to discussing the clinical uses of the vitamin A family of substances, a brief review of vitamin A metabolism may be in order. Vitamin A (retinol) and its naturally-occurring relatives, retinaldehyde and retinoic acid, are members of a large class of fat-soluble compounds known as retinoids. In addition to retinol, retinaldehyde, and retinoic acid, over 1000 other retinoids have been synthesized in the laboratory. Even if no retinoids are eaten in the diet, the human body can synthesize vitamin A from another group of compounds, known as carotenoids, of which beta carotene is the most widely studied. Whereas retinoids are found only in animal-derived foodstuffs (liver, whole milk, eggs), the water-soluble

Table 8-2

Vitamin	Best food sources	Deficiency disease or symptoms	Side effects of megadoses
A	Liver, eggs, dairy products. Some vegetables contain beta-carotene which is converted to vitamin A.	Impaired growth and development. Poor vision (esp. night) and blindness. Dry skin, dry eyes.	Increased pressure inside head, liver damage. Impaired vision, skin rashes, hair loss.
D	Fortified milk, liver, cod liver oil, fatty fish. Also made in the skin upon exposure to sunlight.	Rickets (in children) osteomalacia (in adults).	High serum calcium and calcium deposits in body. Fatigue, headache, nausea, vomiting, diarrhea.
E	Vegetable and fish oils; liver; whole-grain breads and cereals.	Rarely seen in healthy people; may occur in people with malabsorption syndromes (cystic fibrosis).	See Table 8-4 for extensive list. Most of the list has been derived anecdotally so one can't put much confidence in it.
K	Green leafy vegetables; various other vegetables (peas, cauliflower) and liver. Also made in human intestine.	Bleeding problems especially in newborns.	Rarely taken in megadoses.
Thiamine (B$_1$)	Liver, pork, oysters, whole grain breads and cereals, many breakfast cereals are enriched with this (and other) B vitamins.	Beriberi, characterized by neurologic and cardiovascular problems.	None recognized presently.
Riboflavin (B$_2$)	Liver, meat, dairy products, eggs, dark green vegetables; whole grain breads and cereals.	Sore mouth, tongue and throat; cracking skin in these locations and rash of trunk and extremities; anemia; neuropathy.	None recognized presently.
Vitamin Niacin (B$_3$)	Best food sources Liver, poultry, meat, eggs, wholegrain breads and cereals, nuts and legumes (peas, beans).	Deficiency disease or symptoms Pellagra, characterized by dermatitis (rash), diarrhea, dementia (confusion, impairment of memory) and ultimately, death.	Side effects of megadoses See text for niacin side effects.
Pyridoxine (B$_6$)	Whole grain cereals and breads; liver, green vegetables, bananas, fish, poultry, meats, nuts.	Rash and oral lesions (see riboflavin), convulsions (rare).	Nerve damage (see text). Also, become dependent on megadoses—should taper off megadoses slowly.
Cobalamin (B$_{12}$)	Found only in animal foods—liver, kidneys, meat, fish, eggs, milk, nutritional yeast.	Pernicious anemia, characterized by anemia and neurologic symptoms (numbness and tingling in extremities).	None recognized presently.
C	Citrus fruits, melon, tomatoes, strawberries, potatoes, dark green vegetables.	Scurvy, characterized by bleeding gums, poor wound healing, loose teeth, poor skin, irritability.	Diarrhea, bloating, abdominal pain. Serious toxicities not recognized presently.
Folic acid	Liver, dark green vegetables, wheat germ, legumes.	Megaloblastic anemia, mouth lesions (see riboflavin), maybe increased birth defects (see text).	None presently recognized.
Biotin	Eggs, liver, dark green vegetables.	Not known in humans on natural diet.	None presently recognized.
Pantothenic acid	In all plant and animal products, especially liver, whole grain cereals and breads.	Not known in humans on natural diet.	None presently recognized.

Salient characteristics of the 13 vitamins

carotenoids are strictly obtained from plants (carrots, dark green and orange vegetables, corn, soybeans, tomatoes and palm oil).

The RDA for vitamin A can be (and usually is) met by ingesting a combination of retinoids and carotenoids. Vegetarians will obviously obtain all their vitamin A needs through carotenoids only, and this usually does not present any difficulties. The RDA for vitamin A can be obtained either from 1 mg of vitamin A or 6 mg of beta carotene, or some combination of the two. More carotene (6 mg) than retinol (1 mg) is required for the same amount of vitamin A biological activity because beta carotene is not efficiently converted to retinol in the body.

Although this discussion suggests that retinoids and carotenoids are dietarily interchangeable, there are some significant differences in their metabolism and effects in the human body. If vitamin A is ingested, either from the diet or via supplements, in amounts above the daily requirements, the excess is stored in the liver. Those stores may then be utilized when dietary intake is low. If large amounts of vitamin A are chronically ingested, liver storage capacity may be exceeded and the liver (and other organs) may be damaged. Under most circumstances, blood level of vitamin A is unaffected by intake of either retinoids or carotenoids because of the liver's ability to absorb the excess or make up for a short-term (up to several months) dietary deficiency. Thus, in most people, taking extra vitamin A *will not raise* the blood vitamin A level.

The metabolism of beta carotene is quite different from that of vitamin A. Beta carotene is not stored in the liver, and after ingestion, is absorbed directly into the bloodstream. This means that blood level of beta carotene *is directly related* to the amount of carotene in the diet. As a matter of fact, a large intake of beta carotene can lead to a condition known as carotenemia, in which the high circulating levels of carotene lead to a yellowish-orange coloration of the skin. Canthaxanthin, a carotenoid related to beta carotene, works by the same mechanism and is the active ingredient in "tanning pills" (see Chapter 2).

Clinical Uses

Dermatology

Outside the United States, vitamin A deficiency is a very serious problem (16a). Vitamin A is required for proper vision, growth, reproduction, and normal skin. Retinoids have also been used as drugs for various medical conditions. It is in the field of dermatology that retinoids have found their greatest utility so far. Since therapeutic doses of vitamin A cause unacceptable side effects, great efforts have been directed at synthesizing vitamin A analogues with greater beneficial activity and less toxicity. One such drug, 13-cis retinoic acid (Accutane), was approved by the FDA in late 1982, and has revolutionized the treatment of *severe* acne. Another retinoid, etretinate, has been found to be effective in many cases of psoriasis (8). Retinoids have also been used in other (some quite rare) skin diseases, including Darier's disease, palmo-plantar keratoderma and pityriasis rubra pilaris. Since most retinoids studied to date (including the FDA-approved Accutane) have serious side effects, researchers continue to look for equally (or more) effective but less toxic retinoids.

Prevention of carcinogenesis

Perhaps the most exciting effect of retinoids and carotenoids is their potential to block the process of carcinogenesis (10-16). It was noted 60 years ago that vitamin A deficiency led to development of precancerous skin lesions (17), and that its administration prevented this (18-21). For instance, of 46 vitamin A-supplemented hamsters exposed to the carcinogen, benzpyrene, only 2 developed tumors, while 24 of 53 control (unsupplemented) animals developed the tumors (21). Another example: Filipino betel nut and tobacco chewers who were supplemented for 3 months with both vitamin A (100,000 IU/wk) and carotene (300,000 IU/wk) had a lower percentage of precancerous cells in their cheeks (1.4%) than unsupplemented controls (4.8%). Nonchewers, as might be expected, had almost no precancerous cells (22).

In addition to such animal and human experimental evidence, several epidemiological studies have demonstrated an inverse correlation between intake of vitamin A and carotene and risk of cancer, especially lung cancer (23-27b). A more recent and extensive such study, however, showed that dietary intake of beta carotene, but *not* of vitamin A itself, was inversely related to the 19-year incidence of lung cancer. The 488 men who ate the least carotene (bottom quartile in carotene consumption) developed 14 lung cancers, whereas the 488 men in the upper quartile of carotene consumption had only 2 lung cancers (28). Intake of other nutrients (e.g., protein, fat, carbohydrate, calcium, phosphorus, iron, vitamins B_1, B_2, B_3, C, D, or cholesterol) was not associated with cancer risk, and cancers other than lung cancer did not seem to be affected by carotene intake.

These results tend to support the hypothesis, proposed by Peto and colleagues (29), that dietary intake of carotene, but curiously, *not* of vitamin A, decreases the risk of developing lung cancer. The most recent such study, however, suggests that neither factor is related to carcinogenesis (30). In this study, levels of vitamins A and E, and of total carotenoids, were measured in serum obtained in 1973 from 111 participants in a hypertension study who were free of cancer in 1973 but later developed the disease. These measurements were compared to those obtained from 210 matched controls in the same study who remained free of cancer. One might expect that if blood levels of vitamins A or E, or of carotenoids, were related to carcinogenesis, that the levels would be lower in those patients who later developed cancer compared to those who remained free of the disease. In fact, this was not found to be the case. Mean values of vitamins

A and E, and total carotenoids were not different in the cancer patients vs. the controls (67.3 and 68.7 ug/dl; 1.16 and 1.26 mg/dl; 114.5 and 111.6 ug/dl, respectively). These authors concluded that the data did not support hypotheses relating intake or serum levels of vitamin A or E, or beta carotene, to a reduced cancer risk. Another recent study showed that a supplement consisting of riboflavin, zinc, and vitamin A had no effect on precancerous lesions of the esophagus in humans (30a). Finally, to complicate matters even further, it has been shown that risk of colorectal cancer was inversely correlated with dietary vitamin D and calcium intake (30b).

It is admittedly frustrating to choose between the competing hypotheses presented above, but the evidence from the studies which did show a relationship between carotene and cancer risk was felt to be sufficiently compelling to induce the organization of a study. This was a cooperative project of the National Heart Lung and Blood Institute/National Cancer Institute/Harvard, which asked 140,000 male physicians aged 40-75 to take one aspirin (325 mg, for its potential against heart attacks) and one beta carotene capsule (30 mg—5 times the RDA), or similar placebos, daily. As of January, 1983, 27,000 physicians had volunteered for the study (31), and it is hoped that this intervention study will help resolve the question as to whether beta carotene supplementation can decrease the risk of developing cancer.

Side Effects

The reader may wonder whether self-treatment with vitamin A or beta-carotene may be indicated prior to resolution of the above controversy. In order to intelligently address this question, one must look not only at the benefits but also at the potential toxicity of these compounds. It is known that both synthetic retinoids (like 13-cis retinoic acid) and natural vitamin A have significant dose-dependent adverse effects, including skeletal problems (32), birth defects (33-33b), and increased lipid levels (33c). The benefits and side effects of this drug have been recently reviewed (33d). Since 13-cis retinoic acid is used in only certain severe clinical circumstances and under careful medical supervision with informed consent of the potential side effects, these side effects may be acceptable.

Vitamin A supplements, on the other hand, are rarely taken with medical supervision, and even doses only a few times greater than the RDA can be toxic. Toxic effects include liver damage, weakness, increased pressure in the brain, bone and joint pain and damage, and dry, rough skin. It should be noted that vitamin A toxicity can also occur secondary to excessive dietary (not only supplemental) intake of vitamin A. For instance, 5 patients with pseudotumor cerebri were discovered to be eating beef liver several times per week (33e). Two patients disclosed that they routinely bought *6 to 24 pounds* of liver each week!

Pseudotumor cerebri is a condition characterized by high pressure inside the brain, accompanied by headache and papilledema (pressure behind the eye). Although usually not a life-threatening condition, its symptoms can be easily mistaken for those of a brain tumor. Excessive liver intake can cause this because of the high vitamin A content of liver.

Several cases of toxicity with the common "low-dose" vitamin A supplement of 25,000-50,000 IU have been published (34,35), and correspondents have recently suggested that excessive vitamin A may also cause gout (36) and anemia (37). It has also been shown that concurrent alcohol intake can enhance the toxicity of vitamin A supplements (38).

The current scientific consensus on beta carotene is that it, unlike vitamin A, is safe, even in megadoses of several hundred times the RDA of 5 mg (39). There is a recent report, however, that suggests that excessive beta carotene may cause amenorrhea (cessation of menstrual periods) (40). It was reported that 10 vegetarian women who had carotenemia became amenorrheic. In these cases, it was felt that carotenemia was due to excessive dietary intake of carotene, rather than to ingestion of carotene supplements. The patients were encouraged to reduce their dietary intake of carotene. Eight of the ten women were successful in modifying their diet, and resumed menstruation. One of these succeeded temporarily and had several periods; eventually, however, she reverted to her previous diet and amenorrhea recurred. Obviously, this is not a controlled study and is offerred here with the hope that it may alert physicians and patients to look for this potential effect (or even to encourage someone to carry out a controlled trial).

Recommendations

In view of the foregoing evidence, the best approach may be to increase dietary carotene intake. This is preferred to taking a pill supplement because the anti-cancer effect of eating carotene-containing vegetables (if it is real) may be due to some other substance in these food items. Indeed, this concept may apply to other nutrients, and thus it is often recommended to eat the original foodstuff rather than take a purified supplement. In addition, dietary sources of carotene—mostly vegetables and fruits—are recommended anyway for other reasons, such as low calories, low fat, and high nutrients and fiber.

If a supplement is taken, beta carotene is preferable to vitamin A, for two reasons. First, much evidence suggests that beta carotene intake may affect cancer risk more than vitamin A intake. Secondly, beta carotene, at this time, appears to be much safer to take than vitamin A, which even in what is considered a "low dose" (e.g., 25,000 IU/day), can be potentially toxic. A 30 mg beta carotene supplement daily, preferably under medical supervision, might be considered reasonable and would conform with the Harvard physician study described above. In view of the report of amenorrhea, women trying to become pregnant might be unwise to take carotene supplements. Finally, if carotene truly has an anticancer effect, individuals over 50 years of age may benefit more from supplements than younger persons, because the potential benefit at that age would be greater, since cancer is usually more common the older one becomes.

Vitamin D

Vitamin D is rarely the object of attention of megavitamin enthusiasts, and will therefore not be discussed herein. This is not meant to imply that vitamin D is unimportant, because both excess and deficiency of this fat-soluble vitamin can impair health.

Vitamin E

Vitamin E, like vitamins A and C, has been the object of considerable attention in both the lay and scientific press. Indeed, a conference dealing exclusively with vitamin E was recently held and a book on the conference published (41). The interested reader may consult the conference book (41) or another book (42) or review articles (43,44) on vitamin E. The role of vitamin E in many disorders, discussed at the conference, is listed in Table 8-3.

Metabolism

Vitamin E is a member of a family of fat-soluble compounds called tocopherols. It is widely distributed in foods, especially vegetable (corn, cottonseed, safflower and soybean) oils; therefore, deficiency in normal individuals is almost unheard of. On the other hand, individuals with malabsorption syndromes, such as cystic fibrosis, biliary atresia and abetalipoproteinemia, often have severe vitamin E deficiency. Once absorbed into the blood from the GI tract, vitamin E is distributed among the lipoproteins (mostly in LDL). Vitamin E is not stored in any specific organ but the body's supply is distributed in the adipose tissue, liver and muscle. There is a correlation between vitamin E intake and its blood level, although it is not a direct correlation. To double the blood level, the intake must be increased approximately 10-fold, and there seems to be no further increase in blood level at intakes above 2000 IU/day (approximately 150 times the RDA!).

Clinical Uses

Even a brief discussion of all the disorders in which vitamin E is said to be therapeutic is beyond the scope of this book. Therefore, I have selected for

Table 8-3

Neuromuscular diseases
Lung disease
Intraventricular hemorrhage
Retrolental fibroplasia
Neurologic problems in patients with abetalipoproteinemia
Cataracts
Hyperlipidemia
Daunorubicin–induced mammary tumors
Liver damage
Hemolytic anemia
Pancreatitis
Protection against certain drugs and air pollution, cigarette smoking
Shock lung
Adriamycin toxicity
Antioxidant—treat free radicals

Disorders in which vitamin E supplementation has been proposed to be beneficial
From ref. 41.

evaluation only a few of the more common medical and popular uses of vitamin E which have been scientifically evaluated.

Retrolental fibroplasia (RLF)

Hittner and colleagues (45) showed that routine vitamin E administration to preterm infants significantly decreased the incidence of RLF. RLF is a disorder of the eyes which usually affects premature infants who are exposed to high concentrations of oxygen. Severe RLF can cause blindness. Dr. Hittner summarized the data (46) for her study and three other double-blind studies (47-49). These four studies included a total of 467 infants weighing less than 1500 gm; blindness due to RLF developed in 13 of 236 (5.5%) control patients but in only 3 of 231 (1.3%) of the vitamin E-treated neonates (p<0.003 for Dr. Hittner's cases). Thus, treatment with vitamin E led to approximately a 75% reduction in the incidence of RLF. No serious side effects were observed in the vitamin-treated patients, but caution was sounded (50) that the same mistake that was made in the 1950s, namely, assuming that oxygen therapy is innocuous, not be made again.

Apropos to this caution, data were recently presented (51) showing that vitamin E may cause necrotizing enterocolitis (NEC), a life-threatening disorder of neonates. The risk of developing NEC seems to increase as the dose of vitamin

E increases. For instance, the disorder developed in 30 percent of infants with vitamin E levels above 3.5 mg% as compared to only 4 percent of infants with levels below 3.5 mg% (51). It is also noteworthy that although vitamin E supplements work equally well whether given by mouth or by intramuscular injection (52), risk of NEC may be higher when vitamin E is given orally. This may be due to the hyperosmolarity of the commercial vitamin E preparation (53). This author (53) therefore suggests diluting the commercial preparation prior to oral administration. In addition, blood levels of vitamin E between 2-3 mg% may protect against RLF without incurring serious risks of NEC.

More recently, at least 38 deaths and 40 cases of serious effects were reported to occur in preemies who had received the intravenous vitamin E preparation E-Ferol (53a), and this product has since been withdrawn from the market. Affected infants had a tendency toward lower weight and higher vitamin E dose than the unaffected infants. In view of the above, it has been recommended that vitamin E be given judiciously to all infants under 1250 gm who require supplemental oxygen therapy (54).

Intraventricular hemorrhage (IVH)

IVH (bleeding inside the head) is another complication which affects premature infants; like retrolental fibroplasia, IVH may respond to vitamin E supplementation. This was initially suggested in 1982 (55) and a recent controlled trial supported this use of vitamin E (56): in premature infants under 32 weeks gestation, the incidence of IVH was lower in vitamin E-supplemented babies (18.8%) than in control babies (56.3%).

Bronchopulmonary dysplasia (BPD)

BPD refers to lung damage that occurs in premature infants who require supplemental oxygen and assisted respiration. BPD is a third complication of "preemies" which has been proposed, on the basis of an uncontrolled trial, to respond to vitamin E (57). Interestingly, the same authors were unable to confirm this finding in a follow-up randomized study (58). These authors attributed this to other differences in the studies. Thus, this use of vitamin E, like many others described in this chapter, remains undocumented.

Platelet aggregation

Vitamin E added to a test tube containing blood platelets (cells important in the clotting mechanism) inhibited their aggregation (59). In this same study, it was noted that when increasing amounts of vitamin E were given to 5 healthy volunteers, blood vitamin E levels increased until the daily dose reached 1800 IU/day (120 times the RDA!), and then the blood concentration leveled off. The blood vitamin E concentration achieved with this dose may be sufficient to cause a 40-50% reduction in platelet aggregation. In two vitamin E-deficient children who demonstrated a tendency to platelet aggregation, vitamin E therapy normalized platelet aggregation (60).

Since it has been hypothesized that hyperaggregable platelets may play a role in atherosclerosis and heart disease, taking megadose vitamin E has been advised by many vitamin enthusiasts. Such enthusiasm may be unwarranted. One clinical study of 5 patients who recently had a heart attack showed that vitamin E supplementation (1000 IU/day) had no effect on platelet aggregation (61). Although such a small study doesn't exclude the validity of vitamin E use in this setting, there's little evidence in support of such use at the present time. It has also been suggested that vitamin E may exert its anti-clotting effects (if any) by interfering with vitamin K production rather than by its effects on platelets (62). At the present time, and in view of the contradictory evidence, it is impossible to recommend vitamin E intake in the hope of decreasing platelet aggregation.

Peripheral vascular disease and intermittent claudication

Peripheral vascular disease refers to blockage of arteries, which leads to decreased blood flow and pain in the involved extremity. This pain comes with even minimal exertion and is known as intermittent claudication. Peripheral vascular disease is usually due to atherosclerosis, and is very common in the United States. This underscores the importance of the comment made by a recent reviewer "studies have provided more support for megadoses of vitamin E in the treatment of peripheral vascular occlusive disease than in any other therapeutic context" (ref.7, p.42). Although there might be some argument on this, it does suggest that vitamin E may be useful in this setting.

A placebo-controlled trial compared vitamin E, vasodilators (drugs which dilate arteries, to increase blood flow), and anticoagulants ("blood thinners"), in patients with claudication (63,64). Vitamin E was most effective, while the vasodilators and anticoagulants were no more effective than placebo. Fifty-four percent of the vitamin E-treated group were able to walk 1 kilometer without pain compared to 23% of the other groups. Blood flow improved with vitamin E therapy; within 2 years, arterial flow increased by one-third in 29/32 vitamin-treated patients, while the other patients actually had a slight further reduction in blood flow. It should be noted that these improvements were observed only after 4 to 6 months of vitamin E supplementation. Though encouraging, these findings bear replication. Until such time, persons with claudication may benefit from vitamin E supplementation, under medical supervision.

Thrombophlebitis

Thrombophlebitis refers to blood clot formation in, and inflammation of veins, usually in the legs. Studies investigating the efficacy of megadose vitamin

E in preventing thrombophlebitis are mixed. A recent analysis of six studies suggested that vitamin E decreases the incidence of peripheral venous thrombosis, and nonfatal as well as fatal pulmonary embolism (65). There are difficulties, however, in interpreting data pooled from several studies, and a controlled trial is needed before such therapy could be scientifically recommended.

Lipoproteins and coronary heart disease

The role of vitamin E therapy in heart disease is very controversial, primarily as a result of the extravagant claims that were made by two physicians, Drs. Wilfrid and Evan Shute in their popular book, *"Vitamin E for Ailing and Healthy Hearts"*. Most of the claims made in the book have been investigated and remain unproven. Nevertheless, some positive data have emerged and are discussed below.

The original cardiovascular claim for vitamin E, made in 1948, was that this vitamin could control the chest pain (angina) often experienced by individuals with atherosclerosis in the arteries which supply blood to the heart (66). Numerous, mostly uncontrolled, trials have investigated this, with contradictory results. At least one double-blind trial showed vitamin E to be of no benefit in angina (67), and two recent reviews (63,68) have concluded similarly.

Another purported cardiac benefit of vitamin E is that it can raise HDL-cholesterol levels in individuals at high risk for coronary disease (69). When another investigator was unable to confirm these results (70), the original author replied (71) that he also had been unable to replicate his own original findings, and speculated that age and sex differences in the groups studied may have been responsible, an interpretation supported by another study (72). However, although vitamin E deficiency may be associated with lipoprotein abnormalities (73), two more recent studies have again failed to show any effect of vitamin E on any serum lipoprotein level, including HDL (74,75). In view of the above, therefore, it is fair to conclude that "at this time, there is no proved scientific basis for the utilization of megadoses of vitamin E in the management of ischemic heart disease or other cardiac disorders" (7).

Hematologic disorders

Vitamin E supplementation appears to be useful in several uncommon genetic red and white blood cell disorders (44), including glucose-6-phosphate dehydrogenase (G6PD) deficiency, beta-thalassemia major, sickle cell anemia, and glutathione synthetase deficiency. These types of diseases would not constitute a reason for self-administration of vitamin E, since they should be under a physician's care.

Fibrocystic breast disease

The treatment of fibrocystic breast disease with vitamin E, if successful, would certainly constitute a significant use of the vitamin since this condition is very common. A double-blind study suggests that vitamin E does work in this setting (76). Dr. Robert London and his colleagues treated 26 patients with a placebo for 4 weeks, followed by 600 IU of vitamin E daily for the subsequent 8 weeks. Ten patients were good responders, 12 were fair responders, and 4 did not respond to the vitamin E therapy. Since placebo came first, followed by vitamin E, and since the natural history of fibrocystic disease is one of variable manifestations and spontaneous remissions and exacerbations, no firm conclusions can be made. A more rigorous study needs to be done in a larger group of patients.

Antioxidant

It is said that vitamin E is the oldest recognized biologic antioxidant (77). Indeed, it is hypothesized that vitamin E may ameliorate RLF, BPD, and IVH (the conditions which affect preemies) and various inherited red blood cell disorders as a result of its antioxidant properties. These conditions have in common either high local oxygen concentrations (in RLF, BPD and IVH) or the failure of endogenous antioxidant systems (in the genetic red cell abnormalities). One correspondent recently reported that 1600 IU of dl-alpha-tocopherol prevented alopecia (hair loss) in 11 of 16 patients who received doxorubicin (Adriamycin) (77a). It may be reasonable to follow this up in view of the fact that alopecia is an almost universal side effect of this anticancer drug.

In addition to the above conditions, some have hypothesized that aging might be due to unchecked oxidant (free radical) damage, and these individuals have therefore recommended megadosing with vitamin E, and other antioxidants, to extend lifespan. There is no credible scientific evidence to support this use of vitamin E in humans.

Miscellaneous

Vitamin E has been touted as useful in preventing skin problems, enhancing athletic ability and sexual potency, alleviating fatigue, and lowering blood pressure (78). A scientific discussion of these claims is impossible since no data are available. Many of these claims are supposedly logical extensions of known properties of vitamin E, and some conditions in which vitamin E has been claimed to be useful resemble vitamin E deficiency symptoms. The rationale is that, for instance, since lipid abnormalities are seen in vitamin E-deficient individuals, megadose vitamin E should cure lipid abnormalities. This is akin to saying that since anemia is often due to iron deficiency, excess iron will cure all

Table 8-4

Thrombophlebitis
Pulmonary embolism
Hypertension
Fatigue, dizziness
Gynecomastia
Vaginal bleeding
Headache
Nausea, diarrhea, intestinal cramps
Muscle weakness & myopathy
Visual complaints
Hypoglycemia
Stomatitis
Chapped lips
Urticaria (hives)
Aggravation of diabetes mellitus
Aggravation of angina pectoris
Disturbances of reproduction
Decreased rate of wound healing

Purported side effects of vitamin E megadoses
Modified from ref. 79.

types of anemia. This is obviously incorrect, because even large amounts of iron won't cure anemia which is due to sickle cell disease or vitamin B_{12} deficiency.

Side Effects

It is widely held, both among lay and medical personnel (77), that megadose vitamin E therapy is innocuous. Roberts, in a recent commentary, disputes this opinion (79). He has compiled anecdotal reports, from his own experience and from the medical literature, of side effects observed in patients taking megadoses of vitamin E. These side effects are listed in Table 8-4. Although it is likely that vitamin E therapy was only coincidental and not causative of some of these side effects, it is ironic that some conditions for which vitamin E therapy has been recommended (thrombophlebitis, hypertension, fatigue) are thought to be *caused* by vitamin E therapy. Roberts' opinion, however, is not universal among physicians. For instance, Toone found vitamin E to be helpful in angina (80) without any side effects, while Cohen reported "amazing weakness and fatigue" one week after starting to take 800 IU of vitamin E daily (81). Finally, Farrell and Bieri found neither benefits nor side effects in a group of 28 adults (82). It may be that different preparations are responsible for variations in benefits and side effects, an hypothesis supported by a recent study (83).

Recommendations

In view of the foregoing, it is fair to conclude that with the possible exception of retrolental fibroplasia and perhaps peripheral vascular disease, there is insufficient evidence at the present time to recommend megadose vitamin E therapy in any clinical conditions. Since neither RLF nor peripheral vascular disease lend themselves to self-treatment, this implies that there are no circumstances in which the current scientific evidence supports megadosing with vitamin E. This is not to say that researchers shouldn't continue to investigate vitamin E. If they do, however, it would be wise to perform controlled trials, since the vitamin E literature is littered with uncontrolled studies the results of which couldn't be replicated in controlled trials. Furthermore, although vitamin E is less toxic than the other fat-soluble vitamins, sufficient questions have been raised about its side effects that it is not scientifically prudent to recommend it with the thought that "it can't do any harm, and it might do some good". The burden of proof remains with proponents to show that potential benefits outweigh side effects.

Vitamin K

Vitamin K, important in the clotting mechanism, is rarely taken in megadoses. It will therefore not be further discussed here.

WATER-SOLUBLE VITAMINS

Nine water-soluble vitamins are recognized—eight B complex vitamins and vitamin C. Many of the B vitamins (and megavitamins in general) are recommended in the popular literature. It has been widely held that water-soluble vitamins, even in megadoses, are nontoxic. The rationale for this was that any excess vitamin would simply be excreted in the urine. This dogma has been recently shaken by the description of significant neurological damage in 7 patients who took megadoses of pyridoxine (vitamin B_6). The damage was irreversible in some of these patients. Studies which describe complications of megavitamins now appear with greater frequency in the medical literature (84,85), and a recent review article summarizes the toxicities of water-soluble vitamins (86).

In view of the fact that self-treatment with vitamins is so common, it may be perhaps somewhat surprising to realize that the nutritional status of our population, on the whole, is fairly good. For instance, a recent study of 270 free-living (not in institutions) elderly (>60 years of age) subjects showed dietary nutrient intake to be adequate with the possible exception of vitamin D and calcium (87). Average intakes of some nutrients were below the RDA, but for various reasons, this was not considered significant. Average intake of vitamin C in this population was more than twice the RDA. Despite this, several studies have shown that vitamin C is the most commonly taken vitamin supplement (88-91). Thus, there seems to be discordance between the nutrients that our population is deficient in (calcium and vitamin D) and the ones that are most frequently taken in supplements (vitamin C).

Finally, it is of some interest that while the use of vitamin supplements has traditionally been deemed unnecessary by practitioners of orthodox medicine, two studies have shown that nurses and dietitians take just as many supplements as the general population (90,91). Approximately 60% of these medical professionals took some kind of nutrient supplement. The most commonly used supplements were multivitamins, followed by vitamins C and E. This seems to be an example of medical professionals saying "do as I say, not as I do". It should be noted, however, that many of those using supplements were pregnant, lactating, or using them for specific and medically-appropriate reasons (e.g., potassium in subjects taking high blood pressure medications, or calcium in postmenopausal women). Thus, it appears that there are some very good reasons to take certain supplements, and the purpose of this chapter is to delineate and discuss those reasons.

The vitamin-supplement studies quoted above dealt with healthy non-institutionalized individuals. One study has often been quoted as showing that the population at large requires supplemental vitamin C (92); in this study, however, the 80 subjects were chronic nursing home patients, many of whom were confused and bedridden. It is not surprising therefore, that 73 of the 80 patients were vitamin deficient, and benefited from multivitamin supplementation. The findings of this study (92) may apply to the institutionalized population, but they certainly do not apply to healthy free-living individuals.

At this point, I'll briefly discuss the B-complex vitamins as a group, and then deal with each of the B complex vitamins and vitamin C individually.

B Complex

The eight B complex vitamins are grouped together because of similarities in structure and function, and because they are frequently found in the same foodstuffs. In addition, they are often taken as a "B-complex" supplement, rather than individually. Some of the B complex vitamins are also taken in megadoses separately, e.g., pyridoxine and niacin.

Articles in the popular literature often recommend that B complex supplements be taken when a person is under "stress", including during illness, convalescence, pregnancy and prior to and after surgery (78). Another popular writer extends this list of indications to include fatigue, irritability, nervousness, fear, depression and insomnia (93). To my knowledge, there are no scientific studies which support these recommendations, and as pointed out previously, water-soluble vitamins such as the B complex group can have significant and permanent side effects.

Thiamine (Vitamin B₁)

Thiamine is not often taken in megadoses. There are some rare inherited disorders in which megadoses of thiamine must be taken for survival (94), but this hardly provides the rationale for recommending megadoses to normal healthy individuals. Alcoholics are often thiamine-deficient. A recent paper showed that thiamine added to sorghum beer is well absorbed from rat small intestine (and presumably from human intestine as well) (94a). The authors concluded that fortification of beer with thiamine may prevent thiamine deficiency in beer-drinking alcoholics. There are no studies which show that megadoses of thiamine are of any benefit to healthy people. In view of that, it is not recommended that megadoses of this vitamin be taken.

Riboflavin (Vitamin B₂)

As is true of thiamine, megadoses of riboflavin are rarely recommended in the popular literature. Another similarity to thiamine is the recent description of a muscle disease which responded to large doses of riboflavin (95). There is some argument in the medical literature as to whether normal riboflavin intakes are adequate. Some authors believe not (96), while others present data that riboflavin intake in 24 healthy elderly females is adequate (97). One group has concluded that healthy young women require more than RDA amounts of riboflavin, and that aerobic exercise increases riboflavin requirements (98,99). Their recommendations for riboflavin intake of 1.9 mg for normal women and 2.2 mg for exercising women are only slightly higher than the 1980 RDA of 1.2 mg. In view of these studies, a 1 or 2 mg daily supplement of riboflavin (as in a multivitamin tablet) may be beneficial, especially if the person is dieting or eats an inadequate diet.

Niacin (Vitamin B₃)

Two forms of this vitamin exist: nicotinic acid and nicotinamide. Both the salutary actions and side effects of this vitamin depend on the form taken.

Clinical Uses

Hyperlipidemia

The most important clinical use of megadose niacin is in decreasing serum cholesterol, and consequently, the incidence of atherosclerosis (see also Chapter

6 for a further discussion of this topic). Only nicotinic acid (not nicotinamide) lowers serum cholesterol. Patients who received clofibrate and niacin after suffering a heart attack had decreased serum cholesterol and triglyceride levels and somewhat fewer reinfarctions (repeat heart attack) than controls (100). A similar study in which niacin-treated patients were followed for 5 years confirmed a decrease in serum lipids and in the mortality of the treated group (101). Similar findings have been reported in a more recent study of patients with familial hypercholesterolemia (genetic condition characterized by high serum cholesterol) (102).

Miscellaneous

Several other conditions may be potentially treatable with high doses of niacin. One is a rare genetic metabolic condition called Hartnup disease which has been reported to respond to high-dose nicotinic acid (103). Other potential uses of megadose nicotinic acid include certain cases of extreme photosensitivity (104) and reduction of intestinal fluid loss in cholera in humans (105). The case of photosensitivity occurred in a 59 year old white man who had become extremely sensitive even to 5 minutes of sunlight. He had had stomach surgery that may have contributed to niacin deficiency. No other factors were felt to be responsible for the photosensitivity. After 10 days of treatment with 100 mg of nicotinic acid twice daily, he had no reaction to 2 hours of sunlight. The author noted that three other patients with photosensitvity did not respond to nicotinic acid.

Animal studies have suggested that megadose nicotinic acid may reduce plasma loss after burns (106), and decrease the toxicity of paraquat in rats (107). These last two uses of niacin have not been investigated in humans. In addition, very large doses of niacin (from 25 to over 1000 times the RDA!) were administered in the above studies. Such doses of nicotinic acid may be associated with many bothersome and some serious side effects, and consequently, are experimental and should be taken only under medical supervision.

Side Effects

Flushing of the face, neck and chest, headache, and itching are common side effects of megadose niacin (7). More serious side effects include cardiac arrhythmias (heart rhythm abnormalities), hypotension (low blood pressure), aggravation of peptic ulcers, and liver damage.

An interesting case of niacin side effects was recently reported to the Centers for Disease Control (CDC) in Atlanta (108). On April 27, 1983, 14 of 69 persons attending a brunch had acute onset of rash, itching, and sensation of warmth after they ate pumpernickel bagels. None of 44 people who did not eat the bagels became sick. Investigation revealed that in an attempt to enrich the pumpernickel flour, a large quantity of niacin had been accidentally added. Thus, each bagel contained about 190 mg of niacin, approximately 12 times the RDA.

Pyridoxine (Vitamin B₆)

The requirement for pyridoxine, like that for niacin, can be met by ingesting several different forms of the vitamin—pyridoxine, pyridoxal, and pyridoxamine. Vitamin B_6 is popularly recommended for tingling fingers, muscle spasms, numbness in the hands, and edema (fluid accumulation). I am unaware of any scientific evidence which supports these popular uses. Indeed, someone with edema, which can often be due to heart failure, might fatally delay appropriate medical therapy by treating himself with megadose pyridoxine. There are, however, some intriguing potential medical uses for pyridoxine, although none of these have garnered a consensus from the experts.

Clinical Uses

Seizures

There is a rare form of epilepsy (convulsions) which responds only to treatment with megadose vitamin B_6 (109). This is similar to the genetic disorders described above with thiamine, riboflavin and niacin. These rare vitamin-dependent disorders are characterized by a physiologic need for megadoses of vitamins. If such doses aren't taken, various abnormalities occur. In the case of pyridoxine, seizures occur in the absence of megadoses of pyridoxine. It should be emphasized that maybe 1 out of 1000 epileptics fall in this category, and that megadose pyridoxine is of no use in other types of epilepsy.

Hyperkinesis

It has been proposed that pyridoxine supplementation may suppress the symptoms of hyperactivity (110). This study, however, included only six patients, and the effect noted was only a trend, rather than a statistically significant difference. Furthermore, other investigators have shown that megavitamins (including pyridoxine) not only don't ameliorate hyperkinesis, but actually exacerbate the condition (111). It has also been suggested that vitamin supplementation may improve mental performance, but a recent study found no such effect (112).

Oral contraceptives (OCPs)

Women taking OCPs have been shown to have biochemical characteristics suggestive of pyridoxine deficiency, although the clinical significance of this observation is unclear (113). Normal pyridoxine metabolism in OCP users may be achieved with a 5 mg supplement (RDA = 2.0 mg). Pyridoxine has also been reported to ameliorate the symptoms of premenstrual syndrome (114). In this randomized, double-blind, crossover trial, 36 women, most of whom were not taking OCPs, alternated taking 100 mg of pyridoxine with placebo. They were asked to record any changes in symptoms of premenstrual syndrome such as depression, irritability, tiredness, swollen breasts, swollen fingers and ankles, headache and stomach ache. Sixteen of the 36 noticed no difference in their symptoms during the placebo or pyridoxine periods. The other 20 women were all better during the pyridoxine trial, and worse during the placebo. No woman was better relieved of symptoms on placebo than on pyridoxine. This is strong evidence for efficacy of pyridoxine in relieving symptoms of premenstrual syndrome, and the fact that no side effects were reported is encouraging. Nevertheless, in view of recent reports of side effects in the same dosage range (500 mg/d), supplements of 100 mg daily should not be taken lightly.

Miscellaneous

Whereas the pyridoxine RDA for pregnant women is 2.6 mg, a recent randomized double-blind study suggested that pregnancy outcome was improved when total pyridoxine intake (diet plus supplements) was in the 5.5 to 7.5 mg/d range (115). This does not really qualify in the megadose range. Another study showed that individuals with sickle cell anemia have lower plasma pyridoxine levels than controls (116). Supplementation with 100 mg of pyridoxine per day normalized this. In one of the 16 patients studied, there was a reduction in the frequency and severity of sickle crises. Finally, a recent study suggests that pyridoxine function is decreased in asthmatics. Patients reported that pyridoxine supplementation (50 mg twice daily) decreased the frequency and severity of asthmatic attacks (116a). It must be noted, however, that this study involved only 7 patients and that the administration of pyridoxine was not by double-blind or placebo-controlled means.

Side Effects

The foregoing discussion has presented potential uses for megadose pyridoxine supplementation. These promising uses of pyridoxine cannot be said to be scientifically established, and more research will be required. Some had argued, however, that even though these potential applications of megadose pyridoxine weren't "proven", there was little harm in taking large amounts of this vitamin. It has now been clearly shown that this asssumption is erroneous.

Schaumburg and colleagues recently described 7 adults who had severe, and in some cases permanent, nerve damage, due to megadose vitamin B_6 (117). The daily consumption of pyridoxine ranged from 2000 to 6000 mg per day (over 2000 times the RDA!) None were taking the vitamin for any medically-sound reason, or under medical supervision. Several patients started taking pyridoxine at lower doses, and increased their intake with the thought that "more might be better". Since 500 mg pyridoxine tablets are readily available in health-food stores and by mail-order, it would be quite easy to ingest the "minimal" 2000 mg dose which caused this neurologic disorder. In a letter to the editor, Dr. Pauling argued that this study should not preclude megadosing with pyridoxine. Rather, he believes that, "From this report and the evidence quoted above we may conclude that the recommended orthomolecular range should not extend as far as 2000 mg [2 g] per day for a continued period" (118).

The inadvisability of even this dose range (even Dr. Pauling's maximal recommendation of 2000 mg per day is about 1000 times the RDA!) was made clear by an update from Drs. Berger and Schaumburg. They described a 34-year-old woman who had the typical picture of pyridoxine-induced neurologic disorder while taking "only" 500 mg of pyridoxine daily (119). Dr. Schaumburg also informs us that he has now identified a total of over 30 individuals suffering from the same pyridoxine-induced disorder. Since most of the affected individuals were taking this vitamin for unclear reasons and without medical supervision, it seems that the rationale that "it might be useful, and it can't hurt" is no longer tenable.

Cobalamin (Vitamin B_{12})

Vitamin B_{12} is not often self-administered in megadose quantities, although some physicians regularly give B_{12} shots for unspecified (and probably inappropriate) reasons. A study from the United Kingdom found that many of the physician-prescribed B_{12} shots were unnecessary (119a). Little scientific information is available about megadosing with B_{12}. There is a vitamin B_{12}-dependent syndrome (120), as there is for the other water-soluble vitamins discussed above, and various diseases and surgeries (e.g., of the stomach or small intestine) are associated with vitamin B_{12} deficiency (121,122). All of these conditions should be under a physician's care and will therefore not be further discussed herein. Finally, recent reports (e.g., 122a) suggest that mild cobalamin deficiency may be more common than previously thought, and may present without the typical hematologic (e.g., megaloblastic anemia) and clinical features.

Folic Acid

Clinical Uses

Prevention of birth defects

Ironically, although folic acid is infrequently recommended in the lay press, there is increasing evidence that folic acid supplementation may prevent neural tube defects (NTDs). NTDs are defects in the formation of the spinal column which can result in malformation of the brain or spinal cord. In one randomized double-blind trial, the effect of 4 mg of folic acid was tested in women who had previously borne a child with a neural tube defect, and thus are at greater risk of having another (123). There were no recurrences of NTD in 44 women who took the supplement compared to 6 NTD births in the 61 women who did not. One correspondent reported that periconceptional (around the time of conception) supplementation with a multivitamin decreased the incidence of cleft lip (124). Another study showed that a multivitamin supplement decreased the risk of NTD (125). Although this conclusion has been questioned by some (e.g., 126,127), a recent article in a publication which advises British physicians on drug prescription concluded, "It is reasonable to give a multivitamin to women who have previously borne a child with a neural tube defect and who are preparing to become pregnant. Supplements should be started 25 days before the planned conception and continue until the second missed period" (128).

It should be noted that the supplemental amounts of folic acid or multivitamins in these studies were in the RDA range, not megadose amounts. For instance, in one study (125), the daily supplement consisted of:

vitamin A—4000 IU	nicotinamide—15 mg
vitamin D—400 IU	ascorbic acid—40 mg
thiamin—1.5 mg	folic acid—360 ug
riboflavin—1.5 mg	ferrous sulfate (iron)—75.6 mg Fe
pyridoxine—1 mg	calcium phosphate—480 mg

Not exceeding the RDA is important since megadose amounts of some vitamins (e.g., vitamin A) are known to *cause* birth defects.

It is unclear from these studies whether it is folic acid or some other vitamin that is responsible for the beneficial effect of the supplement. It may also be that the women that benefited from the supplement may have been marginally deficient in one of the vitamins, and that this accounted for the benefit observed with the supplement. Thus, women who are very well nourished (as all pregnant women should be) may not derive benefit from a multivitamin supplement. In view of the above studies, however, I believe it would be reasonable for a woman who had had an NTD birth previously to take a multivitamin supplement prior to conception and up to the second missed period. This advice may be moot since most pregnant women in the United States are usually given a multivitamin supplement.

Neurologic conditions

Again, this use of folic acid is in the RDA, not megadose, range. The only reason for discussing this application of folic acid is that it may not be widely appreciated that folic acid deficiency may result in neurologic symptoms even in the absence of megaloblastic anemia (129,130). The neurologic disorder due to folate deficiency was indistinguishable from subacute combined degeneration of the spinal cord, an untreatable disease. Some patients were depressed, and had muscular fatigue, numbness and creeping sensations in the arms and legs with muscle cramps (the "restless legs syndrome"). Most patients responded to 5-30 mg (10-60 times the RDA) of folic acid. Since it has been classically taught that folic acid deficiency is accompanied by megaloblastic anemia, it is important to note that several of these patients had normal red cell indices (as was true of mild vitamin B_{12} deficiency, discussed above).

Miscellaneous

Cervical dysplasia is an abnormality of the cervix (usually found on Pap smear), which may precede the development of cervical cancer. It is unclear as to why cervical dysplasia develops, although sexual activity at a young age and multiple sexual partners are known to increase the risk of developing cervical dysplasia. It is also unknown why some cases of cervical dysplasia progress to cervical cancer while others change back to normal cervical state.

A recent report (131) suggests that folic acid supplementation in current users of birth control pills can arrest the cervical dysplastic process or cause it to regress. In this double-blind, placebo-controlled study, 47 women with mild to moderate dysplasia received either 10 mg of folic acid or a placebo (interestingly enough, the placebo was 10 mg of vitamin C!) daily for 3 months. This amount of folic acid represents 20 times the RDA. Mean biopsy scores (indicative of the degree of dysplasia of the cells) were significantly better in the folate-supplemented group than in the unsupplemented group. Final versus initial cytology scores were also significantly better in supplemented subjects. Although this study is encouraging, further corroboration would be helpful. In addition, it is not known whether the purported benefits of folic acid supplementation would apply to lower doses of folic acid, or to women not taking birth control pills, or would last longer than three months, etc. It is also unknown whether long-term folic acid supplementation might have any potential side effects. Thus, until further evidence becomes available, it is recommended that only women on the pill be candidates for this therapy, and that if they choose to do so, they should do so under medical supervision.

Pantothenic Acid, Biotin

Neither of these essential vitamins are commonly recommended in the popular literature. In addition, there is little research on these substances in the medical literature. In view of this, these substances will not be discussed further herein.

Vitamin C (Ascorbic Acid)

Last, but certainly not least, to be discussed in this chapter is vitamin C, probably the most popular of all vitamins. This may be due to the prestige of one of its primary proponents, double Nobel laureate Dr. Linus Pauling, or to the fact that vitamin C has been proposed to cure one of man's (and woman's, I might add) most common maladies, the cold.

Clinical Uses

The most common conditions in which vitamin C has been proposed to be therapeutic are briefly discussed below. Some popular uses of vitamin C have not even been dealt with in the scientific literature and therefore cannot be discussed.

Cancer

This popular use of vitamin C is discussed first not because it has been most rigorously documented but because if it were correct, it would represent perhaps the most convincing reason to recommend megadose vitamin C. Unfortunately, the current evidence clearly suggests that vitamin C has no role in the treatment of cancer.

Since it is widely accepted that host factors, such as a person's resistance, play a significant role in the development of cancer, and since that vitamin C may be important in immunity, it had been logically proposed that vitamin C (or lack of it) may play a role in cancer. A variety of laboratory evidence (132-134) has in fact suggested such a role for vitamin C. However, although animal and laboratory data are good leads, they are not nearly as convincing as a well-designed clinical trial.

In an attempt to satisfy critics and skeptics, Cameron and Pauling published the results of their clinical trial showing the benefit of vitamin C in terminal cancer patients (135). This trial, however, was *not prospective, randomized, double-blind, nor placebo-controlled*. The treatment group of 100 terminal cancer patients received 10 g of vitamin C daily. The control group, matched for severity and type of cancer, received nothing. The mean survival time for the vitamin C-treated patients was 210 days. This was more than 4 times longer than the control group survival of 50 days.

Others have questioned the validity of uncontrolled trials such as this one (136). To resolve this issue, Creagan and colleagues conducted a prospective randomized placebo-controlled double-blind study involving 150 patients with terminal cancer (137). One group consisting of 60 subjects received 10 g of vitamin C daily, while another group, of 63 patients, received a comparably-flavored placebo. The remaining 27 patients had decided not to participate in the gtudy (i.e., had changed their mind) after randomization. This latter group, which is essentially a non-placebo control group like the control group used in Cameron's study, proved to be rather interesting.

There was no significant difference in survival between the placebo and vitamin C group. There was only one patient in the study who was a long-term survivor—he was alive 63 weeks after entering the study (compared to average survival of 8 weeks for other patients in the study). This patient had received the placebo.

Sixty-three percent of the patients given the vitamin C, and 58% of those given the placebo claimed some improvement in symptoms during treatment (this is a fairly impressive placebo effect). Interestingly, side effects were also similar in both groups, with about 40% of patients experiencing mild nausea and vomiting. There was no excess of heartburn or other gastrointestinal symptoms in patients receiving vitamin C. Most patients, however, did not take vitamin C for a long period of time (due to death).

Of great interest is the third group of patients, who initially volunteered for the study but then changed their mind. These patients, who received neither vitamin C nor placebo had a significantly worse survival than the 123 patients who took *something* (whether vitamin C or placebo). The median survival of this group was 25 days, vs. 51 days for the rest.

In response to this study, Pauling speculated (138) that the vitamin-C-treated patients in Creagan's study did not improve because they had received chemotherapy, which "damage(s) the body's protective mechanisms, and vitamin C probably functions largely by potentiating these mechanisms". Although the scientific basis for this contention (especially in humans) is weak, Creagan's group repeated their double-blind controlled study, except that this time, *none* of the 100 patients assigned to either vitamin C or placebo had received chemotherapy, and only 4 had received radiation therapy (139). The patients in this study were all ambulatory, and overall, in very good general condition, with minimal symptoms. Despite this, vitamin C therapy showed no advantage over placebo. No patients showed objective improvement upon treatment with vitamin C. Although the patients had colorectal cancer, it seems reasonable, as was pointed out in the accompanying editorial, that "additional controlled trials in patients with other types of tumors do not appear warranted" (140).

Thus, these two carefully performed scientific studies showed no benefit of vitamin C in terminal cancer patients, although it is impossible to say what effects ascorbic acid may have on patients with precancerous lesions. Indeed, there is some recent evidence (similar to that quoted above in reference to folic acid) that a low vitamin C intake may predispose women to cervical dysplasia

(141). In this case-control study, a low daily intake (30 mg—one-half of RDA) of vitamin C was associated with a seven-fold risk of cervical dysplasia, compared to above-average vitamin C intake. This association was independent of income, age of first intercourse, and number of sexual partners. Beta carotene (not only vitamin C) intake was also lower in patients who developed cervical dysplasia.

The mean vitamin C intake for the women who had cervical dysplasia was 80 mg, while that for the controls was 107 mg. Although this difference is statistically significant, it is hard to believe that such a small difference could be biologically significant. This may suggest that this finding is coincidental and unrelated to the development of dysplasia. Even if this finding is genuine, it would not be supportive of *megavitamin* therapy since 107 mg is not even twice the RDA of vitamin C. If this finding is confirmed, it might argue for an increase in the RDA.

Infections

The cure of infections, especially the common cold, is probably the best advertised and promoted use of vitamin C today. In fact, Dr. Pauling wrote a book on this topic (142). Many of the published studies which have supported the benefit of vitamin C for the cold, however, have suffered from the same faults— such as lack of controls—as the Cameron and Pauling terminal cancer study described above. In a careful review of this subject (143), Chalmers examined 14 clinical trials of ascorbic acid. He found that only 8 of these 14 studies were scientifically sound enough to be analyzable. These studies suggested that vitamin C led to a slight and insignificant difference in the number and duration of colds. In most studies, the severity of symptoms was significantly worse in the placebo group. In one of these studies, however, many of the patients had tasted their capsules and correctly guessed what group they were in. All differences in severity and duration were eliminated by analyzing only the data from those who did not know which drug they were taking. Chalmers concluded:

> "Since there are no data on the long-term toxicity of ascorbic acid when given in doses of 1 g or more per day, it is concluded that the minor benefits of questionable validity are not worth the potential risk, no matter how small that might be".

The interested reader is strongly encouraged to review this study and pursue the references therein.

Vitamin C has also been used in other infectious diseases, e.g., labial herpes ("cold sores")(144) and even rabies (145). These are, however, isolated reports that obviously cannot establish cause-and-effect relationship, and to my knowledge, no controlled studies of vitamin C in other infectious diseases have been carried out. Until such time, the use of megadose vitamin C in the treatment of any infection appears unwarranted.

Cholesterol and atherosclerosis

It was originally reported in 1950 that large doses of vitamin C could retard atherogenesis in cholesterol-supplemented rabbits. Since then, this topic has remained controversial and unresolved, with evidence supporting both sides of the argument. This has been recently well-reviewed (146).

As this review pointed out, it is clear that vitamin C supplements have no effect on cholesterol levels in normocholesterolemic healthy individuals. In hypercholesterolemic individuals, however, the results are more mixed. Whereas Peterson and colleagues (147) found no effects, Ginter (148) reported significant reductions when hypercholesterolemic patients were given 1 g per day for 12 months. It has been proposed that some patients respond because they are marginally vitamin-C-deficient. The fact that relatively "low" doses (such as 1 g per day) have significantly lowered serum cholesterol would support this interpretation. Alternatively, some have suggested that vitamin C controls the breakdown of cholesterol to bile acids in the liver (149). The latter study, however, compared deficient to normal animals, and therefore would not truly bear on the question of whether vitamin C supplementation of *normal*, not deficient, individuals, has any effect on cholesterol.

In conclusion, it is truly difficult to say whether vitamin C has a significant effect on serum cholesterol in hypercholesterolemic patients. Keeping the potential side effects of vitamin C (discussed below) in mind, it may be reasonable for individuals to attempt moderate vitamin C supplementation (e.g., up to 1 g/day) while monitoring serum cholesterol levels.

Miscellaneous

It is impossible to discuss all the conditions in which vitamin C has been said to be therapeutic. These have been adequately reviewed recently; the interested reader is referred to this 49-page review article (7). These conditions include venous thrombosis, diabetes mellitus, lung damage from smoking or air pollution, sudden infant death syndrome, stress, wound healing, and enhancement of alertness and mental function. None of these conditions have been the object of well-controlled scientific trials which allow for a reasonably unbiased scientific conclusion. It cannot be said that vitamin C is clearly not therapeutic in these conditions, but in the absence of proof that it is, megadosing with vitamin C cannot be recommended.

Side Effects

Vitamin C is widely viewed as being nontoxic, and to a large extent, this is correct. Several recent reports, however, suggest potential toxicities of megadoses of this vitamin. The frequency of these side effects cannot be determined, but it is probably low. These side effects include possible gastritis (150), inter-ference with copper status in men (151), and a recent report of kidney failure (152). The latter case is illustrative of the careless use of megavitamins in gen-eral, and of vitamin C specifically:

A 70-year-old man went to a "chelation therapy" center for treatment of claudication (pain in the legs caused by poor blood supply, due to atherosclerosis). The previous day, he was shown to have poor kidney function (creatinine of 5.0 mg/dl). Despite this, the patient received an infusion of 2.5 g of vitamin C. It is unclear if the patient also received the chelation treatment. Twelve hours after the vitamin C infusion, he experienced severe bilateral flank pain, passed a few drops of bloody urine, and then stopped making urine (his kidneys stopped working), necessitating the initiation of dialysis. His creatinine at this time was 10.0 mg/dl (indicative of kidney failure). Numerous crystals of calcium oxalate (the breakdown product of vitamin C) were found in his kidneys.

Although this is an anecdotal case, it seems likely that the acute deposition of these crystals in an elderly patient with already marginal kidney function was sort of "the straw that broke the camel's back". It is impossible to say what the patient's kidney status would have become in the absence of the vitamin C infusion, but it is likely that the vitamin C infusion did not help matters.

MEGAVITAMINS:THE BOTTOM LINE

With certain exceptions, discussed above, it appears that megavitamin ther-apy is unwarranted in the majority of situations in which it is currently recommended in the popular literature. In addition, even the previously-thought-to-be-safe water-soluble vitamins have been shown to have significant potential toxicities (e.g., pyridoxine). In the absence of more compelling evidence, mega-vitamin supplementation cannot be recommended, except in certain cases, dis-cussed above (e.g., niacin for hypercholesterolemia). It should also be noted that megadosing can, on occasion, occur from unusual eating habits, such as inges-tion of large quantities of liver. As is true of advice about other nutritional practices, moderation is the key.

The question of whether *multivitamin* supplementation is indicated is a bit more difficult to answer. Many nutrition experts do not use a multivitamin sup-plement, and do not recommend them routinely. There are no compelling reasons not to use a multivitamin supplement except for cost, perhaps. Another consid-eration is that the diet of some individuals may worsen if they take a multivitamin supplement because they may argue, "Well, I'm taking a vitamin supplement anyway, so I'm covered". Finally, iron supplements in menstruating women and calcium supplements for women over age 40 seem reasonable, but these topics are covered in the next chapter.

REFERENCES

1. Truswell AS: Vitamins I, Vitamins II. Br Med J 291:1033, 1103, 1985

1a. Food and Nutrition Board: Recommended Dietary Allowances. 10th ed. Washington, D.C., National Research Council, National Academy of Sciences, 1985.

1b. Harper AE: Origin of Recommended Dietary Allowances — an historic overview. Am J Clin Nutr 41:140, 1985

1c. Munro HN: Evolving scientific bases for the Recommended Dietary Allowances — a critical look at methodologies. Am J Clin Nutr 41:149, 1985

1d. Beaton GH: Uses and limits of the use of the Recommended Dietary Allowances for evaluating dietary intake data. Am J Clin Nutr 41:155, 1985

1e. Kamin H: Status of the 10th edition of the Recommended Dietary Allowances — prospects for the future. Am J Clin Nutr 41:165, 1985

2. Brody J: Jane Brody's Nutrition Book, Bantam Press, 1981

3. Kunz RM (ed.): The AMA Family Medical Guide. Random House, N.Y., N.Y., 1982

4. Holmes A: Nutrition & vitamins. Facts On File, Inc. 1983

5. Lehninger AL: Principles of Biochemistry. New York, N.Y., Worth Publishers, 1982

6. Hodges RE: Megavitamin therapy. Primary Care 9:605, 1982

7. Wolliscroft JO: Megavitamin therapy. DM 29:1, 1983

8. Cheripko J, Ehmann CW: Use of retinoids for acne and psoriasis. In: Yetiv JZ, Bianchine JR (eds.): Recent Advances in Clinical Therapeutics, New York, Grune & Stratton, 1983, pp. 295

9. Goodman DS: Vitamin A and retinoids in health and disease. N Engl J Med 310:1023, 1984

10. Bollag W: Vitamin A and retinoids: From nutrition to pharmacotherapy in dermatology and oncology. Lancet 1:860, 1983

11. Sporn MB: Retinoids and suppression of carcinogenesis. Hosp Practice 18:83, 1983

12. Editorial: Vitamin A and cancer. Lancet 2:325, 1984

13. Peto R, et al: Can dietary beta-carotene materially reduce human cancer rates? Nature 290:201, 1981

14. Sporn MB, Newton DL: Chemoprevention of cancer with retinoids. Fed Proc 38:2528, 1979

15. Meyskens FL: Vitamin A and cancer. Arizona Med 37:84, 1980

16. Maugh TH: Vitamin A: Potential protection from carcinogens. Science 186:1198, 1974

16a. Gunby P: 'Mild' vitamin A deficiency now major world problem? JAMA 252:3086, 1984

17. Wolbach SB, Howe PR: Tissue changes following deprivation of fat-soluble A vitamin. J Exp Med 42:753, 1925

18. Rowe NA, Gorlin RJ: The effect of vitamin A deficiency on carcinogenesis. J Dent Res 38:72, 1959

19. Chu EW, Malmgren RA: An inhibitory effect of vitamin A on the induction of tumors of forestomach and cervix in the Syrian hamster by carcinogenic polycyclic hydrocarbons. Cancer Res 25:884, 1965

20. Davies RE: Effect of vitamin a on 7,12-dimethylbenz(a)-anthracene-induced papillomas in Rhino mouse skin. Cancer Res 27:237, 1967

21. Saffioti U, et al: Experimental cancer of the lung. Inhibition by vitamin A of the induction of tracheobronchial squamous metaplasia and squamous cell tumors. Cancer 20:857, 1967

22. Stich HF, et al: Reduction with vitamin A and beta-carotene administration of proportion of micronucleated buccal mucosal cells is Asian betel nut and tobacco chewers. Lancet 1:1204, 1984

23. Bjelke E: Dietary vitamin A and human lung cancer. Int J Cancer 15:561, 1975

24. Hirayama T: Diet and cancer. Nutr Cancer 1:67, 1979

25. MacLennan R, et al: Risk factors for lung cancer in Singapore Chinese, a population with high female incidence rates. Int J Cancer 20:854, 1977

26. Mettlin R, et al: Vitamin A and lung cancer. J Nat Cancer Inst 62:1435, 1979

27. Gregor A, et al: A comparison of dietary histories in lung cancer cases and controls with special reference to vitamin A. Nutr Cancer 2:93, 1980

27a. Salonen JT, et al: Risk of cancer in relation to serum concentrations of selenium and vitamins A and E: matched case-control analysis of prospective data. Br Med J 290:417, 1985

27b. Colditz GA, et al: Increased green and yellow vegetable intake and lowered cancer deaths in an elderly population. Am J Clin Nutr 41:32, 1985

28. Shekelle RB, et al: Dietary vitamin A and risk of cancer in the Western Electric study. Lancet 2:1185, 1981

29. Peto R, et al: Can dietary beta-carotene materially reduce human cancer rates? Nature 290:201, 1981

30. Willett WC, et al: Relation of serum vitamins A and E and carotenoids to the risk of cancer. N Engl J Med 310:430, 1984

30a. Munoz N, et al: No effect of riboflavine, retinol and zinc on prevalence of precancerous lesions of oesophagus. Randomized double-blind intervention study in high-risk population in China. Lancet 2:111, 1985

30b. Garland C, et al: Dietary vitamin D and calcium and risk of colorectal cancer: a 19-year prospective study in men. Lancet 1:307, 1985

31. Editorial: Horde of MDs in aspirin-carotene trial. Med Trib 24:1, 1983

32. Pittsley RA, Yoder FW: Retinoid hyperostosis: skeletal toxicity associated with long-term administration of 13-cis retinoic acid for refractory icthyosis. N Engl J Med 308:185, 1983

33. Young FE (FDA Commissioner): Update on birth defects with isotretinoin. FDA Drug Bull 14:15, 1984

33a. Editorial: Vitamin A and teratogenesis. Lancet 1:319, 1985

33b. Lammer EJ, et al: Retinoic acid embryopathy. N Engl J Med 313:837, 1985

33c. Bershad S, et al: Changes in plasma lipids and lipoproteins during isotretinoin therapy for acne. N Engl J Med 313:981, 1985

33d. Pochi PE: Isotretinoin for acne. N Engl J Med 313:1013, 1985

33e. Selhorst JB, et al: Liver lover's headache: pseudotumor cerebri and vitamin A intoxication. JAMA 252:3365, 1984

34. Herbert V: Toxicity of 25,000 IU vitamin A supplements in "health" food users. Am J Clin Nutr 36:185, 1982

35. reference #3 in Herbert's article

36. Mawson AR: Hypervitaminosis A toxicity and gout. Lancet 1:1181, 1984

37. White JM: Vitamin A-induced anemia. Lancet 2:573, 1984

38. Leo MA, Lieber CS: Interaction of ethanol with vitamin A. Clin Exp Res 7:15, 1983

39. Maclaren DS: Dermatology in General Medicine, 2nd ed. Fitzpatrick TB, et al (eds.) McGraw-Hill, New York, 1979

40. Kemmann E, et al: Amenorrhea associated with carotenemia. JAMA 249:926, 1983

41. Lubin B, Machlin LJ (eds.): Vitamin E: Biochemical, Hematological, and Clinical Aspects. Ann NY Acad Sci 393:1-506, 1982. Based on a conference of the same name, sponsored by the New York Academy of Sciences, held Nov. 11-13, 1981

42. Machlin LJ (ed): Vitamin E. A Comprehensive Treatise. New York, Maral Dekker, 1980.

43. Horwitt MK: Therapeutic uses of vitamin E in medicine. Nutr Rev 38:105, 1980

44. Bieri JG, et al: Medical uses of vitamin E. N Engl J Med 308:1063, 1983

45. Hittner HM, et al: Retrolental fibroplasia: efficacy of vitamin E in a double-blind clinical study of preterm infants. N Engl J Med 305:1365, 1981

46. Hittner HM: Vitamin E in retrolental fibroplasia (letter). N Engl J Med 306:867, 1982

47. Finer NN, et al: A controlled trial to evaluate the role of vitamin E in the incidence and severity of retrolental fibroplasia in the low birth weight neonate. Presented at a conference on Retinopathy in Prematurity, Washington, D.C., December 4-6, 1981

48. Milner RA, et al: RLF in 1500 gram neonates: part of a randomized clinical trial of the effectiveness of vitamin E. Ibid.

49. Ehrenkranz RA, Puklin JE: Lack of effect of vitamin E administration during respiratory distress syndrome in preventing retinopathy of prematurity. Ibid.

50. Weiter JJ: Retrolental fibroplasia: and unsolved problem. N Engl J Med 305:1404, 1981

51. Sobel S, et al: Vitamin E in retrolental fibroplasia (letter). N Engl J Med 306:867, 1982

52. Hittner HM, et al: Retrolental fibroplasia and vitamin E in the preterm infant — comparison of oral versus intramuscular:oral administration. Peds 73:238, 1984

53. Finer NN, et al: Vitamin E and necrotizing enterocolitis. Peds 73:387, 1984

53a. Bove KE, et al: Vasculopathic hepatotoxicity associated with E-Ferol syndrome in low-birth-weight infants. JAMA 254:2422, 1985

54. Vitamin E advised for all infants who need supplemental oxygen. Pediatric News, February, 1983

55. Chiswick ML, et al: Vitamin E and intraventricular hemorrhage in the newborn. An NY Acad Sci 393:109, 1982

56. Chiswick ML, et al: Protective effect of vitamin E (DL-alpha-tocopherol) against intraventricular haemorrhage in premature babies. Br Med J 287:81, 1983

57. Ehrenkranz RA, et al: Amelioration of brochopulmonary dysplasia after vitamin E administration: a preliminary report. N Engl J Med 299:564, 1978

58. Ehrenkranz RA, et al: Prevention of bronchopulmonary dysplasia with vitamin E

administration during the acute stages of respiratory distress syndrome. J Pediatr 95:873, 1979

59. Steiner M, Anastasi J: Vitamin E. An inhibitor of the platelet release reaction. J Clin Invest 57:732, 1976
60. Lake AM, et al: Vitamin E deficiency and enhanced platelet function. Reversal following E supplementation. J Peds 90:722, 1977
61. Gomes JAC, et al: The effect of vitamin E on platelet aggregation. Am Heart J 91:425, 1976
62. Olson RE, Jones JP: The inhibition of vitamin K action by D-alpha-tocopherol and its derivatives. Fed Proc 38:710, 1979
63. Farrell PM: Deficiency states, pharmacological effects and nutritional requirements. In Machlin LJ (ed.): Vitamin E. A Comprehensive Treatise. New York, Maral Dekker, 1980. p.579-94
64. Haeger K: Long-time treatment of intermittent claudication with vitamin E. Am J Clin Nutr 27:1179, 1974
65. Kanofsky JD, Kanofsky PB: Prevention of thromboembolic disease by vitamin E. N Engl J Med 305:173, 1981
66. Shute EV, et al: The influence of vitamin E on vascular disease. Surg Gynecol Obstet 86:1, 1948
67. Anderson TW: Vitamin E in angina pectoris. Can Med Assoc 110:401, 1976
68. Olson RE: Vitamin E and its relation to heart disease. Circulation 48: 179, 1973
69. Hermann WJ, et al: The effect of tocopherol on high-density lipoprotein cholesterol. Am J Clin Pathol 72:848, 1979
70. Hatam LJ, Kayden HJ: The failure of alpha-tocopherol supplementation to alter the distribution of lipoprotein cholesterol in normal and hyperlipoproteinemic persons (letter). Am J Clin Pathol 76:122, 1981
71. Hermann WJ: Reply to above letter. Am J Clin Pathol 76:124, 1981
72. Barboriak JJ, et al: Vitamin E supplements and plasma high-density lipoprotein cholesterol. Am J Clin Pathol 77:371, 1982
73. Meydani SN, et al: Altered lipoprotein metabolism in spontaneous vitamin E deficiency of owl monkeys. Am J Clin Nutr 38:888, 1983
74. Kesaniemi YA, Grundy SM: Lack of effect of tocopherol on plasma lipids and lipoproteins in man. Am J Clin Nutr 36:224, 1982
75. Chapkin RS, et al: Effect of vitamin E supplementation on serum and high-density lipoprotein-cholesterol in renal patients on maintenance hemodialysis. Am J Clin Nutr 38:253, 1983
76. Gonzalez ER: Vitamin E relieves most cystic breast disease; may alter lipids, hormones. JAMA 244:1077, 1980
77. Oski FA: Vitamin E — A radical defense. N Engl J Med 303:454, 1980
77a. Wood LA: Possible prevention of Adriamycin-induced alopecia by tocopherol. N Engl J Med 312:1060, 1985
78. American Health brochure and H&J Products information sheet.
79. Roberts HJ: Perspective on vitamin E as therapy. JAMA 246:129, 1981
80. Toone WM: Effects of vitamin E: Good and bad. N engl J Med 289:979, 1973
81. Cohen HM: Effects of vitamin E: Good and bad. N Engl J Med 289:980, 1973

82. Farrell PM, Bieri JG: Megavitamin E supplementation in man. Am J Clin Nutr 28:1381, 1975

83. Horwitt MK, et al: Serum concentrations of alpha-tocopherol after ingestion of various vitamin E preparations. Am J Clin Nutr 40:240, 1984

84. Editorial: Sensory neuropathy from megadoses of pyridoxine. Nutr Rev 42:49, 1984

85. Davidson RA: Complications of megavitamin therapy. South Med J 77:200, 1984

86. Alhadeff L, et al: Toxic effects of water-soluble vitamins. Nutr Rev 42:33, 1984

87. Garry PJ, et al: Nutritional status in a healthy elderly population: dietary and supplemental intakes. Am J Clin Nutr 36:319, 1982

88. Schutz HG, et al: Food supplement usage in seven Western states. Am J Clin Nutr 36:897, 1982

89. Bowerman SJA, Harrill I: Nutrient consumption of individuals taking or not taking nutrient supplements. J Am Diet Assoc 83:298, 1983

90. Willett W, et al: Vitamin supplement use among registered nurses. Am J Clin Nutr 34:1121, 1981

91. Worthington-Roberts B, Breskin M: Supplementation patterns of Washington State dietitians. J Am Diet Assoc 84:795, 1984

92. Brocklehurst JC, et al: The clinical features of chronic vitamin deficiency. A Therapeutic trial in geriatric hospital patients. Geront Clin 10:309, 1968

93. Mindell E: Handouts obtained in health food store in 1981.

94. Mandel H, et al: Thiamine-dependent beriberi in the "thiamine-responsive anemia syndrome". N Engl J Med 311:836, 1984

94a. Katz D, et al: Intestinal absorption of thiamin from yeast-containing sorghum beer. Am J Clin Nutr 42:666, 1985

95. Arts WFM, et al: NADH CoQ reductase deficient-myopathy: successful treatment with riboflavin. Lancet 2:581, 1983

96. Garry PJ, et al: Nutritional status in a healthy elderly population: riboflavin. Am J Clin Nutr 36:902, 1982

97. Alexander M, et al: Relation of riboflavin nutriture in healthy elderly to intake of calcium and vitamin supplements: evidence against riboflavin supplementation. Am J Clin Nutr 39:540, 1984

98. Belko AZ, et al: Effects of exercise on riboflavin requirements of young women. Am J Clin Nutr 37:509, 1983

99. Belko AZ, et al: Effects of aerobic exercise and weight loss on riboflavin requirements of moderately obese marginally deficient young women. Am J Clin Nutr 40:553, 1984

100. The Coronary Drug Project Research Group: Clofibrate and niacin in coronary heart disease. JAMA 231:360, 1975

101. Rosenhamer G, Carlson L: Effect of combined clofibrate-nicotinic acid treatment in ischemic heart disease. Atherosclerosis 38:129, 1980

102. Kane JP, et al: Normalization of low-density lipoprotein levels in heterozygous familial hypercholesterolemia with a combined drug regimen. N Engl J Med 304:251, 1981

103. Baron DN, et al: Hereditary pellagra-like skin rash with temporary cerebellar ataxia, constant renal amino-aciduria and other bizarre biochemical features. Lancet 2:421, 1956. Also discussed in Nutr Rev 42:251, 1984.

104. Shelley WB, Shelley ED: Nicotinic-acid-responsive photosensitivity. Lancet 2:576, 1984

105. Rabbani GH, et al: Reduction of fluid loss in cholera by nicotinic acid: a randomized controlled trial. Lancet 2:1439, 1983

106. Hilton JG, Wells CH: Nicotinic acid reduction of plasma volume loss after thermal trauma. Science 191:861, 1976

107. Brown OR, et al: Niacin reduces paraquat toxicity in rats. Science 212:1510, 1981

108. Leads from the MMWR: Niacin intoxication from pumpernickel bagels — New York. JAMA 250:160, 1983

109. Bachman DS: Late-onset pyridoxine-dependency convulsions. Ann Neurol 14:692, 1983

110. Coleman M, et al: A preliminary study of the effect of pyridoxine administration in a subgroup of hyperkinetic children: a double-blind crossover comparison with methylphenidate. Biol Psych 14:741, 1979

111. Haslam RHA, et al: Effects of megavitamin therapy on children with attention deficit disorder. Pediatrics 74:103, 1984

112. Coburn SP, et al: Effect of megavitamin treatment on mental performance and plasma vitamin B_6 concentrations in mentally retarded young adults. Am J Clin Nutr 38:352, 1983

113. Review: The vitamin B_6 requirement in oral contraceptive users. Nutr Rev 37:344, 1979

114. Barr W: Pyridoxine supplements in the premenstrual syndrome. Practitioner 228:425, 1984

115. Schuster K, et al: Effect of maternal pyridoxine-HCl supplementation on the vitamin B_6 status of mother and infant and on pregnancy outcome. J Nutr 114:977, 1984

116. Natta CL, Reynolds RD: Apparent vitamin B_6 deficiency in sickle cell anemia. Am J Clin Nutr 40:235, 1984

116a. Reynolds RD, Natta CL: Depressed plasma pyridoxal phosphate concentrations in adult asthmatics. Am J Clin Nutr 41:684, 1985

117. Schaumburg H, et al: Sensory neuropathy from pyridoxine abuse. A new megavitamin syndrome. N Engl J Med 309:445, 1983

118. Letters to the editor: Sensory neuropathy from pyridoxine abuse. N Engl J Med 310:197, 1984

119. Berger A, Schaumburg H: More on neuropathy from pyridoxine abuse. N Engl J Med 311:986, 1984

119a. Middleton J, Wells W: Vitamin B_{12} injections: considerable source of work for the district nurse. Br Med J 290:1254, 1985

120. Shinnar S, Singer HS: Cobalamin C mutation (methylmalonic aciduria and homocystinuria) in adolescence. N Engl J Med 311:451, 1984

121. Dawson DW, et al: Malabsorption of protein bound vitamin B_{12}. Br Med J 288:675, 1984

122. Dawson DW: Diagnosis of vitamin B_{12} deficiency. Br Med J 289:938, 1984

122a. Carmel R, Karnaze DS: The deoxyuridine suppression test identifies subtle cobalamin deficiency in patients without typical megaloblastic anemia. JAMA 253:1284, 1985

123. Laurence KM, et al: Double-blind randomized controlled trial of folate treatment before conception to prevent recurrence of neural-tube defects. Br Med J 282:1509, 1981

124. Tolarova M: Periconceptional supplementation with vitamins and folic acid to prevent recurrence of cleft lip. Lancet 2:217, 1982

125. Smithells RW, et al: Further experience of vitamin supplementation for prevention of neural tube defect recurrences. Lancet 1:1027, 1983

126. Oakley GP, et al: Vitamins and neural tube defects. Lancet 2:798, 1983

127. Editorial: Medical research council vitamin study. Lancet 1:1308, 1984

128. Smithells RW: Rational use of vitamins. Lancet 1:1295, 1984

129. Botez MI, et al: Neurologic disorders responsive to folic acid therapy. Can Med Assoc J 115:217, 1976

130. Manzoor M, Runcie J: Folate-responsive neuropathy: report of 10 cases. Br Med J 1:1176, 1976

131. Butterworth CE, et al: Improvement in cervical dysplasia associated with folic acid therapy in users of oral contraceptives. Am J Clin Nutr 35:73, 1982

132. Watson AF: The chemical reducing capacity and vitamin C content of transplantable tumors of the rat and guinea pig. Br J Exp Pathol 17:124, 1936

133. Siegel BV, Morton JI: Vitamin C and the immune response. Experientia 33:393, 1977

134. Bram S, et al: Vitamin C preferential toxicity for malignant melanoma cells. Nature 284:629, 1980

135. Cameron E, Pauling L: Supplemental ascorbate in the supportive treatment of cancer:prolongation of survival times in terminal human cancer. Proc Natl Acad Sci 73:3685, 1976

136. Herbert V: Nutrition cultism — facts and fiction. George Stickley Co., Philadelphia, 1980, p.103

137. Creagan ET, et al: Failure of high-dose vitamin C (ascorbic acid) therapy to benefit patients with advanced cancer. A controlled trial. N Engl J Med 301:687, 1979

138. Pauling L: Vitamin C therapy of advanced cancer. N Engl J Med 302:694, 1980

139. Moertel CG, et al: High-dose vitamin C versus placebo in the treatment of patients with advanced cancer who have had no prior chemotherapy. A randomized double-blind comparison. N Engl J Med 312:137, 1985

140. Wittes RE: Vitamin C and cancer. N Engl J Med 312:178, 1985

141. Wassertheil-Smoller S, et al: Dietary vitamin C and uterine cervical dysplasia. Am J Epidemiol 114:714, 1981

142. Pauling LC: Vitamin C and the common cold. W.H. Freeman and Co., San Francisco, 1970

143. Chalmers TC: Effects of ascorbic acid on the common cold: an evaluation of the evidence. Am J Med 58:532, 1975

144. Terezhalmy GT, et al: The use of water-soluble bioflavonoids-ascorbic acid complex in the treatment of recurrent herpes labialis. Oral Surg 45:56, 1978

145. Banic S: Prevention of rabies by vitamin C. Nature 258:153, 1975

146. Editorial: Vitamin C and plasma cholesterol. Lancet 2:907, 1984

147. Peterson VE, et al: Quantification of plasma cholesterol and triglyceride levels in

hypercholesterolemic subjects receiving ascorbic acid supplements. Am J Clin Nutr 28:584, 1975

148. Ginter E: Vitamin C and plasma lipids. N Engl J Med 294:559, 1976

149. Ginter E: Cholesterol: Vitamin C controls its transformation to bile acids. Science 179:702, 1973

150. Questions and answers: Vitamin C ingestion, gastritis, and antacid therapy. JAMA 250:3228, 1984

151. Finley EB, Cerklewski FL: Influence of corbic acid supplementation on copper status in young adult men. Am J Clin Nutr 37:553, 1983

152. McAllister CJ, et al: Renal failure secondary to massive infusion of vitamin C. JAMA 252:1684, 1984

CHAPTER 9

And What About Megaminerals?

Sodium and potassium are quantitatively the most important minerals in the human diet, and due to their major presumed role in hypertension, Chapter 10 is devoted to these minerals. Chapter 10 also briefly discusses the role of calcium and some other substances in blood pressure control. This chapter deals with minerals other than sodium and potassium, such as calcium, selenium, iron, zinc, magnesium, chromium and fluoride.

Our understanding of mineral metabolism is still in its infancy, even more so than that of vitamins. One of the main reasons for this is that several minerals are also *trace elements*, which means that they exist in the food supply and in our bodies in very small concentrations. For instance, the RDA for vitamin C (in milligrams) is approximately 600 times greater than that for selenium. Such low quantities make it extremely difficult to measure dietary intake and plasma concentrations of these elements, which has hindered research in this field. Indeed, the technology to make such measurements has only become available in the last decade.

This lack of understanding of minerals seems to have had minimal impact on the supplement-loving public (1). In a survey of 2451 adults in seven states, 67% used some form of food supplement. Although multivitamins and megadose vitamin C were most commonly taken, iron, calcium, zinc and dolomite (bone meal) were also frequently ingested. Some of these should be taken, while the rationale for taking others is obscure. Supplements are often taken with the idea that if "some is good, more must be better", or "it might help, and it certainly won't hurt". The previous chapter has suggested that this may not be true of some vitamins (e.g., pyridoxine). This chapter will examine this question as it applies to minerals.

OVERVIEW OF MINERALS

Minerals are inorganic substances which are important to various functions of the body. Some minerals, such as calcium, iron, phosphorus, magnesium, zinc and iodine, are sufficiently well understood to allow Recommended Dietary Allowances (RDAs) to have been established (2). Others, like chloride, copper, fluoride, chromium, selenium, manganese, and molybdenum have "estimated safe and adequate daily intake" levels established. Finally, some, like sulfur, are insufficiently understood to have either label applied to them, and several, including tin, vanadium, cadmium, and nickel, are not currently recognized as essential nutrients.

Before discussing the individual minerals below, a word about the validity of hair analysis for the determination of mineral and vitamin status may be in order.

HAIR ANALYSIS

Despite inadequate scientific support for this methodology, hair analysis, like cytotoxic testing, has caught the public's fancy. Hair analysis is based on the hypothesis that mineral status (e.g., whether any deficiencies exist) can be determined by assaying concentrations of the mineral in a hair sample. Although this hypothesis may be reasonable, even a cursory examination of the pitfalls of this technique will reveal why hair analysis is not the "ultimate test" it is claimed to be. Health professionals need to be acquainted with this topic primarily so that they can discern fact from fiction and advise their patients accordingly. This of course applies not only to hair analysis but also to many other popular nutritional practices discussed in this book.

The pitfalls of hair analysis were recently lucidly reviewed (3); this review should be consulted by the interested reader. One factor which interferes with the reproducibility and validity of hair analysis is the fact that hair is continuously exposed to the external environment. Since hair grows at a rate of ½" per month, the tip of a one-inch hair has been exposed to shampoo, contaminants in air, etc., for two months or more. Since some shampoos contain zinc or selenium, this may significantly alter the hair content of these minerals. The variability of hair zinc concentration due to environmental factors has been recently demonstrated (4).

Dyeing, bleaching, and permanent waving procedures may also alter hair mineral concentrations. It is interesting to note that natural hair color differences (not only artificial dyeing) can affect hair mineral concentrations. For instance, manganese concentrations have been found to be twice as high in the black hair as in the white hair of the same rabbits (5). Incidentally, such use of hair mineral concentration measurement, namely, the comparison of concentrations in the same animal, or between large groups (5a), *may* be valid. It is possible, though unclear at present, that sex, age, location of the hair, coarseness of the hair, and speed of hair growth may also affect mineral concentrations.

The biggest problem with hair analysis, however, is that very little is known about the extent to which hair concentrations of various elements correlate with concentrations in the blood or other organs. Furthermore, the relevance of hair mineral concentrations to health and disease is unclear. For most minerals, even the normal range of concentration in hair is unknown (contrary to what the hair analysis labs will tell you). In other words, if person X's hair zinc (or chromium, or copper, or whatever) concentration is 30, is that high, low or "normal"? If one were to decide it is "high", what does that mean? Could the shampoo used by the patient account for it? This is assuming that the technique used, can, in fact, accurately measure zinc concentrations in hair, which is doubtful in many cases.

In a recent article entitled, "Commercial Hair Analysis: Science or Scam?", Dr. Barrett describes an experiment wherein he sent identical hair samples from 2 healthy teenagers to 13 commercial hair analysis laboratories (5b). The laboratories disagreed on the mineral content of the identical samples, as well as disagreeing on what "normal" values should be. Most reports also contained computerized interpretations of the presumed mineral "deficiencies" that these two teenagers supposedly had. Six labs recommended various quantities of different supplements. Dr. Barrett concluded that, "commercial use of hair analysis in this manner is unscientific, economically wasteful, and probably illegal". Thus, advice given on the basis of hair analysis is likely to be at best worthless, and at worst, incorrect. This, however, does not seem to deter many commercial labs from offering such advice.

MINERALS

Calcium

This mineral has received much attention in both the scientific and lay press recently, due to the association between calcium (or lack thereof) and the incidence of osteoporosis. A recent Consensus Development Conference was held at the National Institutes of Health to discuss the cause and possible treatment of this condition (6). An excellent article on osteoporosis also appeared recently in Consumer Reports (7). The interested reader is encouraged to consult these references.

Osteoporosis is the scourge of mankind (or more accurately, womankind). Osteoporosis, which means "porous bone", is estimated to affect between 15 and 20 million Americans. Over 1 million fractures attributable to osteoporosis occur annually in people over the age of 45. The most common sites of fracture are the spinal vertebrae, the wrist (Colles' fracture) and the hip. It is estimated that 15-20% of victims of hip fracture over 70 years old will die from complications of the fracture or its treatment (e.g., bed rest leading to pneumonia or blood clots to the lung).

Several factors predispose individuals to osteoporosis, and consequently, to a higher risk of fractures. These risk factors include female sex, age—especially after menopause, white race, and low body weight. Cigarette smoking, lack of exercise, and hereditary factors (e.g., fair-haired women of slight frame seem to be at special risk) have also been implicated.

Part of the explanation for the above is the fact that men have greater initial bone mass than women, and blacks more than whites. Thus, men and blacks can lose a greater amount of bone before their bones approach the "fracture threshold" where a slight mechanical stress on the bone may break it. Estrogen prevents (or slows) the development of osteoporosis. Premature menopause, which can be induced by surgical removal of the ovaries, eliminates the protective effect of estrogen and strongly predisposes the woman to acceleration of bone loss (8). Interestingly, bone loss may also occur if cyclic ovarian function is disturbed (a condition characterized by lack of menstrual periods) by excessive exercise (9). These authors, however, wisely caution that this is strictly a preliminary finding which should be "viewed as an impetus for further research rather than as a signal to amenorrheic athletes to cease their strenuous conditioning programs". This would seem especially reasonable in view of the fact that weight-bearing exercise decreases bone loss (10). It may be, however, that the ideal frequency of exercise, at least in terms of its effects on bone, is that which is just short of inducing any menstrual abnormalities (10a).

In addition to the above, several dietary factors may predispose toward osteoporosis (11). The best-known, of course, is inadequate calcium intake. In addition to calcium, vitamin D deficiency, and phosphate and protein *excess*, appear to predispose to bone calcium loss (11a). High-protein diets produce an acidic urine, which increases urine calcium losses. One paper (12) suggests that sodium bicarbonate ingestion, which alkalinizes the urine, is an effective way to increase calcium retention in women with protein-induced urine calcium losses.

The foregoing discussion now brings us to the topic of the advisability of calcium supplementation, to prevent osteoporosis (13). Such treatment is especially important in postmenopausal women, although some experts recommend calcium supplementation before menopause also. Most studies have shown that calcium supplements improve calcium balance both in normal subjects (14) and in those with osteoporosis (14-16). Such supplements also decrease the risk of fractures in postmenopausal women (17). It is discomfiting to consider, however, that in one report, calcium supplementation for 2 years in postmenopausal women *had no effect* on loss of bone mass. It is unclear why the results of this study contrast with those from studies quoted above.

It has also been proposed that fluoride supplementation (especially if combined with calcium supplements) is useful in the treatment of osteoporosis (17,18). The role of exercise and normal protein intake has also been alluded to.

Finally, it has been shown that estrogen decreases the risk of hip and lower forearm fractures in postmenopausal women (19), and that the rate of bone loss depends on the dose administered (20). Bone is lost if the ethinyl estradiol dose is below 15 ug per day; a net gain of bone is observed at doses above 25 ug per day.

Summary and Recommendations

The decision about treatment of osteoporosis requires serious consideration of the benefits vs. side effects of the various options. Most difficult is the decision of whether to recommend hormonal therapy, in view of concerns about thrombosis (blood clots) and uterine cancer. It appears that these potentially serious effects of estrogen therapy are not as frequent as previously thought, and should not preclude its use. Estrogen therapy, however, should only be given after truly informed consent of the patient, achieved by thorough discussion of the pro's and con's with the patient. Unless there are specific contraindications, women who undergo premature menopause secondary to surgical removal of the ovaries should probably be started on hormonal therapy, because the risk of osteoporosis in the future is greater.

The issue of calcium therapy is more easily decided. A recent consensus conference recommended a daily calcium intake of 1000-1500 mg. Since the average American woman ingests about 500-700 mg of calcium per day, there is a substantial dietary calcium deficiency in the United States. Therefore, all postmenopausal women should probably take a calcium supplement unless they have had kidney stones or other contraindications. Such women especially should seek their doctor's advice about the advisability of calcium supplements.

Most postmenopausal women probably need a 500-1000 mg calcium supplement per day, depending on the dietary intake. According to Consumer Reports, the least expensive calcium supplement is Tums antacid tablets, each of which contain 200 mg of elemental calcium as calcium carbonate. Postmenopausal women who ingest large amounts of calcium, usually in the form of dairy products, may only require a few hundred milligrams of calcium in supplement form. Those who ingest the average amount of calcium for women of this age group (about 500 mg daily) will need a supplement of approximately 1000 mg. Obviously, it would be preferable, but probably not realistic, to obtain this calcium from food sources.

This advice is aimed primarily at perimenopausal (around the menopause) or early (first few years) postmenopausal women. It is at this time that the rate of bone loss is greatest. A recent large-scale epidemiologic study, however, disputes the idea that menopause is the pivotal event in the development of osteoporosis (20a). This study showed that the hip fracture rate for white women starts a steep climb at ages 40-45, about 15 years earlier than previously believed. This would imply that therapies aimed at preventing osteoporosis may need to be begun much before menopause. Most studies suggest that calcium supplementation initiated long after menopause (>10 years) is of little use because by this time,

Food	Weight or Measure	Calcium (Milligrams)
Plain skim and lowfat yogurts	1 cup	
Lowfat flavored and fruited yogurts	1 cup	
Dry nonfat milk	¼ cup	350-450
Sardines, with bones	3 ounces	
Some fruited yogurts	1 cup	
Skim and lowfat milks	1 cup	
Whole milk, chocolate milk and buttermilk	1 cup	250-350
Swiss and Gruyère cheeses	1 ounce	
Hard cheeses such as Cheddar and Edam	1 ounce	
Processed cheeses	1 ounce	
Cheese spreads	1 ounce	150-250
Salmon, with bones	3 ounces	
Collards	½ cup	
Cheese foods	1 ounce	
Soft cheeses such as mozzarella, blue and feta	1 ounce	
Cooked dried beans such as navy, pea and lima	1 cup	
Turnip greens, kale, dandelion greens	½ cup	
Ice creams and ice milks	½ cup	
Evaporated whole milk	1 ounce	50-150
Cottage cheeses	½ cup	
Sherbets	½ cup	
Broccoli	½ cup	
Orange	1 fresh	
Dates, raisins	¼ cup	
Egg	1	
Bread, whole-wheat or white	1 slice	20-50
Cabbage	½ cup	
Cream cheese	1 ounce	

Calcium content of some common foods
From FDA Consumer, Sept. 1984, p. 10.

much bone has already been lost, and the rate of bone loss has slowed down. Furthermore, there is little evidence that supplementation at *any* time can cause bone to be redeposited. For this group (much after menopause) and for younger women, there are not sufficient data to enable recommendation of calcium supplementation in hopes of averting osteoporosis or treating the condition, if it already exists. However, since it may be of some benefit, and in the absence of specific contraindications, it is my opinion that calcium supplementation of all women, up to a total calcium intake (including diet) of 1500 mg daily is reasonable.

Finally, men may wonder about need for supplementation. There is even less evidence on this issue, but my opinion currently is that this isn't necessary, for a couple of reasons. First, the incidence of osteoporosis in men is low. Second, because of their greater average caloric intake, men ingest larger amounts of calcium in their diet. Thus, in the absence of any compelling rationale to supplement their diets, the current evidence does not so dictate. To help the reader, Table 9-1 lists the calcium content of some common foods.

Selenium

Selenium is the second mineral to be discussed in this chapter not because it is the best-understood mineral (that honor certainly goes to iron) but because like vitamins A and E, selenium deficiency has been implicated in the pathogenesis of cancer. In addition, selenium has been the object of considerable attention in the lay and scientific press.

The hypothesis that high selenium intake can decrease the incidence of cancer is supported by several lines of evidence. First are animal studies wherein selenium supplementation decreased the frequency of chemically-induced cancers (21,22) and limited tumor growth (23). The response can be impressive; in one experiment, none of 5 selenium-treated mice had any tumors, whereas all five untreated mice developed massive tumors. It should be noted, however, that the anticancer response was dependent on the chemical form and dose of the selenium supplement.

Secondly, epidemiologic data in humans support the anticancer effect of selenium. People living in areas with high selenium levels have a lower incidence of cancer than individuals who live in low-selenium areas (24,25). Several case-control studies also support this conclusion (26-28). In addition, cystic fibrosis patients with low serum selenium concentrations may be predisposed to cancer (28a).

In the most recent case-control study published (28), serum concentrations of selenium, and vitamins A and E, were measured in 12,000 Finnish people in 1977. The subjects were followed for 4 years, during which 30 men and 21 women died of cancer. Their serum levels were compared to 51 individuals who didn't die of cancer during the same time period. The cases (people dying of cancer) and controls were matched for sex, age, and tobacco use. Patients who died of cancer had a mean selenium level of 53.7 ug/l, compared to 60.9 in the controls who did not die of cancer. This difference was accounted for primarily by differences in serum selenium levels in smokers. The risk of fatal cancer was 5.8-fold higher among subjects with low (lowest tertile) serum selenium compared to those with higher values (highest tertile). Smoking men with cancer had serum vitamin A levels that were 26% lower than smoking controls. Subjects with both low selenium and low vitamin E levels had an 11-fold risk of dying from cancer.

It is of some comfort that selenium intake and serum selenium levels measured in the United States (26) are approximately twice as high as those in the Finnish study quoted above. Furthermore, the increased risk from the lowest tertile to the highest tertile in the American study is only two-fold (rather than six-fold). Thus, as serum selenium levels increase, the marginal benefit of additional selenium in the diet or the blood decreases. Nevertheless, there is a gradient of selenium intake in various geographic parts of the United States (23). For instance, Colorado, Kansas, Nebraska, North and South Dakota and Wyoming are very-high-selenium states, while several of the New England states are low-selenium states. It may be that individuals who have been exposed to very low dietary selenium intakes (e.g., New Zealand residents) have become adapted to them and do not manifest biochemical characteristics of selenium deficiency, such as low glutathione peroxidase activity (23a,b).

It should again be emphasized that epidemiologic data cannot *prove* that selenium supplementation will decrease the incidence of cancer, and as yet, no intervention trial in humans has demonstrated this to be the case. Furthermore, in at least one epidemiologic study (28), the relationship between serum selenium and cancer mortality held for *smokers only* (and for men only, since none of the women smoked). Thus, it is unclear from the current data whether there is a relationship between selenium and cancer in nonsmokers.

It must also be realized that selenium toxicity can occur. A recent report described selenium poisoning resulting in at least one fatality, in China (29). The most common sign of toxicity was loss of hair and nails. The skin, nervous system, and teeth also seemed affected. Daily dietary selenium intakes were estimated to be 4990 ug (compared to about 100 ug in the United States) and serum selenium levels averaged 3.2 ug/ml— approximately 20-50 times higher than levels in the United States! The source of excess selenium was a stony coal of very high selenium content, which entered the soil and was absorbed by crops grown in the soil. Although this report from China may not be relevant to the United States, selenium supplements in pill form can also be toxic.

A case in point is a recent report of a 57-year-old woman who took selenium supplements; the label stated that each pill contained 150 ug of selenium (30). After experiencing hair loss, fingernail abnormalities, nausea, vomiting and increasing fatigue, the lady consulted her physician. He believed her hair loss was due to emotional stress following the death of her husband. Two months later, she heard that the supplements were being recalled due to the fact that they contained approximately 200 times as much selenium as was stated on the label!

Selenium is widely, though unevenly, found in many foods. The major sources of selenium in the American diet include seafood, meat, cereals and grains. Intake in the United States varies from state to state, but average consumption in the United States ranges from 50-150 ug daily (31). Selenium balance can be maintained on about 80 ug/d in men and 60 ug/d in women (32). Although there is no established RDA for selenium, the "estimated safe and adequate daily intake" first established by the RDA committee in 1980, is 50-200 ug.

There are currently no data about potential toxicity of moderate selenium supplements (e.g., a few hundred ug daily). There is also no evidence that such supplements, if taken by individuals who are not selenium-deficient, are beneficial. The epidemiologic data suggest that people who live in selenium-deficient areas may benefit from a supplement, although it is difficult to scientifically recommend such practice at this time. However, I would not consider unreasonable a daily supplement of 100-150 ug in individuals who are interested in doing so. Such individuals would be wise to discuss this with their personal physician, and to read some of the references quoted in this chapter.

Iron

The reader may find it strange that iron is discussed *after* calcium and selenium. It is precisely because the role of iron in disease (primarily anemia) is well understood (33) that it has been neglected until now. This book deals mostly with topics which are controversial or unappreciated by medical and non-medical readers, and that is hardly the case with iron. Nevertheless, some interesting data relating to iron will be briefly discussed.

Iron is important in the formation of hemoglobin, the pigment in red blood cells (RBCs) which carries oxygen to the tissues. When RBCs die after about 120 days in the circulation, their iron content is scavenged and recycled to make new RBCs. Since the body is very efficient in doing this, very little iron is lost from the body. Menstruation in women constitutes a regular loss of iron; this is why most menstruating women require an iron supplement, while men do not.

Iron supplements may be especially needed by vegetarians because the best source of iron is red meat. Iron derived from meat is called heme iron, while iron obtained from plants is known as non-heme iron. Plants are not a good source of iron for two reasons: (1) they do not contain much iron, and (2) their iron is poorly absorbed. Furthermore, some plant foods, e.g., soybeans, inhibit the absorption of the non-heme iron (34,35). Addition of vitamin C or meat to the non-heme iron can reverse some of that inhibition (36,37). In addition to soybeans, other legumes, such as black beans, lentils, mung beans and split peas, are also poor sources of iron (38).

Coffee and tea reduce iron absorption from a breakfast meal, while orange juice, probably due to its vitamin C content, increases it (39,40). In the latter study (40), iron absorption was not affected if coffee was consumed 1 hour before the meal, but absorption was significantly inhibited if the coffee was drunk 1 hour after the meal. Finally, it has been shown that cooking in iron pots increases the amount of iron ingested.

In some developing countries, where iron deficiency may affect half the population, and to some extent in the United States, iron fortification of staples has been implemented. In this country, for instance, most infant formulas are supplemented, as are many breakfast cereals and other foods. The provision of free iron-fortified milk formula to poor American children in the WIC (Women, Infants and Children) program has been shown to be very effective in decreasing the prevalence of anemia (40a). Fortifying salt with iron has been demonstrated to be effective as an iron supplement in some countries (41,42). The logic of encouraging salt intake, however, in view of its potential role in high blood pressure, is questionable. One wonders if the solution of one problem may not be creating another. Since iron deficiency is not currently a major health problem in the United States, it appears unlikely that iron fortification of foods will go beyond its present applications.

Before leaving the topic of iron, some recent data which suggest that iron deficiency can cause cognitive (intellectual) deficiencies will be presented (43-45). Iron deficiency, both with and without anemia, has been associated with cognitive difficulties. The iron-deficient but non-anemic 2-year-olds were identified by decreased mean RBC volumes and/or an increased RBC concentration of protoporphyrin (>30 ug/dl) (43). Impairments in intellectual performance in these non-anemic but iron-deficient children were reversed within 7-10 days of beginning iron supplementation.

In another report, this one dealing with 10-year-old anemic children, a standardized achievement test (mathematics, biology, social science, and language) was given to the anemic children and non-anemic controls (45). The non-anemic controls had significantly higher scores than the anemic children. Iron supplementation for 5 months improved the scores of the anemic children, but had no effect on the scores of the non-anemic controls. Placebo had no effect on the scores of either group.

These studies therefore support the hypothesis that iron deficiency, whether or not it is accompanied by anemia, can adversely affect the learning and problem-solving capacity of children. This finding gives additional impetus to the efforts to find iron-deficient individuals, especially children, and treat them. Table 9-2 lists the iron content of some foods.

Zinc

Zinc, like selenium, is a trace element. Unlike selenium, however, enough is known about zinc for an RDA to have been established for it. The RDA for zinc varies from 3 mg for infants under six months of age to 15 mg for adults and 25 mg for nursing women. It has only been recently appreciated that severe zinc deficiency is very common in the world, although not so much in the United States. Zinc deficiency is associated with skin rashes, loss of hair, impaired immune response, digestive problems, reduced taste perception and loss of appetite, defective wound healing, change in behavior and poor growth (46). In the United States, mild to moderate zinc deficiency is often found in vegetarians, especially females and vegans (47), because seafood, meat, and poultry are the best sources of zinc (48). In addition, plant-derived foods often contain substances which prevent the absorption of zinc (more on this below).

Mild zinc deficiency may be rather subtle; in some cases, zinc deficiency may cause failure to achieve growth potential without any obvious stunting or growth

Meat	Milligrams Per 100 Grams (3.5 oz.)	Non-Meat	Milligrams Per 100 Grams (3.5 oz.)
Beef liver, fried	5.7	Pinto beans, boiled	3.0
Hamburger, cooked, lean	2.7	Chickpeas, boiled	3.0
Lamb chop, broiled	1.8	Spinach, raw	2.7
Shrimp	1.8	Raisins, seeded (Muscat)	2.6
Chicken breast, roasted	1.04	Eggs	2.01
Perch	.92	Soybean curd	1.8
		Bean sprouts	1.6
Non-Meat		Broccoli	1.1
		Romaine lettuce	1.1
Filberts (hazelnuts)	8.1	Avocado	1.0
Pistachios	6.7	Iceberg lettuce	0.57
Cashews	6.4	Apple	.18
Whole-wheat bread	3.2		
Enriched white bread	3.0		
Popcorn (popped with oil)	3.0		
White beans, boiled	3.0	Source: U.S. Department of Agriculture	

Iron content of some foods
From FDA Consumer, Sept. 1984, p. 11.

failure (49). The authors concluded that mild zinc deficiency can limit growth in children. This finding, however, is by no means universal—Aboriginal children who have rates of growth less than those of white children were not helped by a zinc supplement (50). In any case, it must be emphasized that zinc supplementation will only allow the deficient child to achieve his growth potential; there is no evidence that zinc will stimulate growth in a non-deficient child, or in a deficient child, beyond his expected height.

The therapeutic use of zinc, has been proposed in several other clinical conditions. For instance, it has been suggested that since a high zinc intake interferes with copper absorption, zinc supplements may prevent the abnormal copper accumulation that accompanies a genetic metabolic disorder known as Wilson's disease (51-53). The results in these case reports were so impressive that the authors opined that a controlled trial was unnecessary to establish the efficacy of zinc in the treatment of this disease. Another investigator, however, has seen little improvement in his zinc-treated Wilson's disease patients (54). This physician concluded that there are obviously some other factors which determine whether a patient will respond to oral zinc. One of the potential advantages of zinc in this disease is that it is much less toxic than the standard drug of choice, penicillamine.

Zinc supplementation has also been shown to be useful in the treatment of the intellectual deterioration that accompanies liver failure due to cirrhosis (55). In this condition, known as hepatic encephalopathy, the existence of a zinc deficiency provides the rationale for supplemental zinc. Anorexia nervosa is another disease which is characterized by a zinc deficiency and which has been reported to be ameliorated by zinc supplementation (56). Zinc deficiency in anorexia nervosa is due both to inadequate intake and poor absorption of zinc (57).

Zinc has also been proposed as having a role in cholesterol dynamics. Rat studies showed that acute zinc deficiency decreased serum cholesterol; most of the drop was due to a fall in HDL (58). Conversely, cholesterol feeding led to decreases in serum zinc levels (59). Both of these animal studies suggest that there is a relationship between serum zinc and cholesterol levels. Strangely enough, *high* doses of zinc (not only zinc deficiency) have also been shown to decrease HDL (60). This raised the concern that zinc supplementation may be atherogenic via its reduction of the "good" HDL cholesterol. Most recently, however, the effects of a daily supplement of about 30 mg of elemental zinc for 8 weeks were studied in sedentary and trained men (61). This level of supplementation is about twice the RDA; nevertheless, neither cholesterol (including HDL) nor triglyceride levels were affected by this zinc supplement. Although the current data are sketchy, it is fair to conclude at the present time that zinc supplementation in RDA amounts has minimal, if any, effects on lipids or cardiac risk.

Zinc intake below half of the RDA amount has been associated with poor pregnancy outcome (62-64). It has also been proposed that zinc deficiency plays a role in other medical problems, including skin disorders (65,66), and prostate diseases (67). While there appears to be some reasonably scientific evidence in support of the former, there is none for the latter. Although the prostate does contain high concentrations of zinc, there is no evidence that zinc deficiency can cause prostate problems, or that zinc supplements can prevent them.

A classic (though rare) dermatologic disorder called acrodermatitis enteropathica was discovered to be caused by zinc deficiency due to failure to properly absorb zinc. Acrodermatitis enteropathica, however, is a rare reason for failure to absorb zinc. Much more common and clinically-relevant factors may also result in zinc malabsorption. For instance, iron coadministered with zinc decreases zinc absorption (68-70). This is especially relevant because many multivitamin/mineral supplements contain more iron than zinc. This problem can usually be avoided by taking the iron and zinc supplements separately, a few hours apart. Studies of the effect of a high-protein diet have shown conflicting results; a recent study (71) concluded that protein at levels commonly consumed by Americans did not affect zinc and copper status.

The effects of tin on zinc absorption have been studied, with conflicting results. While some have shown that moderate amounts of tin— such as the quantity that might be present in food stored in a tin-alloy can—reduced the absorption of zinc (72) while others have not (69).

Fiber, phytate and oxalate, substances usually in abundance in plant foods, interfere with zinc absorption (46,73). This is exacerbated by the fact that these foodstuffs contain very little zinc. Coffee, cheese and cows' milk also reduce zinc absorption in humans (46). On the other hand, red table wine, even with the alcohol removed (74), and human breast milk, enhance zinc absorption (75,76). This appears to be another example of the better nutritional value of human breast milk versus cows' milk or baby formula.

Finally, a study measuring hair concentrations suggested that consumption of hard water (having high calcium content) may decrease zinc absorption (77). In this study, hair zinc in two groups of children from different parts of Canada were compared. Those living in soft-water areas had higher hair zinc concentrations and were slightly heavier and taller than their counterparts in the hard-water area. Hair copper and manganese levels were similar in the two groups of children. For the reasons discussed previously in the section on hair mineral levels, and due to the epidemiologic nature of this study, it is hard to interpret these findings.

Summary and Recommendations

Several surveys have suggested that the average intake of zinc in the United States is below the RDA of 15 mg for adults. The most rigorous of these surveys showed mean intake of 9.9 mg in 28 adult men and women (78). Although the RDA does allow some margin of safety, if only a small percentage of this already low zinc intake is absorbed, it may result in zinc deficiency. As mentioned previously, this would be especially problematic for vegetarians (47), or individuals ingesting iron supplements or large amounts of plant foodstuffs. Zinc deficiency is also common in individuals on low-calorie diets (78), and in very obese patients who have undergone intestinal bypass surgery (79), due to malabsorption.

Thus, it seems reasonable to encourage these individuals to emphasize zinc-rich foods in the diet, including meat, fish, shellfish, poultry and dairy products (48). Oysters are unusually high, but variable, in zinc content, ranging from 5 to 60 mg per ounce (48). Since vegetarians, especially strict vegetarians, are unlikely to ingest these foodstuffs, it is recommended that they take a 10-20 mg supplement of zinc daily. The zinc will probably be best absorbed if taken on an empty stomach, and at least one hour away from meals or intake of iron.

At present, there are no compelling reasons for megadosing with zinc. Although major side effects have not yet been reported with zinc megadosing, the absence of such reports does not certify such practice as safe. An exception might be Wilson's disease, or acrodermatitis enteropathica, but individuals with these conditions will certainly be under medical supervision and should not self-prescribe without the input of their doctor.

Magnesium

Unlike potassium, selenium and zinc, not much has been written about magnesium in the lay press. There are, however, some interesting data which suggest that magnesium deficiency plays a role in sudden death. The data are only preliminary, and primarily epidemiologic in nature. To my knowledge, no magnesium supplementation studies have been published in support of this hypothesis.

Two articles which review the relationship between mineral intake (and heart content) of magnesium and heart disease illustrate the complexity of this association (80,81). The former article found not only a low magnesium level in the hearts of victims of sudden death, but also low levels of iron and potassium and an elevated level of calcium. Whether any of these findings are causative or merely coincidental is unclear at present. The second article adds chromium, selenium, silicon, cadmium, lead, copper and fluoride as additional potential factors in the development of heart disease. At the current state of knowledge it is hard to determine which of these associations is(are) etiologically important.

As a further example of this difficulty, one report showed that individuals who died from heart disease had lower serum selenium concentrations than controls (82). A later report from the same group showed that people who had a high serum level of eicosapentaenoic acid (see Chapter 6) tended to have high serum levels of selenium (83). Thus, it would appear that individuals with higher serum selenium have less heart disease. It might be argued, however, that these individuals have less heart disease because they have high levels of EPA, and not because of their high selenium levels. This, indeed, was the interpretation of the data by these Finnish researchers in their second paper.

As mentioned previously, there are epidemiologic data which support a role for magnesium deficiency in heart disease. One study showed that men who experienced heart attacks were more likely to drink water with low fluoride and magnesium levels than controls (84). In addition to this epidemiologic data, laboratory studies support a role for magnesium in heart disease. For example, dog coronary arteries (85) and human umbilical vessels (86) constricted when magnesium was withdrawn from the liquid that was bathing them; this was reversed by replacement of magnesium. Low magnesium concentrations also potentiated the contractile effects of norepinephrine, acetylcholine, serotonin, angiotensin, and potassium.

This raises the possibility that magnesium deficiency can cause coronary vasospasm. As mentioned in Chapter 6, coronary vasospasm has been occasionally implicated as the cause of heart attacks and even sudden death. This goes along with the observation that of the minerals that are deficient in soft water, magnesium is the only one that has been found to be lowered in the cardiac muscle of sudden death victims. The role of magnesium in blood pressure regulation is also supported by the common use of magnesium sulfate in the treatment of toxemia of pregnancy.

Magnesium has also been proposed as having a role in physical fitness. Plasma magnesium correlated significantly with maximal oxygen consumption (an indicator of physical fitness) in a group of male university varsity athletes

(87). Although the authors hypothesized that magnesium may facilitate oxygen delivery to working muscle tissue, other interpretations are possible. It may be, for instance, that athletes who do more aerobic exercise (e.g., runners) and are more likely to have higher maximal oxygen consumption, also eat greater amounts of food, which leads to higher magnesium levels. In other words, the correlation could be solely coincidental, and not a cause-and-effect relationship. The reader will recall that the only way to establish a cause-and-effect relationship is to compare the effects of magnesium supplementation versus placebo on the maximal oxygen consumption of athletes with low magnesium levels.

A recent survey suggests that the average magnesium intake in American men and women is less than the RDA. Intake for men averaged 323 mg (RDA = 350 mg) and for women was 234 mg (RDA = 300 mg) (88). In addition, daily magnesium balances were negative for both sexes. None of the subjects had any obvious symptoms which were attributable to the magnesium deficiency. Thus, the clinical relevance of marginally failing to meet the magnesium RDA is unknown.

Whole grain products, nuts, and green leafy vegetables are high in magnesium. Overt deficiency symptoms are unusual in normal individuals, but can occur in alcoholics, those with chronic diarrhea and malabsorption syndromes. There is little information on toxicity of magnesium, but absence of such information does not imply the safety of high-dose supplements. One report suggests that magnesium toxicity can lead to respiratory depression and low blood pressure, with potentially fatal results (88a). At the present time, there is no compelling reason to supplement one's diet with magnesium (with the exceptions noted above), but it is unlikely that a daily supplement of about 300 mg or less would be harmful.

Fluoride

The issue of fluoridation has become not only a scientific battle, but a political and emotional one. It has been argued that people ought to have the freedom to choose whether to drink fluoridated water, and that adding fluoride to the public water supply is an infringement of civil rights. This is more of a philosophical question than a medical one, and I will leave the reader to ponder it. The issue of the medical value of fluoride, however, will be briefly discussed. The interested reader is referred to a recent review for further detail (89).

There is considerable agreement among experts that fluoridation of public water supplies is the main reason why the incidence of caries (cavities) has decreased over the past decade or two (90). One reviewer notes that as of 1977, 35,000 papers had been published verifying the effectiveness and safety of water fluoridation (89). Fluoride ingested at optimal levels before eruption of the permanent molars reduces caries about 50-60%. The optimal level is 1 mg per liter (about a quart) of water. Fluoride continues to have its anti-cavity effect even during adult life, though to a lesser extent than during childhood. Excessive levels of fluoride are said to cause a visible mottling of the teeth by some (91); others state that the dental fluorosis "is not generally discernible to the lay person" (92).

In view of the tremendous costs of dental disease, and in view of the above, it is the opinion of many experts (and this author) that fluoride supplements are indicated for all children and adults unless they are drinking optimally fluoridated water. Community water fluoridation is the simplest, most economical mechanism to provide this fluoride "supplement". The argument that fluoridation of public water supplies is an abridgement of certain freedom appears specious since many other such freedoms are abridged for the collective good of society.

Chromium

Little is known about the role of chromium, one of the essential trace elements, in human metabolism. Chromium is necessary for normal carbohydrate and lipid metabolism. It has been suggested that chromium deficiency may impair glucose tolerance, even to the extent of causing diabetes mellitus. At present, however, there is little evidence to support this view. In fact, when the effect of a chromium supplement on glucose metabolism in diabetics was compared to placebo, no differences were noted (93). Lipid levels also showed no change with chromium supplementation.

In view of the current state of knowledge, no recommendations can be made regarding chromium intake. It is unlikely that chromium deficiency will occur if a balanced diet is taken.

MEGAMINERALS: THE BOTTOM LINE

As the reader has no doubt gleaned from this chapter, the need for mineral supplements depends on the age and sex of the subject, as well as his normal diet and other factors. Postmenopausal and lactating women should probably take a calcium supplement, unless their diet is unusually high in this element. Iron supplements should be taken by most menstruating women, unless their diet is especially iron-rich. Zinc supplements should probably be taken by most vegetarians, and definitely by vegans. Advice about selenium is less certain; individuals living in low-selenium areas may well benefit from a selenium supplement, although the resulting benefit may defy measurement. Advice about magnesium is also hard to support scientifically. Fluoride should be taken by all children, and probably most adults, unless fluoridated water is consumed.

It must be emphasized that at best, the above summary recommends only

RDA amounts (or actually less) of these minerals as supplements. There are no indications for the general public to take mega-supplements of any mineral at the present time. Certain unusual diseases, such as Wilson's disease and acrodermatitis eneteropathica may respond to greater-than-RDA amounts of certain minerals. These diseases, however, should be under the care of a physician, and any plans for nutrient supplements should be discussed with this individual.

REFERENCES

1. Schutz HG, et al: Food supplement usage in seven Western states. Am J Clin Nutr 36:897, 1982
2. Food and Nutrition Board: Recommended Dietary Allowances, 10th edition. Washington, D.C. National Research Council, National Academy of Sciences, 1985
3. Hambidge KM: Hair analyses: worthless for vitamins, limited for minerals. Am J Clin Nutr 36:943, 1982
4. Buckley RA, Dreosti IE: Radioisotopic studies concerning the efficacy of standard washing procedures for the cleansing of hair before zinc analysis. Am J Clin Nutr 40:840, 1984
5. Hambidge KM, et al: Chromium, zinc, manganese, copper, nickel, iron and cadmium concentrations in the hair of residents of Chandigarh, India and Bangkok, Thailand. In: Hemphill DD (ed.). Trace Substances in environmental health. VIII. Columbia, MO, University of Missouri, 1974. pp.39
5a. Saner G, et al: Hair manganese concentrations in newborns and their mothers. Am J Clin Nutr 41:1042, 1985
5b. Barrett S: Commercial hair analysis. Science or scam? JAMA 254:1041, 1985
6. Consensus Conference: Osteoporosis. JAMA 252:799, 1984
7. Anonymous: Osteoporosis. Consumer Reports, October, 1984. pp.576
8. Richelson LS, et al: Relative contributions of aging and estrogen deficiency to postmenopausal bone loss. N Engl J Med 311:1273, 1984
9. Drinkwater BL, et al: Bone mineral content of amenorrheic and eumenorrheic athletes. N Engl J Med 311:277, 1984
10. Dalen N, Olsson KE: Bone mineral content and physical activity. Acta Orthop Scand 45:170, 1974
10a. Editorial: Exercise and osteoporosis. Br Med J 290:1163, 1985
11. Parfitt AM: Dietary risk factors for age-related bone loss and fractures. Lancet 2:1181, 1983
11a. Sowers MR, et al: Correlates of mid-radius bone density among postmenopausal women:a community study. Am J Clin Nutr 41:1045, 1985
12. Lutz J: Calcium balance and acid-base status of women as affected by increased protein intake and by sodium bicarbonate ingestion. Am J Clin Nutr 39:281, 1984
13. Dixon AJ: Non-hormonal treatment of osteoporosis. Br Med J 286:999, 1983
14. Heany RP, et al: Calcium nutrition and bone health in the elderly. Am J Clin Nutr 36:986, 1982

15. Horowitz M, et al: Effect of calcium supplementation on urinary hydroxyproline in osteoporotic postmenopausal women. Am J Clin Nutr 39:857, 1984
16. Recker RR, Heaney RP: The effect of milk supplements on calcium metabolism, bone metabolism and calcium balance. Am J Clin Nutr 41:254, 1985
17. Riggs BL, et al: Effects of the fluoride-calcium regimen on vertebral fracture occurrence in postmenopausal osteoporosis. N Engl J Med 306:446, 1982
18. Editorial: Fluoride and the treatment of osteoporosis. Lancet 1:547, 1984
19. Weiss NS, et al: Decreased risk of fractures of the hip and lower forearm with postmenopausal use of estrogen. N Engl J Med 303:1195, 1980
20. Horsman A, et al: The effect of estrogen dose on postmenopausal bone loss. N Engl J Med 309:1405, 1983
20a. Doepel L:Looking at menopauses's role in osteoporosis. JAMA 254:2379, 1985
21. Shamberger RJ: Relationship of selenium to cancer: I. Inhibitory effect of selenium on carcinogenesis. J Natl Cancer Inst 44:931, 1970
22. Thompson HJ, Becci PJ: Selenium inhibition of N-methyl-N-nitrosourea-induced mammary carcinogenesis in the rat. J Natl Cancer Inst65:1299, 1980
23. Greeder GA, Milner JA: Factors influencing the inhibitory effect of selenium on mice inoculated with Ehrlich ascites tumor cells. Science 209:825, 1980
23a. Thomson CD, et al: Effects of supplementation with high-selenium wheat bread on selenium, glutathione peroxidase and related enzymes in blood components of New Zealand residents. Am J Clin Nutr 41:1015, 1985
23b. Robinson JR, et al: Urinary excretion of selenium by New Zealand and North American human subjects on differing intakes. Am J Clin Nutr 41:1023, 1985
24. Shamberger RJ, et al: Antioxidants and cancer. Part VI. Selenium and age-adjusted human cancer mortality. Arch Environ Health 31:231, 1976
25. Schrauzer GN, et al: Cancer mortality correlation studies — III: Statistical associations with dietary selenium intakes. Bioinorg Chem 7:23, 1977
26. Willett WC, et al: Prediagnostic serum selenium and risk of cancer. Lancet 2:130, 1983
27. Salonen JT, et al: Association between serum selenium and risk of cancer. Am J Epidemiol 120:342, 1984
28. Salonen JT, et al: Risk of cancer in realtion to serum concentrations of selenium and vitamins A and E: matched case-control analysis of prospective data. Br Med J 290:417, 1985
28a. Stead RJ, et al: Selenium deficiency and possible increased risk of carcinoma in adults with cystic fibrosis. Lancet 2:862, 1985
29. Yang G, et al: Endemic selenium intoxication in China. Am J Clin Nutr 37:872, 1983
30. Centers for Disease Control: Selenium intoxication — New York. Morbidity and Mortality Weekly Report 33:157, 1984
31. Welsh SO, et al: Selenium in self-selected diets of Maryland residents. J Am Diet Assoc 79:277, 1981
32. Levander OA, Morris VC: Dietary selenium levels needed to maintain balance in north American adults consuming self-selected diets. Am J Clin Nutr 39:809, 1984
33. Finch CA, Cook JD: Iron deficiency. Am J Clin Nutr 39:471, 1984

34. Hallberg L, Rossander L: Effect of soy protein on non-heme iron absorption in man. Am J Clin Nutr 36:514, 1982

35. Lynch SR, et al: Soy protein products and heme iron absorption in humans. Am J Clin Nutr 41:13, 1985

36. Morck TA, et al: Reduction of the soy-induced inhibition of non-heme iron absorption. Am J clin Nutr 36:219, 1982

37. Gillooly M, et al: The relative effect of ascorbic acid on iron absorption from soy-based and milk-based infant formulas. Am J Clin Nutr 40:522, 1984

38. Lynch SR, et al: Iron absorption from legumes in humans. Am J Clin Nutr 40:42, 1984

39. Rossander L, et al: Absorption of iron from breakfast meals. Am J clin Nutr 32:2484, 1979

40. Morck TA, et al: Inhibition of food iron absorption by coffee. Am J Clin Nutr 37:416, 1983

40a. Vasquez-Seone P, et al: Disappearance of iron deficiency anemia in a high-risk infant population given supplemental iron. N Engl J Med 313:1239, 1985

41. Report of the Working Group on Fortification of Salt with Iron: Use of common salt fortified with iron in the control and prevention of anemia — a collaborative study. Am J Clin Nutr 35:1442, 1982

42. Cook JD, Reusser M: Iron fortification, an update. Am J Clin Nutr 38:648, 1983

43. Anonymous: Iron lack, poor performance tied in very young. Ped News 17(12):2, 1983

44. Tucker DM, et al: Iron status and brain function:serum ferritin levels associated with asymmetries of cortical electrophysiology and cognitive performance. Am J Clin Nutr 39:105, 1984

45. Pollitt E, et al: Cognitive effects of iron-deficiency anemia. Lancet 1:158, 1985

46. Solomons NW: Zinc bioavailability: implications for pediatric nutrition. Pediatric Basics, Gerber Products Co., Fremont, MI 49412. #33, October, 1982 p.4

47. Freeland-Graves JH, et al: Zinc status of vegetarians. J Am Diet Assoc 77:655, 1980

48. Murphy EW, et al: Provisional tables on the zinc content of foods. J Am Diet Assoc 66:345, 1975

49. Walravens PA, et al: Linear growth of low-income preschool children receiving a zinc supplement. Am J Clin Nutr 38:195, 1983

50. Smith RM, et al: Growth-retarded Aboriginal children with low plasma zinc levels do not show a growth response to supplementary zinc. Lancet 1:923, 1985

51. Brewer GJ, et al: Oral zinc for Wilson's disease. Ann Intern Med 99:314, 1983

52. Anonymous: Oral zinc therapy for Wilson's disease. Nutrition Rev 42:184, 1984

53. Hoogenraad TU, et al: Effective treatment of Wilson's disease with oral zinc sulphate: two case reports. Br Med J 289:273, 1984

54. Walshe JM: Treatment of Wilson's disease with zinc sulphate. Br Med J 289:558, 1984

55. Reding P, et al: Oral zinc supplementation improves hepatic encephalopathy. Results of a randomized controlled trial. Lancet 2:493, 1984

56. Bryce-Smith D, Simpson RID: Case of anorexia nervosa responding to zinc sulphate. Lancet 2:350, 1984

57. Dinsmore WW, et al: Zinc absorption in anorexia nervosa. Lancet 1:1041, 1985

58. Koo SI, Williams DA: Relationship between the nutritional status of zinc and cholesterol concentration of serum lipoproteins in adult male rats. Am J Clin Nutr 34:2376, 1981

59. Koo SI, Ramlet JS: Dietary cholesterol decreases the serum level of zinc:further evidence for the positive relationship between serum zinc and high-density lipoproteins. Am J Clin Nutr 37:918, 1983

60. Hooper PL, et al: Zinc lowers high-density lipoprotein-cholesterol levels. JAMA 244:1960, 1980

61. Crouse SF, et al: Zinc ingestion and lipoprotein values in sedentary and endurance-trained men. JAMA 252:785, 1984

62. Mukherjee MD, et al: Maternal zinc, iron, folic acid, and protein nutriture and outcome of human pregnancy. Am J Clin Nutr 40:496, 1984

63. Hunt IF, et al: Zinc supplemental during pregnancy: effects on selected blood constituents and on progress and outcome of pregnancy in low income women of Mexican descent. Am J Clin Nutr 40:508, 1984

64. Tuttle S, et al: Zinc and copper in human pregnancy:a longitudinal study in normal primigravidae and in primigravidae at risk of delivering a growth-retarded baby. Am J Clin Nutr 41:1032, 1985

65. Editorial: Skin disease: the link with zinc. Br Med J 289:1476, 1984

66. Fell GS: The link with zinc. Br Med J 290:242, 1985

67. Questions and Answers: Zinc therapy for enlarged prostate? No supportive evidence. JAMA 250:1099, 1983

68. Solomons NW, et al: Studies on the bioavailability of zinc in humans: mechanism of the intestinal interaction of nonheme iron and zinc. J Nutr 113:337, 1983

69. Solomons NW, et al: Studies on the bioavailability of zinc in humans: intestinal interaction of tin and zinc. Am J Clin Nutr 37:566, 1983

70. Valberg LS, et al: Effects of iron, tin and copper on zinc absorption in humans. Am J Clin Nutr 40:536, 1984

71. Colin MA, et al: Effect of dietary zinc and protein levels on the utilization of zinc and copper by adult females. J Nutr 113:1480, 1983

72. Johnson MA, et al: Effects of dietary tin on zinc, copper, iron, manganese and magnesium metabolism in adult males. Am J Clin Nutr 35:1132, 1982

73. Turnlund JR, et al: A stable isotope study of zinc absorption in young men: effects of phytate and alpha-cellulose. Am J Clin Nutr 40:1071, 1984

74. McDonald JT, Margen S: Wine versus ethanol in human nutrition. Am J Clin Nutr 33:1096, 1980

75. Casey CE, et al: Availability of zinc: loading test with human milk, cow's milk and infant formulas. Ped 68:394, 1981

76. Lonnerdal B, et al: The effect of individual components of soy formula and cows' milk formula on zinc bioavailability. Am J Clin Nutr 40:1064, 1984

77. Patterson KY, et al: Zinc, copper, and manganese intake and balance for adults consuming self-selected diets. Am J Clin Nutr 40:1397, 1984

78. Lowy SL, et al: Zinc balance during protein sparing fasts. Fed Proc 40:856, 1981

79. Anderson KE, et al: Some aspects of intestinal absorption of zinc in man. Eur J Clin Pharm 9:423, 1976

80. Chipperfield B, Chipperfield JR: Differences in metal content of the heart muscle in death from ischemic heart disease. Am Heart J 95:732, 1978

81. Karpanen H, et al: Minerals, coronary heart disease and sudden coronary death. Adv Cardiol 25:9, 1978

82. Salonen JT, et al: Association between cardiovascular death and myocardial infarction and serum selenium in a matched-pair longitudinal study. Lancet 2:175, 1982

83. Miettinen TA, et al: Serum selenium concentration related to myocardial infarction and fatty acid content of serum lipids. Br Med J 287:517, 1983

84. Luoma H, et al: Risk of myocardial infarction in Finnish men in relation to fluoride, magnesium, and calcium concentration in drinking water. Acta Med Scand 213:171, 1983

85. Turlapaty PD, Altura BM: Magnesium deficiency produces spasms of coronary arteries: relationship to etiology of sudden death ischemic heart disease. Science 208:198, 1980

86. Altura BM, et al: Magnesium deficiency-induced spasms of umbilical vessels: relation to preeclampsia, hypertension, growth retardation. Science 221:376, 1983

87. Lukaski HC, et al: Maximal oxygen consumption as related to magnesium, copper and zinc nutriture. Am J Clin Nutr 37:407, 1983

88. Lakshmanan FL, et al: Magnesium intakes, balances, and blood levels of adults consuming self-selected diet. Am J Clin Nutr 40:1380, 1984

88a. Fassler CA, et al: Magnesium toxicity as a cause of hypotension and hypoventilation. Occurrence in patients with normal renal function. Arch Intern Med 145:1604, 1985

89. Richmond VL: Thirty years of fluoridation: a review. Am J Clin Nutr 41:129, 1985

90. Leads from Morbidity and Mortality Weekly Report: Dental caries and community water fluoridation trends — United States. JAMA 253:1377, 1985

91. Hein JW: Fluorides and dental caries. Science 220:143, 1982

92. Leverett DH: Fluorides and dental caries. Science 220:144, 1982

93. Uusitupa M, et al: Effect of inorganic chromium supplementation on glucose tolerance, insulin response, and serum lipids in noninsulin-dependent diabetics. Am J Clin Nutr 38:404, 1983

CHAPTER 10

High Blood Pressure—Salt and Other Substances

High blood pressure is the commonest disease in the United States, affecting more than 60 million Americans. It is also often called the silent killer because hypertension (the medical term for high blood pressure), even if severe, often causes no symptoms until the disease has wrought much organ damage. The good news is that hypertension is easily diagnosed, and there has been significant improvement in hypertension detection and control over the past decade (1). Some believe that these improvements in hypertension detection and control are responsible for the recent decline in cardiovascular disease in the United States, an opinion supported by a recent analysis of the Framingham data (2).

It is now quite clear that untreated moderate or severe hypertension increases the risk of heart disease and death (3); treatment of the blood pressure reduces that risk (3,4). It appears that the *type* of treatment (i.e., *how* the blood pressure is lowered) is less important than the degree to which the blood pressure (BP) is decreased. Thus, it is (or should be) the goal of physicians to use methods of lowering BP that have the least side effects.

For instance, it has been shown that weight loss often eliminates the need for drug treatment of hypertension (5), and weight loss not only has no side effects, but has other beneficial effects in addition to blood pressure reduction (see Chapter 13). Unfortunately, obese individuals often find it difficult to reduce weight, and not all hypertensives are overweight to begin with. Such individuals often end up taking antihypertensive medications, and although drugs currently prescribed for high blood pressure are a vast improvement over those of a decade or two ago, all drugs have side effects. If the same BP-lowering can be achieved in non-pharmacologic (non-drug) ways, that would certainly be preferable. A discussion of non-pharmacologic dietary methods to control high blood pressure is the goal of this chapter. This topic has been reviewed in detail recently (5a,5b).

Although sodium has received the most attention as a dietary component which affects blood pressure, several recent articles have focused on the effect of other dietary constituents on the regulation of blood pressure. These include dietary potassium, calcium, magnesium, and even fat and fiber. Prior to discussing these, however, a brief word about hypertension may be in order.

HIGH BLOOD PRESSURE DOES KILL

In the pioneer Veterans Administration study (3), 143 men with severe hypertension were randomly treated with either a blood pressure medication or a placebo. Four deaths and 23 severe complications—heart attacks, strokes, eye and kidney problems—occurred in the placebo group, compared to no deaths and only 2 severe complications in the treated group. Similar findings were noted in a subsequent publication (4) dealing with moderate hypertension.

Although moderate and severe hypertension are clearly dangerous, it is unclear whether mild hypertension is a risk factor for cardiovascular disease. Diastolic blood pressure refers to the lower of the two pressures usually reported, and is measured while the heart is relaxing. The systolic blood pressure (SBP) is the higher of the two pressures, measured while the heart is contracting. Mild hypertension is usually defined as a diastolic blood pressure (DBP) between 90 and 104 mm Hg, although in practice, most physicians consider a DBP over 99 mm Hg to be in the moderate range.

Several extensive and expensive studies attempting to determine whether mild hypertension should be treated have been published in the last few years, but controversy continues. Full discussion of this question is beyond the scope of this book, but the interested reader is referred to several excellent recent reviews and editorials which eloquently present both sides of this question (6-14). In addition, this extremely important topic will be addressed again in the last section of this chapter where recommendations to the individual with mild or borderline hypertension will be made.

ETIOLOGIC FACTORS IN HYPERTENSION

Sodium

Salt, once traded for gold ounce-for-ounce, is now considered "A New Villain", as Time magazine proclaimed in a cover story in the March 15, 1982, issue. According to a recent national poll conducted by the Roper Organization, salt heads the list of food and beverage items that people are concerned about for health reasons (14a). Seventy percent of the respondents said that they were "very" or "somewhat" concerned about salt. Other items of concern (and the percent concerned in parentheses include cholesterol (65%), sugar (63%), caffeine (53%), saccharin (36%), and aspartame (30%). The evidence against salt has been accumulating over several decades, although this certainly hasn't eliminated controversy about its role in the pathogenesis (development) or treatment of hypertension. Several types of studies have been performed to elucidate the salt-hypertension link:

Animal Studies

Scientists in the hypertension field have studied a strain of rat which is salt-sensitive. In this Dahl rat, hypertension develops only if the animal is exposed to a high salt diet. Once established, however, maintenance of hypertension is no longer dependent on a high salt intake (15). The Dahl model may not be relevant to all (or even most) types of human hypertension, because several types of hypertension in man can occur in the virtual absence of salt. What the animal models do tell us is that genetics can play an important role in hypertension, but this is well accepted anyway. For instance, if both parents are hypertensive, 48% of their children will be hypertensive; if only one parent has high blood pressure, 28% of the offspring will have hypertension, but if neither parent has hypertension, only 3% of the children would develop it (16).

Cross-cultural Comparisons

Much has been made of the fact that in primitive societies, most of whom ingest very little salt, hypertension is rare. In addition, blood pressure in these cultures does not rise with age, as it does in ours. For instance, the Yanomano Indians, a tribe inhabiting the tropical rain forests of Brazil and Venezuela, average an intake of 1 mEq (milliequivalent) of sodium per day (17), compared to 150-200 mEq in the United States! Hypertension is essentially non-existent in the Yanomano tribe. One must consider, however, the many other differences, in addition to sodium intake, which exist between the Yanomano and American societies. These include genetics, other dietary differences, body weight, level of exercise, exposure to pollution, etc. As discussed in Appendix A, these are the weaknesses of epidemiologic methods, such as cross-cultural comparisons.

It should also be kept in mind that primitive societies live under Darwin's "rules" of "survival of the fittest" much more than we do. Thus, if a Yanomano Indian has survived to age 40 or 50, he is likely to be a fairly healthy individual and consequently less prone to develop hypertension or suffer from degenerative disease. These factors make it difficult to ascribe differences in blood pressure between populations to a single dietary or lifestyle difference between the populations.

Comparison of Salt Intake Within Western Populations

In view of the foregoing difficulties in making cross-cultural comparisons, many investigators have turned to studying subgroups within "civilized" societies. Many studies have attempted to correlate sodium intake (estimated from urinary excretion of sodium) with prevalence of hypertension. The results of these studies, however, have been as controversial as those involving cross-cultural comparisons.

Most such studies have failed to find a significant correlation between prevalence of hypertension and sodium intake. For instance, salt excretion was compared in normotensive (normal BP) and hypertensive subjects in Scotland (18). Both groups had a similar high salt excretion; the investigators, however, were careful to note that this "does not disprove the salt hypothesis". Another survey also showed no relation between salt intake and prevalence of hypertension. In the latter study, salt intake was estimated from dietary histories (e.g., how often do you eat processed meat or pretzels?). There was no correlation between this very crude estimate of salt intake and hypertension (19). Since it is widely believed that salt is bad, it is possible that the saltaholics in this study underestimated their salt intake.

In addition to the methodological problems of such surveys, two other reasons may explain why such intra-population studies have failed to reveal a correlation between salt intake and BP. One reason is that even individuals who ingest little salt by Western standards ingest much more salt than the human requirement. For instance, only a few percent of the individuals in the studies described above (18,19) ate less than 70-80 mEq sodium/day. This amount represents 8 to 50 times the human requirement. It has been argued that blood pressure is not sensitive to salt intake at these high levels, and that one must ingest less than 50 mEq sodium/day to achieve blood pressure reduction. If this is true, it is unfortunate because such a low intake is not currently practical in most salt-consuming countries.

The most important and likely explanation for the lack of correlation between salt intake and BP—biologic variability—has been alluded to previously. It appears that approximately one in three persons is sensitive to salt intake in the range of 75-300 mEq/day. The rest of the population is sensitive only to very severe sodium restriction (<10-50 mEq/day). Most likely, this salt sensitivity is genetically determined, but current methods cannot identify the sensitive individuals. When a group of subjects is studied, the salt-sensitive individuals are outnumbered by the salt-insensitive individuals, and this is probably responsible for the lack of correlation which has been noted in several studies. Even investigators who do not embrace the salt hypothesis concede the existence of a salt-sensitive subgroup. What has been debated is whether salt restriction for the *whole* population is appropriate if only 20 to 30% of all individuals are likely to benefit.

Human Interventional Studies

This type of study is the "gold standard" in terms of establishing a cause-and-effect relationship between salt intake and hypertension. It is also the least common because it is the most demanding of investigator time and money. Selected studies of this type, in which a group of hypertensive individuals modified their salt intake, are summarized in Table 10-1. These and other studies are also briefly reviewed below.

Kempner, who is usually credited as the pioneer of sodium interventional studies (20), developed a diet which was subsequently modified by Watkins (21,22). Kempner's diet contained 5 g of fat and less than 10 mEq of sodium daily. Patients ate 1/2 to 3/4 pounds of rice per day, prepared in water or juice, with no milk or salt added. All fruits and fruit juices (which are high in potassium and low in sodium) were allowed, except for nuts, dates, avocados, dried or canned fruit. Only one banana was allowed per day, while sugar could be taken without limit, with up to a pound being eaten daily. Most of the patients taking this diet were severely hypertensive and had not responded to the (admittedly limited) medical therapy available in the 1940s.

The results, especially for the mid-1940s, were astounding. About 2/3rds of the 500 patients, who had an average initial BP of 199/116 responded, their BP decreasing to 152/95. It often took 40-50 days for the blood pressure to decrease, and some patients did not respond. There was one major problem with this diet: it is said that no one in his right mind could stick with it for a long period of time. Many investigators were unable to duplicate these results, presumably because of their inability to motivate their patients as Kempner had done (apparently, he had a very authoritarian style, and his patients did exactly what they were told).

Kempner's studies were important, but a diet containing <10 mEq of sodium does not constitute a realistic method of dietary control of blood pressure. The studies in Table 10-1 reduced sodium in a more practical range. Several of these studies are double-blind and placebo-controlled, which increases confidence in their findings. Most of these studies dealt with mild hypertensive patients. One, however, involved normotensive individuals whose parents are hypertensive (26) and another involved normal newborns (30). Of the 9 studies in Table 10-1, 7 showed BP to be significantly lower on a sodium-restricted diet. One study (29) attempted to eliminate or reduce the need for blood pressure medications by reducing sodium intake. By decreasing daily sodium intake from 161 to 37 mEq (an impressive reduction), 80% of the experimental patients were able to either reduce the dose of, or discontinue altogether, their blood pressure medications.

Two studies (31,32) showed no decrease in blood pressure despite a significant reduction in sodium intake. Both had few patients (18 and 12) and short intervention periods (4 weeks). In addition, the mean BP in one study (31) was in the normotensive range (137/83). All of these factors make it more difficult to demonstrate a significant effect of sodium restriction.

Perhaps differences in the cooperation of patients in various studies may also account for negative results. For instance, 5 patients in the Watt (31) study excreted an equal amount or more sodium in their urine while they were supposedly taking placebo pills compared to when they were taking sodium pills.

Table 10-1

Author, year	Ref #	# of subjects	Length of exper. period	Change in Na intake (mEq)	Change in BP (mm Hg)	Does ↓ Na intake ↓ BP?	Comments
Parijs et al, 1973	23	17	1 month	191 to 93	167/113 to 159/109*	YES	Subjects asked to reduce sodium intake on their own. Diurectics reduced BP even further.
Morgan et al, 1978	24	31	2 years	195 to 157	157/101 to 150/94*	YES	Subjects asked to reduce Na intake to <100 mEq/day (but reduction was less). One-third of patients on sodium restriction achieved normal BP.
Parfrey et al, 1981	25 27	15	3 mos.	228 to 123 (K changed from 61 to 123 at same time)	156/103 to 142/94*	YES	During low Na period, subjects also received K supplement, so it is impossible to separate their effect on BP.
Parfrey et al, 1981	26 27	12	2–4 wks.	304 to 164 (K changed from 76 to 179 at same time)	128/75 to 117/64*	YES	Subjects were students whose parents were hypertensive. Note that again, low Na period was supplemented with K.
MacGregor et al, 1982	28	19	4 wks.	162 to 86	154/97 to 144/92*	YES	Subjects asked to reduce Na intake. Then, sodium pills were added to diet in double-blind, placebo-controlled design.
Beard et al, 1982	29	45 per group	3 mos.	161 to 37	133/83 to 131/82*	YES	90 patients on blood pressure medicines were divided into 2 groups. One group was advised to reduce dietary Na intake, and 4 out of 5 people in this group either stopped or reduced the dose of blood pressure med.
Hofman et al, 1983	30	240 per group	6 mos.	417 to 148 (these intakes are per month)	116 vs. 114* (only systolic BP was reported)	YES	One group of newborns was assigned to a low-Na diet, the other to a normal-Na diet from birth. At 6 mos, BP was 2.1 mm lower in the low-Na group than the normal-Na group.
Watt et al, 1983	31	18	4 wks.	143 to 87	137/83 to 136/82	NO	Patients with mild HBP were asked to restrict Na intake. Then sodium pills were added in double-blind placebo-controlled fashion. No change in BP seen.
Richards et al, 1984	32	12	4 wks.	180 to 80	152/102 to 149/102	NO	12 patients were put on 3 diff. diets—reg, low Na, high K (see table 10-2). No change in BP.

Summary of recent studies investigating the effect of dietary sodium on blood pressure

This suggests either a mistake in pill administration or the failure of the patients to restrict their dietary sodium intake.

Another explanation for the lack of response to sodium restriction is the significant variability among patients. For instance, in MacGregor's study (28), despite a reduction in sodium intake in all 19 patients, 5 had no change in BP and one actually had a slight *increase* ! This finding underscores the importance of regular follow-up of hypertensive patients because it is currently impossible to predict who will and who won't respond to various therapeutic maneuvers.

In terms of the amount of blood-pressure-lowering effect, sodium restriction (in sensitive individuals) is usually equal to taking a single Step 1 blood pressure medication (23,24). Beta blockers like propranolol, and diuretics ("water pills") such as hydrochlorothiazide, are the most commonly prescribed Step 1 medications. The effects of sodium reduction and blood pressure pills are additive. Thus, decreasing dietary sodium in responsive patients may eliminate or reduce the need for taking BP medications.

As mentioned previously, sodium isn't the only dietary constituent that may affect blood pressure. A discussion of the blood pressure effects of potassium, calcium, magnesium, fat and fiber, follows. The last section of this chapter will summarize the studies and translate the sometimes difficult-to-understand scientific message into simple recommendations for the reader.

Potassium

Much animal and some human epidemiologic and experimental evidence has suggested that potassium supplementation can decrease blood pressure. Some authorities believe that the hypotensive effects that have been attributed to low-sodium diets may actually be due to the high potassium content of such diets. Interestingly, most unprocessed foods naturally contain little sodium; many such foods (e.g., fruits and some vegetables) contain large amounts of potassium. Thus, diets consisting mainly of unprocessed foods are usually low in sodium and high in potassium. That is perhaps why our body has evolved complex mechanisms (e.g., the aldosterone system) to excrete potassium and conserve sodium. It is only due to the ready availability of salt and its use for curing, preserving and flavoring food that the ratio of sodium to potassium in the diet has changed.

It was actually suggested in the mid-1950s that potassium supplements might lower BP (33). This idea is supported by recent epidemiologic evidence (34,35). Plasma potassium level (34) and estimated dietary potassium intake (35) are inversely related to BP in both men and women. This means that as the dietary intake of potassium or plasma level increases, blood pressure tends to fall.

It is only very recently, however, that the first controlled study of the effect of supplemental potassium on BP in humans was published (36), and only 6 other such studies have been published to date (37-41,32). These are summarized in Table 10-2 and are discussed briefly below.

Six of these seven studies have shown that potassium supplementation decreases blood pressure. The seventh study did not, but drew significant criticisms from several correspondent. One of the major criticisms was that only 12 subjects were studied. In view of biologic variability, as discussed above, such a small sample size may not allow significant effects of potassium supplementation to be seen. This aspect of biologic variability was well demonstrated in MacGregor's study (37), which *did* show potassium to have hypotensive effects. In that study, while 16 of 23 patients had a fall in BP (one had a decrease from a mean arterial pressure of 116 to 92 mm Hg!), 6 patients had essentially no change in BP and one patient's BP *increased* from 103 to 114 mm Hg despite potassium supplementation. If MacGregor's study group had contained only 12 subjects, it is quite possible that the results might not have shown significance.

These studies suggest, therefore, that not all individuals will respond to potassium supplementation (or sodium restriction), emphasizing the importance of follow-up. Furthermore, since all four studies were short-term, it is unclear whether the effects of potassium supplements would remain the same, decrease or even increase with chronic administration.

One of the seven studies (39) investigated normotensive subjects; potassium supplements lowered BP in these individuals also. This suggests that potassium plays a role in normal blood pressure regulation (42). Another finding of these studies was that sodium restriction and potassium supplementation work synergistically in lowering BP. One recent paper suggests that potassium supplementation may decrease BP by enhancing the excretion of sodium (43).

This group of articles on potassium stimulated several letters to the editor. One correspondent (44) noted that Western food preparation methods eliminate much of the natural potassium in food, and add sodium. For instance, boiling potatoes in salted water leaches out 40% of their natural potassium, while steaming them preserves the potassium. One way of preserving natural potassium in potatoes (or any other foodstuff) is to boil them in water containing a potassium-based salt substitute (45). This maneuver can actually *increase* the potassium content of the vegetable. To demonstrate the applicability of this technique, five healthy volunteers were asked to use a salt substitute at home in this manner, without otherwise changing their diet (45). Their urinary potassium excretion (a measure of potassium intake) increased from 67 to 115 mEq/day. If the diet had been further modified to increase intake of fruits and vegetables, potassium intake would have been even higher. Even with this simple modification, however, the increase in dietary potassium was similar to that achieved in the studies listed in Table 10-2. It should also be kept in mind that the use of the potassium salt substitute simultaneously decreases the sodium intake.

Table 10-2

Author, year	Ref #	# of subjects	Length of exper. period	Change in K intake (mEq)	Change in BP (mm Hg)	Does ↓ K intake ↓ BP?	Comments
Iimura et al, 1981	36	20	10 days	41 to 124	114 to 103 (mean art. pressure)	YES	Patients were on normal-Na diet during study, and authors speculated that hypotensive effect of K was due to increased urinary excretion of sodium.
MacGregor et al, 1982	37	23	4 wks.	62 to 118	155/99 to 148/95	YES	Patients were supplemented with K or placebo in double-blind fashion. Fall in BP was not related to sodium excretion.
Morgan, 1982	38	8	4 wks.	46 to 113	158/101 to 148/93	YES	Two weeks of K supplement given to hypertensive subjects. Open design (not double-blind)
Khaw & Thom 1982	39	20	2 wks.	78 to 130	116/72 to 115/70	YES	Subjects were 20 healthy male volunteers who were given K supplement and placebo in double-blind fashion. DBP was significantly lower on K supplement.
Smith et al, 1983	40	10	2 wks.	65 to 128	156/93 to 148/91	YES	Two weeks of supplement in open design, given to hypertensive volunteers.
Overlack et al, 1983	41	16	4wks.	66 to 153	152/98 to 135/88	YES	Non-blind study of potassium supplement.
Richards et al, 1984	32	12	4 wks.	60 to 180	152/102 to 149/100	NO	Patients received K suppl. in unblind fashion. Change in BP was not significant. K suppl. resulted in variable changes in BP.

Summary of recent studies investigating the effect of dietary potassium on blood pressure

An editorial in The Lancet has reviewed the potassium literature and speculated on the potential mechanisms by which potassium might decrease BP (45a).
It pointed out that in hypertensive patients taking diuretics, potassium supplements not only improved diuretic-induced hypokalemia but also decreased BP
(45b). The editorial concluded that "a logical move would be to correct diuretic-
induced hypokalemia in hypertensive patients" and that "if hypokalemia aggra-
vates hypertension, perhaps diuretics should not be used routinely as first-line
treatment".

Several companies have recently introduced low-sodium versions of their
products. Bay and Hartman (46) were concerned that Campbell's new low-
sodium soup had a high potassium content. Their concern was prompted by the
finding that several of their kidney dialysis patients had developed hyperkalemia
(high level of potassium in the blood), which can be dangerous. A representative
of the Campbell Soup Company stated that no potassium is added to the new low-
sodium soup, and that the increased potassium is due to "increased amounts of
vegetables, noodles, chicken . . . all natural products (which) contain potassium". This emphasizes the importance of having absolutely normal kidney
function before embarking on a diet which is high in potassium.

Calcium and Magnesium

Although sodium and potassium are the minerals most often associated with
blood pressure control, recent evidence suggests that it is calcium that is directly
responsible for changes in the blood pressure. It is believed that minerals such as
sodium and potassium influence BP by altering concentrations of calcium in the
cells of the blood vessels. Calcium entry into blood vessel cells makes the blood
vessels constrict, which increases BP. Indeed, three drugs known as "calcium
channel blockers" (verapamil— Calan, Isoptin; nifedipine—Procardia, Adalat;
diltiazem—Cardizem), which block the entry of calcium into these blood vessel
cells, can be used to control high blood pressure.

Several epidemiologic studies have suggested an association between calcium
and blood pressure in humans. Some investigators have found a positive correlation between BP and the calcium level in the blood (47,48), while others have
found the opposite—that individuals with low serum calcium levels (49) or low
dietary calcium intake (50) tend to have higher blood pressure. The latter is
supported by direct experimental evidence that calcium supplementation reduces
BP in spontaneously hypertensive rats (51,52).

This epidemiologic and animal evidence has now been buttressed by several
randomized, double-blind, placebo-controlled studies. One was in normal pregnant women (52a) and another in healthy (normotensive) adults (53). A daily
supplement of 1 gram of elemental calcium led to a significant decrease (5.6% in

women, 9% in men) in diastolic BP (53). The hypotensive effects of calcium supplements have also been demonstrated in hypertensive individuals (53a,b). In both of these controlled trials, about half of the patients responded to approximately 1 g of elemental calcium. It has been proposed that the primary abnormality in essential hypertension is that too much calcium is allowed *into* the cells of blood vessels. For instance, calcium levels in platelets of hypertensive patients were higher than those in platelets of normotensive individuals (54). Treatment of the hypertensive patients with calcium channel blockers decreased calcium levels within the platelets, and this correlated with the fall in the patient's BP (54). Interestingly, two other types of drugs which are used to treat high blood pressure (beta blockers and diuretics) also resulted in a reduction in intracellular calcium. This again suggests that calcium is the mediator or "final common pathway" by which various factors alter BP.

The mechanism by which supplemental calcium might decrease BP is unclear. Indeed, in view of the foregoing discussion, one might expect that a calcium supplement would increase the amount of calcium in the blood, and that consequently more calcium would enter the blood vessel cells and cause them to contract. However, if most of the supplemental calcium stays in the bloodstream *outside* the blood vessel cells, this may actually *relax* the blood vessels (54,55) and consequently, lower BP. Thus, the *ratio* of calcium in the bloodstream to inside the blood vessel cells may be a more important determinant of BP than the absolute calcium concentrations in either compartment.

Though less is known about it, magnesium has had a long history of use in the treatment of conditions characterized by high blood pressure. In fact, magnesium sulfate is the drug of choice for treating preeclampsia, an abnormal condition during pregnancy characterized by hypertension.

Only a few studies of magnesium in essential hypertension have been published. One showed an inverse correlation between serum magnesium concentrations and BP in normal elderly Danish subjects (57). Magnesium may act as a calcium antagonist and an excess of magnesium may prevent calcium entry into cells. On the other hand, magnesium deficiency may lead to increased concentrations of calcium in the blood vessel cells, which results in contraction of the blood vessels (58). Another study (59) and the accompanying editorial (60) suggest that although magnesium sometimes antagonizes the actions of calcium, it can also mimic them. It has also been proposed that the changes in mineral level may vary with the type of hypertension (61).

Only two studies have investigated the effects of magnesium supplementation (62,62a). In the first, 20 hypertensive patients on diuretics ("water pills") received a daily supplement of 360 mg (=RDA) of magnesium, while 19 hypertensive patients served as controls. Systolic and diastolic BPs decreased significantly in the experimental group, by a mean of 12/8 mm Hg. Only one of the 20 patients had no decrease in BP. The controls had no change in BP. The mechanism by which magnesium decreased the blood pressure was not readily apparent, but it is possible that magnesium would have this effect only in patients receiving diuretics.

The second study (62a), unlike the first, was a double-blind study; it showed that magnesium supplementation had no hypotensive effect in 17 mild to moderate essential hypertensives. One major difference is that these patients, unlike those in the first study, were not taking diuretics or any other antihypertensive drugs. However, bias also is possible in the first study since it was neither double-blind nor placebo-controlled. The second study lasted only one month, and therefore, no definite conclusions can be drawn about longer periods of supplementation. This issue must be considered to be unsettled at this time, pending the performance of additional controlled studies.

For further detail, the interested reader should consult a recent editorial on the role of magnesium as the body's own "calcium blocker" (63).

Vegetarian Diet, Fat, and Fiber

Several epidemiologic studies have suggested that vegetarian diets can lower BP (64-66). Many of these studies have compared vegetarian Seventh Day Adventists and omnivorous Mormons; the two faiths are said to be similar in their avoidance of stimulants, tobacco and alcohol, but differ in their dietary habits. As mentioned previously, however, epidemiologic studies cannot establish cause and effect.

A recent randomized controlled trial assessed the effects of vegetarian diet on BP in a group of 59 healthy (normotensive), normally omnivorous volunteers (67). The subjects ate the lacto-ovo-vegetarian diet (no animal flesh allowed, but eggs and dairy products were ingested) for six weeks. Systolic and diastolic BP fell an average of 5-6 and 2-3 mm Hg, respectively, and rose after resuming the omnivorous diet.

This study showed that the vegetarian diet does lower BP, although the factor(s) responsible for this is(are) unclear. Urinary sodium and potassium excretion did not change, suggesting that neither of these minerals were responsible for the decrease in BP. Two recent studies (68,69) also showed that vegetarians do not have a different sodium intake from non-vegetarians, but both studies suggested that vegetarians do have a somewhat greater intake of potassium than omnivorous subjects. Identification of the dietary factor responsible for the lower BP in vegetarians will have to await further studies (70).

Some have suggested that the BP-lowering effect of the vegetarian diet is due to its lower fat content, or the higher ratio of polyunsaturated to saturated fat (71-73). Only recently, however, has a controlled clinical trial directly examined the effect of dietary fat on blood pressure (74,75). Fifty-seven couples consisting of both hypertensive and normotensive individuals were randomized to three groups. Group I followed a low-fat (high polyunsaturated fat) diet, group II reduced sodium intake, and group III maintained the usual diet. After a 6-week intervention period, groups I and II reverted to their usual diet. BP in the low-fat group (group I) decreased from 138/89 to 130/81; BP returned to baseline after switching back to the regular diet. This study suggests that the low fat content and the high P/S ratio of the vegetarian diet may be responsible for the hypotensive effect of this diet.

It has also been suggested that the hypotensive effect of the vegetarian diet may be due to its high fiber content (76). This is a complicated question because there are many different types of dietary fiber (see Chapter 11 for a more detailed discussion of this). The data at this point are not sufficiently clear to determine whether fiber does indeed have independent hypotensive effects. In a sense, identifying the specific factor responsible for the hypotensive effect is an academic question because the vegetarian diet is simultaneously high in polyunsaturated fat, potassium and fiber, and low in sodium. It may be that all these factors contribute to the BP-lowering effect of the vegetarian diet.

Weight Loss

It has been appreciated for quite some time that weight reduction is accompanied by decreased blood pressure. The mechanism of the fall in BP is not clear. It may be due to decreased intake of sodium which accompanies the decrease in general food intake, but weight reduction can result in decreased BP even if sodium intake is unchanged (77). Thus, weight reduction and decreased salt intake appear to have independent and additive effects in reducing blood pressure (78). As is true of the maneuvers discussed above, several simultaneous dietary alterations are more likely to decrease BP than a single change; thus, it is sensible to reduce sodium intake as well as weight while attempting to decrease BP.

Alcohol

Although not well appreciated even by physicians, there is significant evidence that alcohol, even in small amounts, raises blood pressure. The evidence is both epidemiologic (79,80) and experimental (81,81a). Alcohol did not affect blood pressure in normotensive volunteers, but increased the BP in both hypertensive non-drinkers and habitual drinkers (81a). In another study, however, alcohol increased BP in normotensive habitual drinkers (81b). The hypertensive effect of alcohol is noted even at a moderate level of consumption, e.g., 1-2 drinks per day. As mentioned in Chapter 6, alcohol does appear to increase HDL, and some have argued that moderate intake of alcohol should be recommended.

However, alcohol does not seem to raise the more beneficial type of HDL (HDL$_2$), and in addition, there is no direct evidence that raising HDL decreases cardiac risk. In view of the other detrimental effects of alcohol, it is this author's opinion that at present, alcohol intake should not be recommended to individuals who do not already imbibe. Furthermore, those who do drink should be advised to cut down or eliminate their intake if they are hypertensive.

Miscellaneous

Many factors other than those discussed above have been proposed as either risk factors, or potentially therapeutic in hypertension. For instance, snoring has been shown to be a risk factor for hypertension and angina pectoris (82). Chewing tobacco has been shown to contain large amounts of sodium, which may contribute to hypertension (83). Since anxiety may be potentially contributory to hypertension (84), several papers have been published on the use of relaxation therapy and biofeedback to treat hypertension (e.g., 85). A 16-week aerobic exercise program significantly reduced BP in hypertensives (85a). A recent position paper by the American College of Physicians concludes that biofeedback and relaxation therapies may be useful in the treatment of hypertension.

THE BOTTOM LINE: SUMMARY AND RECOMMENDATIONS

Many studies linking diet to blood pressure regulation in both normotensive and hypertensive individuals have been presented. Some of the data are seemingly contradictory, although upon closer examination, differences in study goals and designs may account for the discrepancies. For instance, it may seem perplexing that one study (31) has failed to confirm the hypotensive effect of a low-sodium diet until it is noted that (1) the degree of hypertension was milder than in most of the other studies, (2) the experimental periods lasted only 4 weeks (most of the positive studies lasted 8 to 12 weeks, and one lasted 2 years), (3) only a mild degree of sodium restriction was achieved, and (4) 4 of the 18 subjects demonstrated essentially no reduction in sodium intake. Any one of these reasons could by itself account for the lack of positive results; all four factors operating in concert virtually ensure negative results.

The effects of diet on BP have been reviewed in some detail above. The extensive and sometimes-contradictory discussion may have left the reader confused. This final section of the chapter will translate the multiple studies presented into simple and practical suggestions for the reader. The interested reader is also encouraged to consult several excellent reviews (5a,14,87,88) which deal with this question in more detail.

A review of the literature suggests that a person of (1) normal weight (2) who ingests a diet moderate in sodium (<2 g sodium = 5 g sodium chloride = 88 mEq) (3) low in fat, especially the saturated type (4) high in fresh fruits and vegetables (5) normal to high in calcium and magnesium, is very unlikely to develop hypertension. In normotensive patients, these maneuvers may prevent hypertension that might otherwise have developed, or may minimize the degree of blood pressure elevation if hypertension does develop. My guess is that a person pursuing such a diet would have less than a 5% life-long risk of developing hypertension, compared to the national average risk of 30-40%. In addition, probably 75% of individuals already hypertensive can achieve normal blood pressures by following the 5 dietary maneuvers noted above.

All hypertensive individuals, including those with mild hypertension, should be counseled on these five dietary points. Since it has been shown that physicians' knowledge of sodium content of foods is no greater than that of the general public (89), physicians who treat many hypertensive and diabetic patients may choose to incorporate the services of a dietitian in their practice. Furthermore, a dietitian may be invaluable in teaching and motivating patients who have diseases which are potentially diet-responsive (90). Utilizing a dietitian's services is also much more cost-effective than using physicians' services for this purpose.

It is worth noting that all the dietary recommendations discussed above are beneficial not only in their effects on blood pressure, but also in other ways. For instance, eating vegetarian and low fat diets, drinking little alcohol, and losing weight are all healthy lifestyle modifications. The more benefits that an individual obtains from an alteration in lifestyle, the more likely he is to maintain that new lifestyle, even though it may be difficult. For example, an obese, hypertensive hypercholesterolemic patient may correct all of these abnormalities without the need for drug therapy simply by changing his diet and losing weight.

Some general comments and recommendations can be made about sodium. It is clear that severe dietary sodium restriction (<10 mEq/day), while unrealistic (in the United States, at least) is effective in decreasing BP in most hypertensive patients. It is also clear that approximately one-third of hypertensive individuals will respond to much milder dietary sodium restriction (70-100 mEq/day). In hypertensive patients who require BP medication, sodium restriction will likely potentiate the effects of the medication, or possibly eliminate the need for the drug altogether. Since there are no side effects of a moderately-sodium-restricted diet, and in view of our inability to identify the salt-sensitive patients, all hypertensive patients (and probably *most* individuals) should strive for such a diet.

Eating a low-sodium diet does not have to be unpleasant. Indeed, hypertensive patients taking blood pressure pills in one study (quoted above (29)) decreased their sodium intake from 161 to 37 mEq per day; 80% of these patients were able to reduce the dose or stop taking high blood pressure medications altogether. Despite the drastic reduction in sodium intake, "The diet group reported feeling happier, less depressed and less dependent on analgesics [pain medicines]. Two thirds of the diet group intend to continue the [low-sodium] diet indefinitely" (29).

All individuals, including healthy non-hypertensive persons, can benefit from the low-sodium, low-fat high-fiber diet described above. Individuals with cardiac risk factors such as hypertension, diabetes, hypercholesterolemia, and smoking, should be especially encouraged to pursue this prudent diet. Those with mild hypertension, however, may be treated somewhat differently than those with moderate to severe hypertension.

In patients with documented moderate to severe hypertension, non-pharmacologic therapy should be initiated simultaneously with drug therapy to bring blood pressure rapidly under control. As BP is controlled, drug therapy may be tapered or discontinued totally, especially if the patient is complying well with non-drug therapy. This is obviously simplistic, in that many other factors may affect actual treatment decisions.

The approach to mild hypertension is more controversial than that described above for moderate to severe hypertension. Current evidence suggests that sustained mild hypertension (DBP between 90 and 100 mm Hg) may be a risk factor for heart disease, especially if other risk factors— smoking, overweight, diabetes mellitus, family history of severe hypertension, stroke or cardiovascular disease—are also present. Since all drugs have side effects, non-pharmacologic treatment of mild hypertension should be vigorously pursued before drug therapy is recommended. This is underscored by the findings of the MRFIT (Multiple Risk Factor Intervention Trial). This study showed that in people with abnormal electrocardiograms, drug treatment of hypertension with thiazide diuretics ("water pills") was associated with *increased* mortality (there is still much controversy over this point).

Thus, individuals with mild hypertension should initially be aggressively counseled on non-drug means of controlling BP. As emphasized previously, regular follow-up is very important, since some patients won't comply, and not all those that comply will respond to therapy. In addition, follow-up visits present an opportunity to reinforce and expand upon recommendations given previously.

Without pharmacologic treatment, up to one-half of mild hypertensive patients will revert to a normal BP with non-drug therapy. One-quarter will remain mildly hypertensive and the remaining quarter will advance to more severe hypertension and require more vigorous treatment.

Most physicians, upon discovering that a patient has mild hypertension, will advise on non-pharmacologic means of BP-control and recheck BP in 3 months. A consultation with a dietitian may be helpful at this stage. If BP has normalized in the interim, the patient should be encouraged to continue his apparently-successful non-drug efforts and his BP should be rechecked every six months. On the other hand, if BP remains in the mild hypertensive range, non-pharmacologic means of controlling BP should be reviewed with the patient and his BP checked again in another three months. If BP remains elevated at that point, the patient should probably be given the option of drug therapy, taking his lifestyle and other cardiovascular risk factors into account. Each individual has to make a value judgement as to how difficult he would find it to comply with drug therapy versus the hope of obtaining probable but not certain benefits. If drug therapy is initiated, frequent BP checks are warranted initially, to ensure that adequate but not excessive BP-lowering-effect is achieved. Furthermore, even if drug therapy is initiated, the patient should continue to be encouraged to pursue non-drug therapy. For instance, continued weight loss may obviate the need for drug therapy in the future.

The astute reader will note that I have not included magnesium, calcium or potassium supplementation as first-line therapy for high blood pressure. There are several reasons for this:

(1) Only a few studies of potassium, magnesium and calcium supplementation have been published. Some of these studies dealt only with normotensive individuals, making it difficult to extrapolate the conclusions to hypertensive patients. Thus, neither the benefits nor the risks of such therapy are well known.

(2) I believe the maneuvers presented above have less risk, and have benefits other than blood pressure control, and therefore should be tried first.

(3) Since potassium, magnesium and calcium have only recently been studied in humans, side effects of large supplements are not yet well appreciated. It is known, however, that excessive potassium can be lethal in individuals with marginal kidney function (a condition to which hypertensive patients are predisposed). We also know that calcium supplements can increase the risk of kidney stones in susceptible individuals.

This opinion may change in the near future, if further controlled studies support the safety and efficacy of supplementationwith these minerals. In addition, there are certain circumstances in which supplementation with these minerals would be appropriate. For instance, it is known that the majority of postmenopausal women do not get their RDA of calcium, and it would be especially reasonable (in fact, recommended) for a hypertensive postmenopausal (or close to it) woman to take a 500 to 1000 mg daily supplement of elemental calcium. It may also be reasonable for hypertensive patients on diuretics to take up to 360 mg of magnesium per day (and perhaps potassium) since some diuretics promote excretion of these minerals from the body. It should also be kept in mind that persons who use salt substitutes are actually taking a potassium supplement.

These supplements should be taken under physician supervision, especially for patients already under a physician's care. Some suplements can interact with prescription medications, with potentially dangerous results. For instance, one type of diuretic which is given to hypertensive patients markedly decreases the urinary excretion of potassium. Taking a potassium supplement in addition to such a drug can lead to dangerous levels of potassium in the blood. People with certain forms of cancer or other medical conditions may already have very high levels of calcium in their blood and obviously, a calcium supplement would not be in order. Thus, self-treatment with these minerals is ill-advised, and careful follow-up, with appropriate laboratory monitoring, is essential.

REFERENCES

1. Folsom AR, et al: Improvement in hypertension detection and control from 1973-1974 to 1980-1981. The Minnesota Heart Survey experience. JAMA 250:916, 1983
2. Hofman A, et al: Does change in blood pressure predict herta disease? Br Med J 287:267, 1983
3. Veterans Administration Cooperative Study Group on Antihypertensive Agents: Effects of treatment on morbidity in hypertension: Results in patients with diastolic blood pressure averaging 115 through 129 mm Hg. JAMA 202:1028, 1967
4. Veterans Administration Cooperative Study Group on Antihypertensive Agents: Effects of treatment on morbidity in hypertension: Results in patients with diastolic blood pressure averaging 90 through 114 mm Hg. JAMA 213:1143, 1970
5. Kannel WB, et al: The relationship of adiposity to blood pressure and development of hypertension. The Framingham Study. Ann Intern Med 67:48, 1967
5a. Kaplan NM: Non-drug treatment of hypertension. Ann Int Med 102:359, 1985
5b. Truswell AS: Diet and hypertension. Br Med J 291:125, 1985
6. Freis ED: Should mild hypertension be treared? N Engl J Med 307:306, 1982
7. Pickering TG: Treatment of mild hypertension and the reduction of cardiovascular mortality: the "of" or "by" dilemma. JAMA 249:399, 1983
8. Kaplan NM: Therapy for mild hypertension. Toward a more balanced view. JAMA 249:365, 1983
9. Paul O: Hypertension and its treatment. JAMA 250:939, 1983
10. Editorial: Hypertension, risk and left ventricular hypertrophy. Lancet 1:941, 1984
11. Goldsmith M: 'Blood Pressure Month brings recommendations. JAMA 251:2193, 1984
12. Moser M: Clinical trials, diuretics, and the management of mild hypertension. Ann Intern Med 144:789, 1984
13. Kaplan NM: Response to Dr. Moser's commentary. Ann Intern Med 144:792, 1984
14. JNC: The 1984 Report of the Joint National Committee on Detection, Evaluation and Treatment of High Blood Pressure. Arch Intern Med 144:1045, 1984
14a. Update: Salt heads health concerns. FDA Consumer, Dec, 1984-Jan, 1985, pp.3
15. Dahl LK, et al: Effects of chronic excess salt ingestion: evidence that genetic factors play an important role in susceptibility to experimental hypertension. J Exp Med 115:1173, 1962
16. Ayman D: Heredity in arteriolar (essential. hypertension: a clinical study of blood pressure of 1524 members of 277 families. Arch Intern Med 53:792, 1934 17. Oliver WJ,

et al: Blood pressure, sodium intake, and sodium related hormones in the Yanomano Indians, a "No Salt" culture. Circulation 52:146, 1975

18. Beevers DG, et al: Salt and blood pressure in Scotland. Br Med J 281:641, 1980
19. Holden RA, et al: Dietary salt intake and blood pressure. JAMA 250:365, 1983
20. Kempner W: Treatment of hypertensive vascular disease with rice diet. Am J Med 4:545, 1948
21. Watkin DM, et al: Effects of diet in essential hypertension. I. Baseline study: Effects in eighty-six cases of prolonged hospitalization on regular hospital diet. Am J Med 9:428, 1950
22. Watkin DM, et al: Effects of diet in essential hypertension. II. Results with unmodified Kempner rice diet in fifty hospitalized patients. Am J Med 9:441, 1950
23. Parijs J, et al: Moderate sodium restriction and diuretics in the treatment of hypertension. Am Heart J 85:22, 1973
24. Morgan T, et al: Hypertension treated by salt restriction. Lancet 1:227, 1978
25. Parfrey PS, et al: Blood pressure and hormonal changes following alteration in dietary sodium and potassium in mild essential hypertension. Lancet 1:59, 1981
26. Parfrey PS, et al: Blood pressure and hormonal changes following alteration in dietary sodium and potassium in young men with and without a familial predisposition to hypertension. Lancet 1:113, 1981
27. Holly JMP, et al: Re-analysis of data in two Lancet papers on the effect of dietary sodium and potassium on blood pressure. Lancet 2:1384, 1981
28. MacGregor GA, et al: Double-blind randomized crossover trial of moderate sodium restriction in essential hypertension. Lancet 1:351, 1982
29. Beard TC, et al: Randomized controlled trial of a no-added-sodium diet for mild hypertension. Lancet 2:455, 1982
30. Hofman A, et al: A randomized trial of sodium intake and blood pressure in new-bormn infants. JAMA 250:370, 1983
31. Watt GCM, et al: Dietary sodium restriction for mild hypertension in general practice. Br Med J 286:432, 1983
32. Richards AM, et al: Blood pressure response to moderate sodium restriction and to potassium supplementation in mild essential hypertension. Lancet 1:757, 1984
33. Meneely GR, et al: Chronic sodium chloride toxicity: the protective effect of added potassium chloride. Ann Int Med 47:263, 1957
34. Bulpitt CJ, et al: Blood pressure and plasma sodium and potassium. Clinical Science 61:85s, 1981
35. Khaw KT, Barrett-Connor, E: Dietary potassium and blood pressure in a population. Am J Clin Nutr 39:963, 1984
36. Iimura O, et al: Studies on the hypotensive effect of high potassium intake in patients with essential hypertension. Clinical Science 61:77s,1981
37. MacGregor GA, et al: Moderate potassium supplementation in essential hypertension. Lancet 2:567, 1982
38. Morgan TO: The effect of potassium and bicarbonate ions on the rise of blood pressure caused by sodium chloride. Clin Sci (suppl)63:407S, 1982
39. Khaw KT, Thom S: Randomized double-blind cross-over trial of potassium on blood-pressure in normal subjects. Lancet 2:1127, 1982

40. Smith SJ, et al: Does potassium lower blood pressure by increasing sodium excretion? A metabolic study in patients with mild to moderate essential hypertension. J Hypertension 1(suppl 2):27, 1983

41. Overlack A, et al: Long-term antihypertensive effect of oral potassium in essential hypertension. J Hypertension 1 (suppl 2:165, 1983

42. Letters to editor: Potassium supplements and hypertension. Lancet 1:1189, 1984

43. Voors AW, et al: Relation between ingested potassium and sodium balance in young Blacks and whites. Am J Clin Nutr 37:583, 1983

44. Henningsen NC, et al: Hypertension, potassium and the kitchen. Lancet 1:133, 1983

45. Smith SJ, et al: Potassium: The kitchen revisited. Lancet 1:363, 1983

45a. Editorial: Dietary potassium and hypertension. Lancet 1:1308, 1985

46. Bay WH, Hartman JA: High potassium in low-sodium soups. N Engl J Med 308:1166, 1983

47. Bulpitt CJ, et al: The relationship between blood pressure and biochemical risk factors in a general population. Br J Prev Soc Med 30:158, 1976

48. Kesteloot H, Geboers J: Calcium and blood pressure. Lancet 1:813, 1982

49. McCarron DA: Low serum concentrations of ionized calcium in patients with hypertension. N Engl J Med 307:226, 1982

50. Ackley S, et al: Dairy products, calcium and blood pressure. Am J Clin Nutr 38:457, 1983

51. Ayachi S: Increased dietary calcium lowers blood pressure in the spontaneously hypertensive rat. Metabolism 28:1234, 1979

52. McCarron DA: Age-dependent attenuation of hypertension in the spontaneously hypertensive rat by dietary supplementation. Proc 4th Internat Symp on Rats with Spontaneous Hypertension. Stuttgart:Schattauer Verlag, 1982. p. 122-125.

52a. Belizan JM, et al: Preliminary evidence of the effect of calcium supplementation on blood pressure in normal pregnant women. Am J Obstet Gynecol 146:175, 1983

53. Belizan JM, et al: Reduction of blood pressure with calcium supplementation in young adults. JAMA 249:1161, 1983

53a. Resnick L, et al: Outpatient therapy of essential hypertension with dietary calcium supplementation (abstract). J Am Coll Cardiol 3:616, 1984

53b. McCarron DA, Morris C: Oral calcium in mild to moderate hypertension: a randomized, placebo-controlled trial (abstract). Clin Res 32:335A, 1984

54. Erne P, et al: Correlation of platelet calcium with blood pressure. Effect of antihypertensive therapy. N Engl J Med 310:1084, 1984

55. Bohr DF: Vascular smooth muscle: dual effect of calcium. Science 139:597, 1963

56. Webb RC, Bohr DF: Mechanism of membrane stabilization by calcium in vascular smooth muscle. Am J Physiol 225:C227, 1978

57. Petersen B, et al: Serum and erythrocyte magnesium in normal elderly Danish people. Acta Med Scand 210:31, 1977

58. Altura BM, Altura BT: Role of magnesium ions in contractility of blood vessels and skeletal muscles. Magnesium Bulletin 1a:102, 1981

59. Cholst IN, et al: The influence of hypermagnesemia on serum calcium and parathyroid hormone levels in human sunjects. N Engl J Med 310:1221, 1984

60. Levine BS, Coburn JW: Magnesium, the mimic/antagonist of calcium. N Engl J Med 310:1253, 1984

61. Resnick LM, et al: Divalent cations in essential hypertension. Relations bewtween serum ionized calcium, magnesium and plasma renin activity. N Engl J Med 309:888, 1983

62. Dyckner T, Wester PO: Effect of magnesium on blood pressure. Br Med J 286:1847, 1983

62a. Cappuccio FP, et al: Lack of effect of oral magnesium on high blood pressure: a double-blind study. Br Med J 291:235, 1985

63. Iseri LT, French JH: Magnesium: Nature's physiologic calcium blocker. Am Heart J 108:188, 1984

64. Sacks FM, et al: Blood pressure in vegetarians. Am J Epidemiol 100:390, 1974

65. Anholm AC: The relationship of a vegetarian diet and blood pressure. Prev Med 4:35, 1975

66. Rouse IL, et al: Vegetarian diet, lifestyle and blood pressure in two religious populations. Clin Exp Pharmacol Physiol 9:327, 1982

67. Rouse IL, et al: Blood-pressure-lowering effect of a vegetarian diet: controlled trial in normotensive subjects. Lancet 1:5, 1983

68. Armstrong B, et al: Urinary sodium and blood pressure in vegetarians. Am J Clin Nutr 32:2472, 1979

69. Ophir O, et al: Low blood pressure in vegetarians: the possible role of potassium. Am J Clin Nutr 37:755, 1983

70. Editorial: Diet and hypertension. Lancet 1:1344, 1983

71. Iacono JM, et al: Reduction in blood pressure associated with high polyunsaturated fat diets that reduce blood cholesterol in man. Prev Med 4:426, 1975

72. Harsha RR, et al: Effect of polyunsaturated rich vegetable oils on blood pressure in essential hypertension. Clin Exp Hypertens 3:27, 1981

73. Enholm C, et al: Effect of a low-fat high P/S diet on serum lipoproteins in a free-living population with a high incidence of coronary heart disease. N Engl J Med 307:850, 1982

74. Puska P, et al: Controlled, randomized trial of the effect of dietary fat on blood pressure. Lancet 1:1, 1983

75. Iacono JM, et al: Effect of dietary fat on blood pressure in a rural Finnish population. Am J Clin Nutr 38:860, 1983

76. Wright A, et al: Dietary fibre and blood pressure. Br Med J 2:1541, 1979

77. Reisin E, et al: Effect of weight loss without salt restriction on the reduction of blood pressure in overweight hypertensive patients. N Engl J Med 298:1, 1978

78. Fagerberg B, et al: Blood pressure control during weight reduction in obese hypertensive men: separate effects of sodium and energy restriction. Br Med J 288:11, 1984

79. Klatsky AL, et al: Alcohol consumption and blood pressure: Kaiser-Permanente Multiphasic Health Examination data. N Engl J Med 296:1194, 1977

80. Cooke KM, et al: Blood pressure and its relationship to low levels of alcohol consumption. Clin Exp Pharmacol Physio 10:229, 1983

81. Potters JF, Beevers DG: Pressor effect of alcohol in hypertension. Lancet 1:119, 1984

81a. Malhotra H, et al: Pressor effects of alcohol in normotensive and hypertensive subjects. Lancet 2:584, 1985

81b. Howes LG: Pressor effect of alcohol. Lancet 2:835, 1985

82. Koskenvuo M, et al: Snoring as a risk factor for hypertension and angina pectoris. Lancet 1:893, 1985

83. Hampson NB: Smokeless is not saltless. N Engl J Med 312:919, 1985

84. Page EW: Hypertensive disorders of pregnancy. Thomas Springfield, Illinois, 1953

85. Little BC, et al: Treatment of hypertension in pregnancy by relaxation and biofeedback. Lancet 1:865, 1984

85a. Duncan JJ, et al: The effects of aerobic exercise on plasma catecholamines and blood pressure in patients with mild essential hypertension. JAMA 254:2609, 1985

86. Health and Public Policy Committee, American College of Physicians: Position paper: Biofeedback for hypertension. Ann Intern Med 102:709, 1985

87. Tillotson JL, et al: Critical behaviors in the dietary management of hypertension. J Am Diet Assoc 84:290, 1984

88. Boon NA, Aronson JK: Dietary salt and hypertension: treatment and prevention. Br Med J 290:949, 1985

89. Heidrich FE, Bergman JJ: Physician knowledge of sodium content of common foods. J Fam Pract 14:693, 1982

90. Lang C, et al: Dietary counseling results in effective dietary sodium restriction. J Am Diet Assoc 85:477, 1985

CHAPTER 11

Should You Eat Like a Bantu? (Or, The Role of Fiber in Health and Disease)

The role of fiber in health and disease has received considerable attention in the lay and scientific press in the past decade, although the information obtained via this research is still not widely appreciated by physicians. Instead, the health food movement seems to have been captivated by fiber and roughage, and probably rightly so. Nevertheless, orthodox medicine is beginning to recognize some of the physiological effects of fiber. Indeed, a symposium on fiber was held in Washington, D.C., in 1981; a summary of that meeting was published the following year (1). More recently, two fiber-related reviews appeared in the prominent journal, The Lancet (2,3).

High-fiber diets have been touted as beneficial in individuals with hypercholesterolemia, diverticulosis, diabetes mellitus, and obesity, and have been proposed as potentially useful in preventing the second most common cancer in the United States, colorectal cancer (4). Furthermore, side effects of reasonable high-fiber diets are usually mild. In addition, a high-fiber diet can be palatable, and may even be more economical than other diets. Last but not least, most foods that are high in fiber, e.g., fruits, vegetables, cereals and legumes, are also healthy for other reasons besides their fiber content. For instance, most high-fiber foods tend to be low in calories, cholesterol, saturated fat, and sodium, and high in vitamins and some minerals. Therefore, high fiber foods appear to be one of the few true "bargains" in meal planning.

Before examining the evidence that supports the foregoing statements, definition of some terms may be in order.

DEFINITION OF FIBER

Although the term "fiber" suggests a single homogeneous substance, it actually comprises at least six categories—cellulose, hemicellulose, lignin, pectin, gums and mucilages (2). While most people would clearly identify the stringy, insoluble material (cellulose) in celery as fiber, the water-soluble material in apples (pectin) is also a type of fiber. Thus, the term fiber is a misnomer because some of these substances are water-soluble and not at all "fibrous".

If the various fibers do not share the common property of stringiness, what properties do the fibers share? Dietary fibers are defined as plant cell wall materials which are indigestible by the human gastrointestinal (GI) machinery. Ruminants like the cow, however, are able to digest these materials, and as a result of this, to the cow, a piece of cellulose is as fattening as a piece of cake would be to us! Both starch in cake and cellulose in celery are made of glucose subunits (see the section on carbohydrate metabolism in Chapter 7). The difference is that we can't digest cellulose to get the glucose out of it, while cows can.

Although human enzymes cannot digest dietary fiber, some of the bacteria in the human GI tract produce enzymes which can digest fiber and release gases and volatile fatty acids (2). These gases contribute to the "intestinal gas" which is one of the unpleasant, but usually temporary, side effects of a high fiber diet. These fatty acids can be absorbed and actually used by the human host for energy-requiring processes (i.e., they constitute calories). Not all types of fiber, however, can be metabolized by bacteria in this fashion, and in reality, the number of calories that can be obtained from fiber in this way is very small (maybe 20-30 calories per day).

Since there are at least six different categories of fiber with variable effects, it is extremely important when reading the literature to identify the type of fiber studied. For instance, it appears that pectin and gums decrease serum cholesterol levels, while cellulose does not. Cellulose, on the other hand, significantly increases fecal bulk, while pectin and gums do not. In this chapter, the purported benefits of fiber in various diseases will be reviewed. Other chapters of this book should be consulted for information on other dietary manipulations that may be indicated in these diseases. Before discussing the effects of fiber in disease, a quick review of the effects of fiber in the healthy human may be warranted.

EFFECTS OF FIBER IN HEALTHY INDIVIDUALS

Probably the best known effect of a high roughage diet is its influence on stool quality and quantity. Most types of fiber act as laxatives, mainly by increasing the bulk and water content of the stool. These effects tend to soften the stool and increase the motility of the GI tract, which leads to decreased intestinal transit time. Transit time refers to the number of hours that it takes for food to travel from the mouth to the anus. Transit time is significantly shortened in individuals (like rural Africans) who ingest a high fiber diet (5). For instance, whereas a normal American may have a transit time of 60-90 hours, that of the rural African might be 30 hours or less.

It has been hypothesized that the shortened transit time of Africans accounts for their low incidence of colon cancer. The hypothesis goes like this: many foods contain substances which are potentially carcinogenic, either in their natural state or after "activation" in the gastrointestinal tract. The tendency of these compounds to promote cancer is related to their duration of contact with the cells lining the colon. A slow transit time allows for longer contact of these substances with the colon cells, whereas rapid transit allows rapid clearance. I personally don't find this to be a very satisfying hypothesis because the speed of transit doesn't necessarily affect contact time. A cell in the colon may be in continuous contact with carcinogenic materials regardless of whether transit time is 30 or 90 hours. In addition, although rural Africans are often used as examples, Eskimos, who eat almost no carbohydrate and presumably have a prolonged transit time have a very low cancer rate (6). This points out the difficulty with developing hypotheses from epidemiologic data (e.g., comparing colon cancer in Africans and Americans without controlling for many other factors which may be relevant).

Another possible explanation for the finding that Africans have a low incidence of colon cancer is that dietary fiber may, due to its water absorptive and bulking effects, "dilute" the concentration of the carcinogenic substances. Again, one would have to explain why Eskimos don't have a high incidence of colon cancer. It is quite likely that many other dietary, genetic, physiological and perhaps even psychological factors play a role in the development of colon cancer, and to ascribe the difference in cancer incidence strictly to differences in dietary fiber is probably simplistic.

It is interesting to note that although fiber increases the overall speed of intestinal transit, it may actually slow down the first part of the trip, from the mouth to the small intestine. By delaying the entry of food into the small intestine, fiber may modify the rate of absorption of nutrients. This may account for the beneficial effects of fiber in diseases like diabetes (see below). Despite a slowdown in passage of food in the upper GI tract, total transit time is significantly decreased by fiber due to faster movement in the lower GI tract.

Different types of fiber affect fecal weight and transit time to various degrees. For instance, in one study, fecal weight increased 127% with bran fiber, but only 20% with guar gum fiber (7). In addition, individual responses to identical dietary fiber intake varied greatly. Even two very similar soybean seed fibers can have different effects (8). Bran, pectin and guar (gum) fibers even affect the structure of the lining of the GI tract differently (9).

POTENTIAL CLINICAL USES OF FIBER IN HUMAN DISEASES

Diabetes Mellitus (DM)

The story of dietary recommendations in the treatment of DM is a fascinating one, and quite instructive for our purposes. DM has simplistically been assessed as a dysfunction of carbohydrate metabolism characterized by excess sugar and insulin shortage. Consequently, the recommendation used to be to restrict carbohydrate and to give insulin. Since this recommendation was so logical, it was never really tested scientifically. Severely limiting carbohydrate calories to 15% of total (as used to be recommended) was accompanied by a high fat intake, which is unfortunate since diabetics already have a propensity toward cardiovascular diseases. In view of this and of the fact that severe carbohydrate restriction hadn't really been proven to be therapeutic in diabetics, the carbohydrate restriction has been relaxed to 30-40% of total calories over the past couple of decades. Relaxing the carbohydrate restriction has been accompanied by a decrease in fat intake (see references 10 and 11 for a review of this topic).

Over the past decade, it has been shown that a *high* carbohydrate diet actually *improves* diabetic control. For instance, 13 diabetic men were switched from a 43% carbohydrate 5 gram fiber diet to a 75% carbohydrate 14 gram fiber (HCF) diet (12). Initially, these diabetic men required either insulin or oral antidiabetes drugs to control their blood sugar. On the HCF diet, oral antidiabetes drugs were discontinued in the five men taking them, and insulin was discontinued in 4 of the other 8 men. Thus, diet alone eliminated the need for drugs in 9 of 13 men. Cholesterol and triglyceride values also decreased significantly.

Although this study is exciting, it did not separate the effects of the high fiber from those of the increased carbohydrate. It appears that each is independently beneficial in improving diabetic control. A recent study showed impressive effects of fiber supplementation on metabolic control in 12 obese poorly controlled non-insulin-dependent diabetics (13). These individuals received 20 grams of guar gum and 10 grams of wheat bran daily for two months. Urinary excretion of glucose decreased from 30.5 to 8.3 g/day, and fasting plasma glucose concentration decreased from 301 to 184 mg/dl. Plasma cholesterol decreased from 277 to 193 mg/dl. No significant changes were observed in the patients' weight, or plasma levels of triglycerides, HDL or insulin. Unlike previous studies, this was a relatively longterm study (2 months compared to a week or two in others) in poorly controlled diabetics.

Quite a few other studies support these findings (14-18, see also bibliography in reference 18), and indeed, I am unaware of any well-controlled studies that haven't confirmed, at least to some degree, the benefits of fiber in improving diabetic control.

The situation in healthy, nondiabetic individuals is somewhat different, in that some studies have shown effects of fiber on glucose levels (8), while others haven't (19). It should be noted, however, that the fiber preparations tested were different, and even slight differences in physical form (e.g., whole seed vs. ground, or cooked vs. raw) may be responsible for differences in physiological effects.

Hypercholesterolemia and Heart Disease

As has been previously emphasized, some types of fiber (but not others) alter lipid levels, and consequently, we hope, cardiovascular risk. For instance, no changes in plasma cholesterol or triglycerides were noted in 6 healthy individuals ingesting large amounts of unprocessed wheat bran (20). The same authors, on the other hand, noted a 15% decrease in plasma cholesterol in individuals taking increased amounts of pectin. Other studies also suggest that some types of fiber have little or no effect on plasma lipids (21,22). All these studies, however, involved normal healthy people.

To compare the effects of different types of fiber, Jenkins and his colleagues added 20 g of fiber from either carrot, cabbage, apple, bran, guar gum or pectin, to controlled diets of 22 healthy volunteers (23). Addition of guar gum and pectin resulted in a 13% decrease in serum cholesterol, while other fibers had small and inconsistent effects. It is impressive to note that the 13% decrease was from *normal*, not hypercholesterolemic, baseline levels. This finding has been supported by another study in normal men who received gum arabic. Although this fiber has little effect on glucose tolerance and stool bulk, it did decrease serum cholesterol (24).

One of the beneficial effects of increasing fiber in the diet is that this change usually also increases the amount of complex carbohydrate, and consequently, decreases fat intake. In fact, this may be partially responsible for decreases in plasma lipids in individuals who increase their intake of fiber. Most of the controlled studies, of course, do not allow a change in the lipid intake, and this would only be relevant to patients who are encouraged to alter both fiber and fat intakes at home.

The foregoing studies have dealt mostly with purified fibers. Of more value to the reader, no doubt, would be studies of supplementation with commercially available, high-fiber foodstuffs. Cluster bean pods, a vegetable commonly consumed in India, contains 20% guar gum (dry weight). Effects of incorporating this vegetable, both in its natural form and purified subfractions, were studied in rats eating a high cholesterol diet (25). All subfractions as well as the whole vegetable lowered serum cholesterol. In addition to these animal findings, locust bean gum (similar to guar gum) has been recently tested in 18 hyperlipidemic and 10 healthy individuals (26,27). Both total cholesterol and LDL fell significantly in both groups. HDL/LDL ratios increased, and acceptance of the locust bean gum supplement was good. In one longterm (4 month) study, hyperlipidemic patients substituted 140 g of dried beans (complex carbohydrate as well as fiber) daily for other sources of starch. Fasting serum triglyceride levels decreased 25%, while cholesterol fell 7%. Two more recent studies further support these findings. In one (28), both oat bran and beans decreased serum cholesterol by 19% in hypercholesterolemic patients. In the other study, guar gum lowered both cholesterol and triglyceride levels without decreasing the "good" cholesterol—HDL.

The hypolipidemic effect of fiber appears to apply only to the pectin and guar gum types of fiber, but not to the cellulose types. While some types of bran have been shown not to affect serum lipids (e.g., reference 20), others have shown significant effects (e.g., reference 28). This may be due to differences in soluble fibers (e.g., pectin and gums) in the different types of bran.

These studies suggest, therefore, that the high complex carbohydrate-high fiber diet has the potential to decrease serum lipids in both normal and hyperlipidemic individuals. In view of the high levels of lipids in the United States, such a dietary modification may be wise for the general population, not just for "officially" hyperlipidemic individuals.

Obesity

It has been suggested that increased fiber in the diet contributes to sensations of satiety and consequently decreases food intake. It is reasonable to assume that 100 calories of apple or bran cereal would be more filling than 100 calories of chocolate. High-fiber foodstuffs have other properties, such as high nutrient content, which enhance their usefulness in a reducing diet. Thus, the HCF diet is also useful as part of a weight-loss plan (see Chapter 13—the F-Plan Diet).

Diverticulosis

Diverticulosis refers to outpouching of the intestinal tract. The little pouches (diverticuli) usually don't cause any problems until they become infected and/or inflamed, a painful condition known as diverticulitis. A *low* fiber diet used to be recommended for both diverticulosis and diverticulitis, the rationale being that the fibrous strands would be irritating to the inflamed diverticuli. It is now believed, however, that the high pressure generated in the GI tract of individuals who eat a *low* fiber diet is responsible for the development or exacerbation of diverticulosis. In fact, increased dietary fiber actually decreases the chance of developing diverticulosis, and is therapeutic in diverticulitis (30). Some gastrointestinal diseases, however, may still be properly treated with a low-fiber diet (e.g., Crohn's disease, ulcerative colitis), although the soluble fibers such as gums and pectin may be acceptable in these disorders. In any case, it is advised that individuals suffering from these disorders consult their physician before making any changes in their diet.

SIDE EFFECTS OF HIGH FIBER DIET

Side effects of a high-fiber diet have been previously alluded to in this chapter. Increased production of intestinal gas is usually temporary. If fiber intake is very high (>50 g/day), bloating or abdominal pain may occur. It has also been suggested that high-fiber diets may lead to malabsorption of some minerals, like calcium and magnesium (31,32). This may be due, however, to other constituents of the high-fiber foods, e.g., oxalic acid in spinach (33), rather than the fiber itself. Wingate has raised the possibility that excessive bran fiber and wheat germ may predispose to coeliac disease (34). As was true of their beneficial effects, it is likely that the adverse effects vary for the different types of fiber. As always, moderation is the key. Thus, "It can be stated with confidence that people who increase their fiber intake up to 50 g/day, double the amount usually present in the British [and American] diet, run no risk of any serious effects on their health" (2).

HIGH FIBER DIETS: THE BOTTOM LINE

Americans can probably benefit from an increase in their fiber intake. It appears that this change is already occurring in the United States. Increased fiber intake is of benefit in carbohydrate intolerance (e.g., diabetes mellitus), hyperlipidemia, obesity, and some gastrointestinal diseases. As noted above, however, moderation is the key. Table 11-1 is a list of rich and moderately rich sources of fiber, taken from the NCI's book, "Diet, Nutrition and Cancer Prevention: A Guide to Food Sources" (also found in reference 35). The dietary fiber content of many foods is still unknown, and the reader should also recall that the *type* of fiber is of importance. With regard to cereals, the brand-name products listed are representative of the fiber content of simiar types of cereals.

REFERENCES

1. Vahouny GV: Conclusions and recommendations of the symposium on "Dietary Fibers in Health and Disease," Washington, D.C., 1981. Am J Clin Nutr 35:152, 1982

RICH SOURCES OF FOOD FIBER

4 grams or more per serving
(Foods marked with an * have 6 or more grams of fiber per serving)

	Serving
Breads and cereals	
* All Bran	⅓ cup-1 oz
* Bran Buds	⅓ cup-1 oz
Bran Chex	⅔ cup-1 oz
Corn bran	⅔ cup-1 oz
Cracklin' Bran	⅓ cup-1 oz
* 100% Bran	½ cup-1 oz
Raisin bran	¾ cup-1 oz
* Bran, unsweetened	¼ cup
Wheat germ, toasted, plain	¼ cup-1 oz
Legumes (Cooked portions)	
Kidney beans	½ cup
Lima beans	½ cup
Navy beans	½ cup
Pinto beans	½ cup
White beans	½ cup
Fruits	
Blackberries	½ cup
Dried prunes	3

MODERATELY RICH SOURCES OF FOOD FIBER

1 to 3 grams of fiber per serving

	Serving
Breads and cereals	
Bran muffins	1 medium
Popcorn (air-popped)	1 cup
Whole-wheat bread	1 slice
Whole-wheat spaghetti	1 cup
40% bran flakes	⅔ cup-1 oz
Grapenuts	¼ cup-1 oz
Granola-type cereals	¼ cup-1 oz
Cheerio-type cereals	1¼ cup-1 oz
Most	⅓ cup-1 oz
Oatmeal, cooked	¾ cup
Shredded wheat	⅔ cup-1 oz
Total	1 cup-1 oz
Wheat Chex	⅔ cup-1 oz
Wheaties	1 cup-1 oz
Legumes (cooked) and Nuts	
Chick peas (Garbanzo beans)	½ cup
Lentils	½ cup
Almonds	10 nuts
Peanuts	10 nuts
Vegetables	
Artichoke	1 small
Asparagus	½ cup
Beans, green	½ cup
Brussels sprouts	½ cup
Cabbage, red and white	½ cup
Carrots	½ cup
Cauliflower	½ cup
Corn	½ cup
Green peas	½ cup
Kale	½ cup
Parsnip	½ cup
Potato	1 medium
Spinach, cooked	½ cup
Spinach, raw	½ cup
Summer squash	½ cup
Sweet potato	½ medium
Turnip	½ cup
Bean sprouts (soy)	½ cup
Celery	½ cup
Tomato	1 medium
Fruits	
Apple	1 medium
Apricot, fresh	3 medium
Apricot, dried	5 halves
Banana	1 medium
Blueberries	½ cup
Cantaloupe	¼ melon
Cherries	10
Dates, dried	3
Figs, dried	1 medium
Grapefruit	½
Orange	1 medium
Peach	1 medium
Pear	1 medium
Pineapple	½ cup
Raisins	¼ cup
Strawberries	1 cup

Fiber content of foods
From FDA Consumer, June 1985, p. 32.

2. Eastwood MA, Passmore R: Dietary fiber. Lancet 2:202, 1983
3. Acheson RM, Williams DRR: Does consumption of fruit and vegetable protect against stroke? Lancet 1:1191, 1983
4. Fink D: Facts about colorectal cancer detection. Ca-A Cancer J for Clinicians 33:366, 1983
5. Burkitt DP, et al: Effects of dietary fiber on stools and transit times and its role in the causation of disease. Lancet 2:1408, 1972
6. Editorial: Eskimo diets and diseases. Lancet 1:1139, 1983
7. Cummings JH, et al: Colonic response to dietary fiber from carrot, cabbage, apple, bran and guar gum. Lancet 1:5, 1978
8. Schweizer TF, et al: Metabolic effects of dietary fiber from dehulled soybeans in humans. Am J Clin Nutr 38:1, 1983
9. Jacobs LR: Effects of dietary fiber in mucosal growth and cell proliferation in the small intestine of the rat: a comparison of oat bran, pectin, and guar with total fiber deprivation. Am J Clin Nutr 37:954, 1983
10. Yetiv JZ: Recent advances in diabetes research and therapy. In: Recent Advances in Clinical Therapeutics, Yetiv JZ, Bianchine JR (eds.), Academic Press, 1981, pp. 141-173
11. Mann JI: Diet and diabetes. Diabetologia 18:89, 1980
12. Kiehm TG, et al: Beneficial effects of a high carbohydrate, high fiber diet on hyperglycemic diabetic men. Am J Clin Nutr 29:895, 1976
13. Kay TK, et al: Long-term effects of dietary fiber on glucose tolerance and gastric emptying in non-insulin-dependent diabetic patients. Am J Clin Nutr 37:376, 1983

14. Jenkins DJA, et al: Treatment of diabetes with guar gum. Lancet 2:779, 1977

15. Jenkins DJA, et al: Guar crispbread in the diabetic diet. Br Med J 2:1744, 1978

16. Chenon D, et al: Effects of dietary fiber on postprandial glycemic profiles in diabetic patients submitted to continuous programmed insulin infusion. Am J Clin Nutr 40:58, 1984

17. Parsons S: Effects of high fiber breakfasts on glucose metabolism in noninsulin-dpendent diabetics. Am J Clin Nutr 40:66, 1984

18. Thorne MJ, et al: Factors affecting starch digestibility and the glycemic response with special reference to legumes. Am J Clin Nutr 38:481, 1983

19. Tsai AC, et al: Effects of soy polysaccharide on gastrointestinal functions, nutrient balance, steroid excretions, glucose tolerance, serum lipids, and other parameters in humans. Am J Clin Nutr 38:504, 1983

20. Truswell AS, Kay RM: Absence of effect of bran on blood lipids. Lancet 1:922, 1975

21. Ullrich IH, Albrink MJ: Lack of effect of dietary fiber on serum lipids, glucose and insulin in healthy young men fed high starch diets. Am J Clin Nutr 36:1, 1982

22. Liebman M, et al: Effects of coarse wheat bran fiber and exercise on plasma lipids and lipoproteins in moderately overweight men. Am J Clin Nutr 37:71, 1983

23. Jenkins DJA, et al: Hypocholesterolemic action of dietary fiber unrelated to fecal bulking effect. Am J Clin Nutr 32:2430, 1979

24. Ross AH, et al: A study of the effects of dietary gum arabic in humans. Am J Clin Nutr 37:368, 1983

25. Sarathy R, Sarawsathi G: Effect of tender cluster bean pods (Cyamopsis tetragonoloba) on cholesterol levels in rats. Am J Clin Nutr 38:295, 1983

26. Zavoral JH, et al: The hypolipidemic effect of locust bean gum food products in familial hypercholesterolemic adults and children. Am J Clin Nutr 38:285, 1983

27. Jenkins DJA, et al: Leguminous seeds in the dietary management of hyperlipidemia. Am J Clin Nutr 38:567, 1983

28. Anderson JW, et al: Hypocholesterolemic effects of oat-bran or bean intake for hypercholesterolemic men. Am J Clin Nutr 40:1146, 1984

29. Bosello O, et al: Effects of guar gum on plasma lipoproteins and apolipoproteins C-II and C-III in patients affected by familial combined hyperlipoproteinemia. Am J Clin Nutr 40:1165, 1984

30. Painter NS: Treatment of diverticular disease. Br Med J 2:156, 1971

31. Kelsay JL: Effect of diet fiber level on bowel function and trace mineral balances of human subjects. Cereal Chem 58:2, 1981

32. Kelsay JL: Effects of fiber on mineral and vitamin bioavailability. In: Vahouny GV, Kritchevsky D (eds.). Dietary Fiber in Health and Disease. New York, N.Y., Plenum Press, 1982, pp. 91-103

33. Kelsay JL, Prather ES: Mineral balances of human subjects consuming spinach in a low-fiber diet and in a diet containing fruits and vegetables. Am J Clin Nutr 38:12, 1983

34. Wingate DL: Is fiber always harmless? Lancet 1:876, 1983

35. Stephenson M: Fiber: Something healthy to chew on. FDA Consumer, June 1985, pp.31

CHAPTER 12

Vegetarian Diets

This chapter logically follows the chapter on fiber because vegetarian diets and high-fiber diets are similar in many respects. Much of what has been said of high-fiber diets applies to vegetarian diets, although lack of animal protein in the strict vegetarian diet does raise other concerns.

DEFINITIONS

Three types of diets are loosely described as vegetarian, although only one is strictly so:

1) Vegan (or strict vegetarian)—no animal flesh or animal byproducts, e.g., dairy products or eggs, are eaten.

2) Ovolactovegetarian—no animal flesh is eaten, but animal products are ingested.

3) Semi-vegetarian—usually no red meat is eaten, but poultry or fish may be ingested occasionally, in addition to the normal ovolactovegetarian fare. Although this diet can't really be described as vegetarian, many people do pursue this type of diet, either on the way to becoming ovolactovegetarians or just for the health benefits of eliminating red meat from the diet.

It is likely that the vast majority of "vegetarians" in the United States belong in groups 2 and 3; true vegans are rather rare. The distinction is important because nutrient intakes and deficiencies of vegans are quite different from those of ovolacto- or semi-vegetarians. Indeed, whereas all three types of vegetarian diets may confer health benefits, vegan diets also present risks of deficiencies, whereas the other types of vegetarian diets usually do not.

ADVANTAGES OF VEGETARIAN DIETS

Decreased Risk of Heart Disease

There is evidence that vegetarians have a lower risk of cardiovascular disease that non-vegetarians (1). A prospective study which examined this issue was recently published (2). A screening questionnaire was distributed to more than 10,000 customers of health food stores in Wales (Great Britain), who were then followed up for seven years. It was noted that vegetarians had lower mortality from heart disease. These data are considered preliminary; the investigators are continuing to follow this group of subjects.

There are several reasons why vegetarians might experience lower mortality from heart disease. They have lower plasma cholesterol than non-vegetarians, and more of their cholesterol tends to be in the high-density (HDL) fraction (2-5, see also Chapter 6). Vegetarians are also less likely to be overweight or have high blood pressure than non-vegetarians (6). Interestingly, the subjects in reference 6 were ovolactovegetarians and not vegans. This means that one does not have to be a strict vegetarian to enjoy the better mortality experience of vegetarians.

It has also been suggested that vegetarians might have less heart disease because they often pursue healthier lifestyles than nonvegetarians— they rarely smoke, and many drink neither alcohol nor caffeine-containing beverages. It is hard to evaluate the separate effects of these habits, although most studies which have examined this question have controlled for these other factors. For instance, Mormons have been used as a control group (e.g., reference 2) because while they abstain from tobacco, alcohol and caffeine, they do eat an omnivorous diet.

Although most studies have examined subjects who have been vegetarians for several years, one recent study looked at what happens to omnivorous individuals who adopt vegetarian diets (7). Presumably this is of more relevance to the reader who is considering switching to vegetarian fare. The effects of 3 weeks of a vegan diet (except that skim milk was allowed) on serum lipids and lipoproteins were studied in 15 healthy free-living subjects in crossover fashion. LDL (the "bad" cholesterol) increased significantly upon switching from the vegetarian diet to the regular diet.

Thus, although the exact reasons which account for it are unclear, it appears that a vegetarian diet does decrease the risk of cardiovascular disease, or at least alters risk factors beneficially.

Better Management of Diabetes Mellitus

Since diabetics are especially prone to heart disease, vegetarian diets are likely to be of benefit to diabetics. Vegetarian diets, which are rich in complex carbohydrates and fiber, also improve the quality of metabolic control in this disease. This topic is discussed in more detail in Chapters 7 and 11.

Decreased Severity of Colonic Disease

Since vegetarian diets are high in fiber, they can be useful in diverticulosis, constipation, and other colonic diseases. This has been discussed in Chapter 11.

Decreased Obesity

As mentioned above, vegetarians are less overweight than age-matched non-vegetarian controls. Since vegetarian diets tend to be bulky and low in fat, it is hard to exceed caloric requirements while eating vegetarian foods. The advantages of achieving ideal body weight are numerous and are discussed in Chapter 13.

Modify Hormonal Status—Breast Cancer and Osteoporosis

It has been hypothesized that estrogen status can affect the incidence of breast cancer. A recent study showed that vegetarian women have an increased fecal output of estrogen hormones, and a 20% lower plasma concentration of estrogen compared to controls (8). It should be noted that the difference in estrogen levels between the two groups of women was not statistically significant. Whether this finding is relevant to the development of breast cancer has been questioned (9), and should certainly be considered speculative at the present time.

It has also been suggested that postmenopausal women who eat red meat may experience greater bone mineral loss than ovolactovegetarian subjects (10); this has not been shown to be the case in men (11). These findings are also quite preliminary, and should not be a major factor in deciding on the type of diet to ingest. What is likely, however, is that diet may indeed affect hormone levels, and we are only beginning to understand this aspect of dietary manipulation.

Miscellaneous

There is some evidence which suggests that a vegetarian diet can reduce the incidence of diabetes (11a). Another study showed that vegetarian women are less than half as likely to develop gallstones or require gallbladder surgery as omnivorous women (11b). This was partially due to the fact that obesity is a risk factor for gallstones, and vegetarians are less likely to be obese. This factor, however, did not account for all the difference between the two groups. There are also economical reasons for pursuing a vegetarian diet in the United States since vegetarian diets are usually cheaper than omnivorous diets.

Some vegetarians believe that eating meat is a wasteful way of utilizing the earth's production of protein, and consequently deprives poorer countries of badly needed protein. This is because a steer needs to eat 5 pounds of vegetable protein to make one pound of meat protein. It is not clear, however, how improved utilization of plant protein in the United States will help the starving in poorer countries. To a large extent, malnutrition in Third world countries is due to difficulties with food *distribution*, not of global food *production*.

Finally, some vegetarians feel on philosophical grounds that it is wrong to kill animals for food (or other) purposes if we can subsist on vegetarian fare. Each reader will, of course, have to consider these factors for himself.

DISADVANTAGES OF VEGETARIAN DIETS

Inadequate Nutritional Intake

This is the major, and perhaps only, real disadvantage of vegetarian diets. It would be more accurate to say "potential disadvantage" because with careful food planning, inadequate nutrition need not be a complication of a vegetarian diet. This difficulty occurs primarily in strict vegetarians. Ovolactovegetarians rarely experience significant nutritional deficiencies. The nutrients which may be deficient in vegetarian diets are outlined below, and are discussed in more detail in the next section:

Protein

Much has been said of requirements for protein, but in the United States, we tend to eat more than adequate amounts of protein. Whereas most animal proteins are *complete* proteins, no single plant protein is complete. A complete protein contains all 8 essential amino acids which the human body requires in order to function properly. An incomplete protein is missing one or more of these essential amino acids. Combining two incomplete but "complementary" proteins in the same meal may yield a complete protein. Complementary refers to the ability of one incomplete protein to "fill in" the amino acid deficiencies of the other incomplete protein.

Once the two incomplete but complementary proteins are broken down to amino acids in the intestine, the body doesn't care whether those amino acids came from one complete protein or two incomplete proteins. Although much is made of this concept in the nutritional literature, it is difficult not to eat complementary proteins unless one follows a very strict unbalanced diet. Most studies that have examined protein intake in vegetarians have found it to be adequate (see also last section in this chapter). This is especially true for ovolactovegetarians since both egg white and milk protein are complete proteins.

Vitamin B_{12}

Deficiency of this vitamin, like most other deficiencies in vegetarians, is found almost exclusively in vegans (12), and rarely in ovolactovegetarians. This is because no plant food is a good source of vitamin B_{12}. Nutritional yeast, grown in a medium containing B_{12} is a good source, but other types of yeast are not. A syndrome due to vitamin B_{12} deficiency, consisting of neurological, gastrointestinal, and hematological manifestations, was recently described in Rastafarian vegans (13). Rastafarianism is a cult-like religious sect that started in Jamaica in the 1930s; its members usually eat a very restrictive vegetarian diet. Although most of the manifestations of the syndrome described above were reversible with vitamin B_{12}, at least one of the patients had residual motor (muscle use) defects due to subacute combined degeneration.

Vitamin D

As was true for other nutrients, ovolactovegetarians can meet the requirement for this nutrient through intake of fortified milk and eggs. In addition, vitamin D is made in the skin upon exposure to sunlight. Approximately 20-30 minutes of sunlight per day is all that is necessary. Vegans who are not exposed to regular sunlight should take a supplement.

Several cases of rickets, a disease of bones due to deficiency of vitamin D, have been reported in strict vegetarians (e.g., 14,15). The latter reference describes other nutritional deficiencies in this group as well. Most of these patients responded to supplementation with vitamin D and to introduction of adequate feeding practices. Rickets, in simple terms, is a disease in which bones are not adequately made due to improper calcium deposition, which is secondary to lack of vitamin D. Strict vegetarians are especially hard hit because their diets are usually low both in vitamin D and in calcium (see next section).

Calcium

Dairy products, which are included in lactovegetarian diets, are excellent sources of calcium. Most plant foodstuffs are poor sources of calcium. Vegans can maximize their calcium intake by eating broccoli, collards, kale, mustard and turnip greens (16). Vegetables high in oxalic acid (like spinach and chard) should be eaten sparingly, even by budding Popeyes, since oxalic acid binds calcium and prevents its absorption into the body. In view of the above, vegans should probably take a calcium supplement.

Iron

This mineral is in short supply in both vegetarian and in omnivorous diets, especially for menstruating women and growing children. Soybeans are one of the best vegetarian sources of iron, and the high intake of vitamin C in vegetarian diets increases the absorption of iron (16). Cooking in cast iron pots also increases the intake of this nutrient.

Summary

Several nutrients are inadequately supplied by vegan diets, but not in ovolactovegetarian diets, especially vitamins B_{12} and D, and calcium and iron. For vegan or otherwise strict vegetarians, a daily mutivitamin which contains these nutrients, plus a calcium supplement, would seem indicated.

VEGETARIAN DIETS IN INFANTS AND CHILDREN

Much of the foregoing discussion also applies to children. For instance, it appears that children on carefully administered ovolactovegetarian diets are no worse off than their omnivorous counterparts, while vegan children tend to be smaller than omnivorous children (17). Therefore, unsupplemented vegan diets are *not* recommended for infants and children.

A recent study dealt with this issue in detail (18). Thirty-nine children who were following different types of vegetarian diets were carefully evaluated. Protein intakes of the vegetarian children were similar to those suggested in the Dietary Goals for the United States, and amino acid composition was adequate. The intakes of animal protein, and of sugar, cholesterol, fat and salt, were lower than those specified in the Goals. All the vegetarian children had been breastfed for some time during infancy; the mean duration of breastfeeding was 12.7 months, with a range of 0.5 to 55 months! Nine of the 39 children were vegans, and essentially all the rest were ovolactovegetarians.

The intakes of the non-vegan vegetarians (mainly ovolactovegetarians) met or exceeded the RDA for most nutrients. The most notable exception for the non-vegan vegetarians was vitamin D, the mean intake of which was less than half of the RDA. This was probably due to the fact that there were 18 macrobiotics in the group of 30 non-vegan vegetarians. Macrobiotics in general, and especially vegan macrobiotics, had lower-than-RDA intakes of vitamins B_{12} and D, as well as calcium and riboflavin. It is interesting to note that whereas 53% of non-macrobiotic vegetarians took vitamin and mineral supplements, only 22% of the vegan macrobiotics (who really needed them) took them.

Although the children's measurements fell in the normal range, there was a disproportionate number (80%) of subjects under the 50th percentile for length. More than 2/3rds of the subjects were above the 50th percentile of both weight for length and skinfold (triceps) thickness, indicating greater fatness than expected. In addition, retarded bone age was present in a quarter of the macrobiotic subjects for whom bone age x-rays were available. Bone age of non-macrobiotic vegetarians was not measured. Finally, immunization schedules were lacking for 59% of the macrobiotics compared to 25% of the other vegetarians.

This study suggests that vegan and macrobiotic diets, which are more restricted than ovolactovegetarian diets, are associated with nutrient deficiencies and shorter-than-normal stature and growth delay (retarded bone age). The nutrient deficiencies were more marked for the vegan macrobiotics, indicating that such diets are inadequate for infants and children. These sentiments are shared by the authors of two recent editorials (19,20), and the interested reader should consult references 15 and 17-21 for further details. The last reference listed (21) must be read by anyone skeptical of the bad effects of very strict vegetarian diets in childhood. In this study, 3 of 25 hospitalized vegan children died on arrival to the hospital, and 5 more died a few hours after admission. The diagnosis was death due to malnutrition.

IMPLEMENTING A VEGETARIAN DIET

As the reader has undoubtedly surmised, vegetarian diets offer several benefits, but very strict vegetarian diets present risks that outweigh their advantages. My recommendation, therefore, is a shift from an omnivorous diet to a semi-vegetarian or ovolactovegetarian diet. Vegetarian cooking may seem foreign to a "meat and potatoes" person, and as always, moderation and slow change is the key. One should not attempt to "go veggie" in one week. A slow elimination of the fattiest meats first, and their replacement with cereals, fruits, and vegetables, will be most easily tolerated. An effort to eliminate all meat in the diet overnight is more likely to end in failure than a gradual introduction of the vegetarian way. Some may choose to eliminate red meat, but continue to eat fish and poultry occasionally, and such a diet is also to be encouraged (see Chapter 6 for a discussion of the benefits of eating fish.)

For the reader interested in going "veggie", there are many excellent vegetarian cookbooks available. A recent review (17) recommends *Laurel's Kitchen* (22) as a particularly thorough and pleasant resource, with tables that are more detailed than those from the usual government sources.

REFERENCES

1. Phillips RL, et al: Coronary heart disease mortality among Seventh-Day Adventists with differing dietary habits: a preliminary report. Am J Clin Nutr 31:191, 1978
2. Burr ML, Sweetnam PM: Vegetarianism, dietary fiber and mortality. Am J Clin Nutr 36:873, 1982
3. West RO, Hayes OB: Diet and serum cholesterol levels: a comparison between vegetarians and non-vegetarians in a Seventh-Day Adventist group. Am J Clin Nutr 21:853, 1968

4. Gear J, et al: Biochemical and hematological variables in vegetarians. Br Med J 1:1415, 1980

5. Burr ML, et al: Plasma cholesterol and blood pressure in vegetarians. J Hum Nutr 35:437, 1981

6. Rouse IL, et al: Vegetarian diet, lifestyle and blood pressure in vegetarians in two religious populations. Clin Exp Pharmacol Physiol 9:327, 1982

7. Cooper RS, et al: The selective lipid-lowering effect of vegetarianism on low-density lipoproteins in a crossover experiment. Acta Med Scand 213:171, 1983

8. Goldwin BR, et al: Estrogen excretion patterns and plasma levels in vegetarian and omnivorous women. N Engl J Med 307:1542, 1982

9. Korenman SG: Estrogen excretion and plasma levels in vegetarian and omnivorous women (letter). N Engl J Med 308:1360, 1983

10. Marsh AG, et al: Cortical bone density of adult lacto-ovovegetarian and omnivorous women. J Am Diet Assoc 76:148, 1980

11. Marsh AG, et al: Bone mineral mass in adult lacto-ovovegetarian and omnivorous males. Am J Clin Nutr 37:453, 183

11a. Snowdon DA, Phillips RL: Does a vegetarian diet reduce the occurrence of diabetes. Am J Pub Health 75:507, 1985

11b. Pixley F, et al: Effect of vegetarianism on development of gall stones in women. Br Med J 291:11, 1985

12. Abdulla M, et al: Nutrient intake and health status of vegans. Chemical analysis of diets using the duplicate portion sampling technique. Am J Clin Nutr 34:2464, 1981

13. Campbell M, et al: Rastafarianism and the vegans syndrome. Br Med J 285:1617, 1982

14. Dwyer JH, et al: Risk of nutritional rickets among vegetarian children Am J Dis Child 133:134, 1979

15. Zmora E, et al: Multiple nutritional deficiencies in infants from a strict vegetarian community. Am J Dis Child 133:141, 1979

16. Krey SH: Alternate dietary lifestyles. Primary Care 9:595, 1982

17. Christoffel K: A pediatric perspective on vegetarian nutrition. Clin Ped 20:632, 1981

18. Dwyer Jt, et al: Nutritional status of vegetarian children. Am J Clin Nutr 35:204, 1982

19. Purvis GA: Vegetarian nutrition in infancy. Getting Down to Basics, Issue #34, December 1982, distributed by the Gerber Products Co., Fremeont, MI 49412

20. Fineberg L: Human choice, vegetable deficiencies and vegetarian rickets. Am J Dis Child 133:129, 1979

21. Shinwell ED, Gorodischer R: Totally vegetarian diets and infant nutrition. Peds 70:582, 1982

22. Robertson L, et al: Laurel's Kitchen: A Handbook for Vegetarian Cookery. Nilgiri Press, Petaluma, CA, 1976.

CHAPTER 13

Obesity: The Battle of the Bulge

Obesity is widely accepted as the commonest nutritional disorder in the United States. Approximately 34 million Americans are considered to be overweight (1). Although much lip service has been paid to this topic within the medical establishment, research in the obesity field is in its infancy, and the success rate of organized medicine in achieving permanent weight reduction is less than 10%. This failure of orthodox medicine has made it easy for the weight-loss field to be overrun by a myriad of self-styled "experts" pandering their "new" weight loss discoveries; many of these "experts" know less about obesity and nutrition than their clients. This, however, does not seem to deter either the enrollment of willing customers or the commercial success of these ventures.

The key is that the diet gurus are *perceived* to know their stuff, and the gullible public eats it up (pun intended). If this were not so, how else could 800,000 hardcover copies be sold in one year, of a book which states that,

> "As long as food is fully digested, fully processed through the body, you will not gain weight. It's only undigested food that is stuck in your body, for whatever reason, that accumulates and becomes fat."

This is an excerpt from *The Beverly Hills Diet* by Judy Mazel, discussed in reference 2. More fascinating than the fact that someone could write this is the fact that 800,000 people spent their hard-earned money on this book!

This chapter will scientifically discuss both the background of the obesity problem as well as evaluate some of the more popular weight-loss diets. It is hoped that the latter may be of use both to the medical professional and to the lay reader who is contemplating one of the weight-loss schemes.

DEFINITIONS

Several terms must be defined at the outset to facilitate understanding of the ensuing discussion. Most of these definitions are widely, though not universally, accepted (3,4):

Table 13-1

	Weight (pounds)					
	Small Frame		Medium Frame		Large Frame	
Height	Men	Women	Men	Women	Men	Women
4′10″	—	102–111	—	109–121	—	118–131
4′11″	—	103–113	—	111–123	—	120–134
5′0″	—	104–115	—	113–126	—	122–137
5′1″	—	106–118	—	115–129	—	125–140
5′2″	128–134	108–121	131–141	118–132	138–150	128–143
5′3″	130–136	111–124	133–143	121–135	140–153	131–147
5′4″	132–138	114–127	135–145	124–138	142–156	134–151
5′5″	134–140	117–130	137–148	127–141	144–160	137–155
5′6″	136–142	120–133	139–151	130–144	146–164	140–159
5′7″	138–145	123–136	142–154	133–147	149–168	143–163
5′8″	140–148	126–139	145–157	136–150	152–172	146–167
5′9″	142–151	129–142	148–160	139–153	155–176	149–170
5′10″	144–154	132–145	151–163	142–156	158–180	152–173
5′11″	146–157	135–148	154–166	145–159	161–184	155–176
6′0″	149–160	138–151	157–170	148–162	164–188	158–179
6′1″	152–164	—	160–174	—	168–192	—
6′2″	155–168	—	164–178	—	172–197	—
6′3″	158–172	—	167–182	—	176–202	—
6′4″	162–176	—	171–187	—	181–207	—

1983 Metropolitan Height and Weight Tables for Men and Women
Weight is with indoor clothing (5lbs. for men, 3 lbs. for women)
Height is with one-inch heels.
From Metropolitan Life Insurance Company, 1983.

Adipose tissue—fat tissue

Adiposity—degree of fatness

Obesity—excessive amount of body fat. In normal young adult males, approximately 15% of body weight is fat; the corresponding figure for women is 22%. A fat percentage over 20% for men and over 25% for women is usually considered obese. Percent body fat is most accurately measured by underwater (hydrostatic) weighing; more frequently, it is estimated from skinfold measurements.

Overweight—although this term is often used synonymously with obese, this is incorrect. Overweight actually means greater than normal weight for a certain height and body frame size. "Normal" weight has been traditionally defined by reference to the Metropolitan Life Insurance table published in 1959. This table was revised in 1983 (Table 13-1). Weights in this table are often referred to as "ideal body weight" (IBW), because the insurance company found that mortality of their insured clients was lowest at these weights. From the above two definitions, one can see how "obese" and "overweight" could differ. For instance, a 260 pound football player would definitely be considered "overweight" according to the insurance company tables, but his percent body fat is likely to be low, and thus he could not be considered "obese". It is realistic, however, to say that most overweight individuals are obese and vice versa.

Relative weight (RW)—the ratio of actual weight to ideal body weight, usually expressed as a percentage. For example, a woman whose IBW is 100 pounds but who actually weighs 120 pounds has a relative weight of 120%. "Overweight" is often defined as a relative weight above 120%.

Body mass index (BMI)—this is another way of measuring the degree of overweight. BMI is calculated by dividing weight (in kilograms) into height squared (in meters). For example, a 70 kg man who is 180 cm tall (about 5'11", 154 pounds) has a BMI of $70/1.8^2 = 21.6$. This BMI is in the middle of the acceptable range. A BMI above 25 or 26 usually coincides with a relative weight>120%, and is considered mild overweight, while a BMI>30 coincides with a RW above 130% and signifies moderate overweight. The BMI correlates fairly well with other techniques of measuring overweight, but is subject to the same weaknesses as relative weight (remember the football player who was "overweight" but not obese).

MEASUREMENT OF OBESITY

Some methods of quantitating obesity have been alluded to in the definitions above. More detailed explanations are provided below.

Although obesity is defined in numerous ways, all definitions and measurements should ideally refer to the amount of body *fat* rather than *weight*. Some methods directly measure, while others indirectly estimate, the amount of fat. As might be surmised, the most accurate methods are also the most expensive and time-consuming, and are usually employed only in research.

Methods of measuring obesity can be arbitrarily divided into 2 types:

Whole-body methods—carcass analysis, underwater weighing, dilution of ^{40}K and other isotopes, and electrical conduction

Body-sampling methods—primarily skinfold measurement, either in one, or more than one, location(s). Tables are available which convert skinfold thicknesses in various locations to percentage body fat. Body sampling methods also include research techniques such as CAT scanning, ultrasound and infrared interactance.

Whole-body Methods

Carcass Analysis

Carcass analysis is the "gold standard" of assessing body fat content, but obviously is not useful in living humans. Other methods have been validated against this method.

Hydrostatic (Underwater) Weighing

This technique, based on the Archimedes Principle, depends on placing a person in a water tank and accurately assessing the body's specific gravity. This technique has been shown to correlate highly with the carcass analysis method (5). In fact, hydrostatic weighing is sufficiently well-validated that it is often used as the "gold standard" against which other methods are compared.

Estimation of Body Water

Several methods estimate body water (6-8) which yields an estimation of lean body mass. If lean body mass is known, it can be subtracted from total weight; the difference is fat weight. Estimation of body water usually depends on dilution of a substance that is distributed exclusively in body water, such as ^{40}K or deuterium.

Electrical Conductivity

This method is based on the principle that electrical conductivity is greater when there is more lean mass, because lean mass contains electrolytes which can conduct electricity (9,10). Comparative studies in 19 adults of widely varying fatness demonstrated excellent correlation between electrical conductivity and total body water methods (9).

Body Sampling Methods

Approximately one-third of the body's fat is in the subcutaneous tissue (tissue just under the skin). Although evolution may have placed this layer of fat to serve as an insulator and shock absorber, obesity scientists have taken advantage of the accessibility of this fat to measure it (11). Skinfold thickness correlates with percentage body fat fairly well, and many tables are available for this purpose (12,13). Skinfold thickness has also been used as a measure of malnutrition (14).

Skinfold Measurement

Skinfold measurement has achieved popularity both in medical and non-medical (e.g., health spa) settings, primarily due to the simplicity of the method. There is no consensus on which skinfold is best to measure, or if a sum of several skinfolds might be an even better indicator of adiposity. If only one or two skinfolds are to be measured, it appears that the triceps or subscapular skinfolds correlate best with percent body fat (12). There is, however, considerable site-to-site variation in skinfolds, especially during the prepubertal years, and in young adults and middle-aged women (13). More definitive recommendations will have to await further research.

Skinfold measurements yield data not only on total body fat content but also on its distribution. Some research suggests that central obesity is more closely correlated with diabetes, hypertension and hypercholesterolemia than is peripheral obesity (1). If this hypothesis is borne out by future research, this would suggest that central obesity is more dangerous to health than peripheral obesity, even if the percent body fat is identical. It is also thought that obesity which is carried from childhood into adulthood is more likely to be of central distribution while weight gain in adult years is more likely to be peripherally distributed.

A variation of the skinfold technique to evaluate adiposity is aptly known as the adipomuscular ratio (AMR). In this technique, the skinfold thickness and the circumference at the same location along the limb are compared (3, p.28). The circumference is presumed to be an index of muscle mass, while the skinfold evaluates adiposity. Another variation is the comparison of two circumference measurements (15). Ratio of waist to thigh circumferences in obese women was used to classify obesity as central or peripheral.

Miscellaneous

Several body sampling techniques were referred to above, including CAT scanning (16,17), ultrasound (18), and a spectrophotometric method (19). These methods are able to measure skinfold thickness relatively accurately in one or more than one location.

Frame Size Measurement

Finally, a brief discussion of frame size assessment may be in order. Although the life insurance company tables are subdivided according to frame size, there is no widely accepted way of determining frame size. Recently, some quantitative techniques have been proposed. Elbow breadth seems to be one possible index of frame size (20), since it is not affected by adiposity. Bony chest breadth on routine chest x-rays may be another possibility (21). A more formal mathematical model for determining frame size, termed the "HAT" model, has been proposed (22). It is based on the relationship between height and the sum of measurements across the shoulders and hips (biacromial and bitrochanteric diameters.) As these estimates become better validated, it is hoped that they will replace the current technique of frame assessment, namely, asking the individuals what frame size he thinks he is, a relatively poor measure (23).

Summary

There is no shortage of measurement techniques in the obesity field. There is, however, a shortage of data to validate these techniques. Perhaps even more lacking is a demonstration that the parameters being measured are worth measuring. Thus, little can be said of the long-term value of measuring skinfolds, or utilizing other methods. It does seem likely, however, that the detrimental effects of obesity would be clear regardless of the technique used to measure it. The section below examines some of the health hazards of obesity. Most of these data have been collected utilizing the relative weight measurement popularized by the availability of the insurance company tables.

HEALTH IMPLICATIONS OF OBESITY

It is accepted as an article of faith both among medical practitioners and the lay public that obesity is detrimental to health. This section evaluates some of the studies that led to this conclusion. While it is clear that severe or morbid obesity is dangerous to health, the effects of mild obesity (approximately 20-30% above ideal body weight) are more controversial. This is very important, because mild obesity is much more common than severe obesity (as is true of hypertension).

As mentioned previously, mild obesity affects approximately 40 million Americans. A report on obesity from the Royal College of Physicians of London has shown that up to 30% of the population of the United Kingdom is overweight to some degree (24), including many children and teenagers (25). Obesity beginning in childhood unfortunately often sets the stage for obesity in later life.

Most of the studies which have analyzed the relationship between obesity and mortality have shown that severe obesity (defined here as a relative weight>150%) is associated with a mortality rate about double that of the average-weight individual. These studies include the huge ones of the life insurance company (both 1959 (26) and 1983 (27)) and the American Cancer Society (28). Although most other reports (e.g., Framingham (29)) have noted the same trend, the number of severely obese individuals in the smaller studies was inadequate for statistical analysis.

A recent study from Denmark (30) followed a group of 1239 severely obese (RW>145%) men for up to 37 years. These men were selected from a population of 331,919 men liable for military service. Compared to controls, the obese men had significantly greater mortality. This may be due to a greater prevalence of hyperlipidemia (31,32), hypertension (32), diabetes (33), and certain types of cancer (28) in obese individuals.

As mentioned above, however, severe obesity is relatively rare, at least compared to mild obesity. Thus, a clinically more relevant question is whether mild obesity is detrimental to health. A recent review of the largest and best-performed studies (34) does suggest that even mild obesity increases mortality. This review includes the findings of the insurance company (26,27), the American Cancer Society (28), and the Framingham studies (35), totaling nearly 5 million subjects.

The opinion that mild obesity increases mortality, however, is not universal. Andres (36) has argued, in fact, that there might even be some *benefits* to mild obesity. Most of the studies quoted by Andres, however, are small studies and often included many older individuals. Since the studies are small, the chance of a beta error (inability to find a statistically significant result because the number of subjects is small) is great. The inclusion of many older individuals (e.g., Palmore's study at Duke of 60 to 94-year-olds) may introduce another bias: if someone in his 70s has already survived that long despite his obesity, he probably won't die at this age as a result of his obesity.

Such individuals may be retrospectively referred to as "healthy obese". The problem, of course, is that we are unable to predict which of the young obese patients will turn out to be "healthy obese" and which will succumb to their obesity or one of its complications. This finding, namely that risk factors decrease in importance with increasing age, has been observed for other risk factors, such as hypercholesterolemia and hypertension.

Assessing the relationship between obesity and cancer presents a different problem. Cancer is often associated with weight loss before it becomes clinically apparent. Thus, a significant percentage of older people who are at or below ideal body weight may be at such a weight because of subclinical cancer (cancer which is present but which hasn't been diagnosed yet). When they are enrolled in studies such as those of the life insurance company, a spurious correlation between their leaness and cancer incidence may be noted. This may be interpreted as suggesting that low body weight predisposes individuals to cancer, whereas another interpretation is that subclinical cancer decreases body weight. Distinguishing between the two is impossible at the present time.

It is not really surprising that underweight individuals also have increased mortality compared to those at "ideal" body weight. Underweight individuals (RW<80%) are probably malnourished, either intentionally or unintentionally. This may be due to peculiar nutritional habits (e.g., strict vegetarianism) or to disease (cancer, anorexia nervosa). The exact factors which account for the underweight status in most underweight persons may not be clear, but one can surmise that this malnutrition state is not healthy. For instance, it has been hypothesized that deficiencies of various vitamins and minerals may predispose individuals to cancer. It is likely that severely underweight subjects will be deficient in one or more of these nutrients.

Summary

With respect to the effects of obesity on health, it is probably fair to say that there is a consensus among experts about the following points:

1) Severe obesity (RW>150%) increases the risk of diabetes, hypertension,

hyperlipidemia, gout, arthritis, gallbladder disease, and cardiovascular disease. If an obese individual already suffers from one or more of these conditions, weight loss is *very* likely to ameliorate or resolve the problem. There is disagreement as to whether milder obesity, *in the absence of these other conditions*, is an independent risk factor.

2) Longer term obesity, especially if present since childhood, increases mortality more than later-onset obesity.

3) Mild obesity (120%<RW<140%), at least according to the largest studies, is also associated with increased mortality. Smoking complicates the picture since lean individuals smoke more than obese individuals. If an individual must smoke to maintain leanness, he is subjecting himself to more risk than if he quit smoking and gained some weight. Ideally, of course, one can stop smoking and also maintain an acceptable weight.

4) In practice, appearance and social factors may play a much more important role in motivating individuals to lose weight than the health considerations discussed above. Thus, morbidity and mortality considerations may only be secondary in encouraging obese individuals to lose weight. Therefore, argument about the health risks of obesity may be academic. Of more use to obese individuals is the provision of a reasonable plan for weight loss and its maintenance. Before these topics are dealt with, however, brief discussions of eating disorders and the cause of obesity are in order.

EATING DISORDERS—ANOREXIA NERVOSA AND BULIMIA

Ours is an extremely weight-conscious society. Although this societal pressure toward weight maintenance may have its advantages, when carried too far, the result may be short stature and delayed puberty (37) or an eating disorder such as anorexia nervosa or bulimia. These two eating disorders have become "fashionable" diseases in the 1980s. Much has been written about anorexia and bulimia, both in the scientific (38-40) and in the lay (41) press.

Although eating disorders have been recognized since the ninth century (42), it has only recently been appreciated how common these diseases are. Approximately 1% of teenaged and young adult women suffer from anorexia, while the incidence of bulimia in the same population is 10-15%. The prevalence of the eating disorders is thought to be on the rise. These diseases affect females primarily; less than 10% of the patients are male.

Anorexia Nervosa

The typical anorectic patient has been a model girl, a high achiever with good grades, and good family and socioeconomic background. The typical bulimic is not a good student, and half have demonstrated acting out behaviors such as alcohol or drug abuse, stealing or promiscuous sexual behavior (43). Feigner et al (44) have outlined the following diagnostic criteria for anorexia nervosa:

(1) Onset before 25 years of age

(2) Loss of at least 25% of original body weight

(3) A distorted body image—they believe that they are fat even though they are emaciated—and bizarre attitudes toward eating

(4) No other known medical or psychiatric illness which would account for the weight loss

(5) At least two of the following conditions—amenorrhea, lanugo, bradycardia, hyperactivity, binge eating and self-induced vomiting.

The primary clinical feature of anorexia, of course, is severe weight loss due to either inadequate food intake, or adequate food intake followed by self-induced vomiting. Approximately 40% of patients with anorexia are also bulimic (binging/purging). Laxative or diuretic abuse may also be observed. It is interesting to note that anorectic patients are often preoccupied with food, and they enjoy preparing meals for others.

Bulimia

Bulimia is characterized by powerful urges to overeat, especially carbohydrates, followed by self-induced vomiting or periods of starvation. This results in a weight that is usually close to ideal body weight. The binge-eating episodes are associated with great distress, and marked by feelings of loss of self-control, self-disgust, anger and depression.

Treatment

Treatment of these eating disorders is aimed at restoring normal eating patterns and body weight, especially in anorexia. If the anorexic patient weighs 25% less than ideal body weight, hospital admission is mandatory. This degree of emaciation is a *medical* emergency, and anorexia has been associated with sudden death (45), as have liquid protein diets. Other conditions associated with anorexia include hormonal problems, such as failure to menstruate, improper temperature regulation, poor thyroid function, etc. Recent reports suggest that osteoporosis is also a frequent complication of anorexia (46,47).

A multifaceted approach to treatment, including medical management, psychotherapy, behavior modification, and family therapy, is thought to be ideal. Weight gain should not be encouraged at too rapid a pace, because medical (edema, congestive heart failure, gastric dilatation) or psychiatric (depression, suicide) side effects may occur. Usually oral refeeding is all that is necessary, but on occasion, intravenous feeding may be called for.

Close followup after discharge is important, since the relapse rate is high (48), as is mortality of untreated (or inadequately treated) anorexia nervosa.

ETIOLOGY OF OBESITY

Although understanding the etiology of obesity may not eliminate the problem of obesity, this knowledge may be useful in motivating the patient. Recent studies suggest that the old concept that "fat people are fat because they eat more than skinny people" may not be entirely correct. Some recent evidence has called this classical concept into question, and it is now apparent that obesity has multiple causes.

It used to be held that two people of identical body size and composition and who have similar activity patterns have identical caloric requirements. Recent data suggest that this is not always true. Recognition of this fact, however, does not invalidate the First Law of Thermodynamics, which states that calories ingested must be either burned or stored (usually as fat). Several studies have now shown that obese individuals may lose weight at markedly different rates, despite identical degrees of caloric restriction (e.g.,49). In this study, obese patients were placed on an 800 calorie daily diet. Total weight loss over the 3-week study period ranged from 1.6 to 9.8 kg (3.5 to 21 pounds). Another study (50) has shown that two people of the same age, sex, body weight and composition, and pattern of activity may differ by up to 40% in energy expenditure. Thus, it is likely that some of the overweight people who always complained that they ate less than their next door neighbor but still gained weight were telling the truth. It is true that obese people often underestimate their caloric intake, but it is becoming quite clear that this is not the only explanation.

Although the existence of this phenomenon (different people losing weight at different rates) is undisputed, the reasons for it are far from clear. This phenomenon is often attributed, especially by lay people, to "hormones". Although hormones may play a role in this diffrence among individuals, invoking the word "hormones" does no more to clarify this issue than saying "genetics". The latter is probably more accurate, but hardly any more enlightening.

Several factors may account for these inter-individual variations. For instance, different people may have different efficiencies in absorbing calories from the gastrointestinal tract. Another difference may be the composition of the calories in the diet. It is known, for example, that fat calories are more efficiently processed in the body (and thus contribute more calories) than carbohydrate or protein calories (51).

The bottom line, however, is that even though these differences exist among individuals, people who have this tendency to gain weight (or not to lose it) will still have to match calorie intake to their unique expenditure. In other words, for each person, there is a caloric intake below which a weight loss *will* occur. That caloric intake may be markedly different for two individuals, but each person has his own "break-even" point. In view of other biologic differences (height, hair color, etc.) which exist among people, it is not surprising that such a difference exists.

The outlook is not totally bleak, however. For instance, it has been suggested that there may be ways (e.g., increased exercise level) of altering the break-even point. Furthermore, as noted above, some foods may be less efficiently metabolized, and consequently, would lead to less weight gain than other foods containing the same number of calories. At our current state of knowledge, trial and error is the best way of finding out the level of caloric restriction which may be necessary for weight loss.

MANAGEMENT OF OBESITY

As mentioned previously, obesity is extremely hard to treat, and it has been said that obesity, like alcoholism, can only be put into remission, never cured. Multiple approaches have been used in the treatment of obesity, including diet, surgery, drugs, and behavior modification, as well as various combinations of these modalities. The success of a treatment plan for obesity ought to be judged on the basis of the following criteria:

1) Does it work? In other words, does the participant lose weight? Although most diets focus on this aspect, it is probably the *least* reliable way to judge weight-loss therapies. Indeed, the cheapest, simplest diet I can think of, which also "works" the best in terms of weight loss, can be stated in one word— starvation. This approach, however, is not a realistic solution to the obesity problem.

2) Can the diet be followed easily, with some difficulty, or is it damn near impossible to adhere to? This is one of the major downfalls of the starvation diet.

3) As a corollary to #2, can the diet be followed for a long period of time? Many diets can be followed for a few weeks, but relatively few obese individuals can achieve ideal body weight that quickly. If a diet "works" initially, but can't be followed for a sufficient length of time to achieve adequate weight reduction, then the diet cannot be considered very effective.

4) Is it safe and relatively free from side effects? Although often brought up as a failure of many diets, very few diets currently practiced are dangerous. Starvation and the liquid protein diets popular in the late 1970s *are* dangerous, but are not utilized much today.

5) Can weight loss be *maintained* after the diet period is over? This aspect is

probably the most important and least appreciated criterion by which weight loss schemes should be judged. This is where starvation and formula diets fail miserably. Although such diets may be tough to follow, a surprising number of people do stick with them and lose significant amounts of weight. However, when the formerly obese individual reaches ideal body weight, he has learned little (if *anything*) about altering the eating habits which led to his obesity in the first place. This accounts for the miserable statistics that less than 10% of obese patients who lose weight will maintain the weight loss for more than 7 years (52). Thus, it is important for the weight-loss program to teach coping skills which will alter the habits which led to the obese state in the first place. This was the role originally envisioned for behavior modification, but the results have been nowhere near those initially hoped for.

One should reflect on the above 5 criteria when one evaluates an ad for a diet which promises a painless 20-pound weight loss in two weeks. The last criterion is especially important, since such diets rarely lead to permanent weight loss.

Discussed below are several approaches which have been used to produce weight loss. These include various types of diets, drug therapy, and even surgical solutions.

Dieting

Sensible Low-Calorie Diets

The most reasonable way to lose weight is to decrease caloric intake and increase physical activity. This remains true even though we recognize that various individuals will have different "break-even" points, as discussed above. Since fats are the most calorically-dense foods, and have other negative health effects, they should be primary candidates for elimination or reduction. This is especially true of saturated fats, because their elimination would have a tendency to lower serum cholesterol. Intake of refined sugars should also be reduced, because sugars contain no nutrients; this is why they are referred to as "empty calories."

At the same time, high-carbohydrate, high-fiber (HCF) foods should be emphasized in the reducing diet. Such foods are bulky and filling, and will have a tendency to decrease sensations of hunger which often accompany weight-loss diets. HCF diets are also rich in nutrients anf fiber, and are usually low in fat.

Finally, there is much evidence that physical activity significantly increases weight loss, and increases the likelihood that weight loss will be maintained (53). Thus, regular aerobic exercise, such as daily walking, jogging or bicycling, is also recommended.

The major disadvantage of this balanced diet is that the rate of weight loss is often slow, and thus compliance tends to be poor. This disadvantage has led to the development of the modified fast diets, discussed below.

Very Low Calorie Diets (Modified Fasts)

Since neither total fasting nor the low-calorie diet described above are considered practical in the treatment of severe obesity, the protein-supplemented modified fast (PSMF) diet was proposed in the early 1970s (53). The objective of all diets is to promote primarily the loss of body fat while conserving lean (usually muscle) tissue. This objective is the raison d'etre of PSMF diets, which have been shown to conserve lean tissue while maximizing fat loss (54-58). The topic of very low calorie diets has been recently comprehensively reviewed (59), and the interested reader is encouraged to consult this review for further detail.

The composition of the various PSMF diets has been the object of extreme controversy. For instance, some have suggested that carbohydrate-free PSMF diets promote greater weight loss and spare body protein better than carbohydrate-containing PSMF diets (60). It has also been proposed that the carbohydrate-free diet promotes greater weight loss because it induces a greater degree of ketosis (breakdown of fats in the body), and that the ketosis suppresses appetite and elevates mood (61). Neither of these potential advantages of carbohydrate-free PSMF diets have been substantiated (62,63). In fact, significant decreases in muscle glycogen (muscle energy source) and endurance were observed on a carbohydrate-free hypocaloric diet (64), and another study showed that nitrogen balance was improved on a carbohydrate-containing hypocaloric diet (65).

The content and form of PSMF diets varies considerably among investigators. Whereas some include actual foods as the protein source (e.g., a high quality protein such as milk, lean meat/poultry/fish, or egg white), others use a powdered formula diet (usually based on milk or egg protein) which is drunk by the patient. Proponents of the former approach contend that eating actual food helps the patient make the transition to a regular diet after the PSMF period is over. Those who favor the formula diet argue that it enhances compliance, thereby fostering a faster weight loss, which further reinforces compliance. There are no controlled trials comparing the two approaches, and it is likely that the form of the PSMF is less important than the type of protein and other aspects of the diet.

The caloric content of most PSMF diets varies from about 300 to 500 calories/day. Protein accounts for most of the calories, with the balance coming from fat and/or carbohydrate. All reputable weight-loss programs also include a vitamin and mineral supplement, which usually contains a multivitamin preparation plus sodium, potassium, and calcium.

PSMF diets should not be followed by prepubertal or pregnant subjects, nor by those with significant heart, liver or kidney disease. Many programs also

won't accept growing teenagers or individuals with potentially hazardous oc-
cupations, e.g., bus drivers. In order to ensure that patients are medically fit to be
enrolled, most centers administer a battery of tests to their prospective patients.
The battery usually includes an ECG (heart rhythm test), chest x-ray, complete
blood count, urinalysis, and blood chemistry panel (usually includes electrolytes, glucose, BUN, creatinine, uric acid, cholesterol, triglycerides, liver
enzymes, albumin and globulin).

Most patients experience a 5-10 pound weight loss the first week, with weight
loss decreasing (to about 3-5 pounds/wk) in the ensuing weeks. The amount of
weight lost and the ability to conserve body protein are quite variable among
individuals (66). One study suggests that greater weight loss may be achieved if
the diet is ingested in the morning than in the evening (67). Hunger is said to be
maximal the first day and tapers off rapidly. Individuals usually follow the PSMF
diets as outpatients except for diabetics, who may be hospitalized to adjust their
insulin or other medications. Most scientific researchers follow their patients
closely, often once a week, although the commercial programs may not. Ideally,
the PSMF diet is only a part of a comprehensive program, which might include
nutrition teaching and learning low-cal cooking, behavior modification, exercise,
and group and individual counseling. Side effects of a well-planned PSMF diet
program are usually mild; they include possible low blood pressure and/or dizziness, especially when getting up quickly, cold intolerance, and constipation.

Despite the efficacy (in terms of short-term weight loss) and simplicity of the
PSMF diet, the long-term success of this weight-loss method is deplorable.
Attrition rates from PSMF programs (and in fact, from most weight-loss programs) are very high. For instance, in one study quoted previously (54), only
about half the patients were able to continue for more than 16 weeks. Only 17
(33%) out of 52 patients came within 33 pounds of their ideal body weight. And
in fact, the results of this study are probably better than those of most other
similar studies. In another study (57), 22 patients *finished* the study still 61%
overweight (they had started an average of 86% overweight).

The long-term results of PSMF diets are even worse (68), although this study
involved fasting in addition to PSMF. Of 207 patients who were initially enrolled
in the program, only 121 (58%) were available at follow-up an average of 7.3
years after enrollment. Regain to original weight occurred in half of this group,
and only 7 subjects (3% of the originally enrolled group, or 6% of the follow-up
group) remained reduced for the duration of follow-up.

Thus, the discussion of the PSMF diet underscores the importance of the
criterion discussed previously—that a weight-loss remedy must show long-term
maintenance of weight loss. In fact, some have suggested that to lose and regain
weight repeatedly may be worse physically (and certainly psychologically) than
to remain overweight.

Drug Therapy

Although this book deals primarily with nutritional topics, the reader has noted that I have digressed several times to discuss non-nutritional topics. In this spirit, I will briefly discuss drug treatment of obesity because it is my perception that most obese individuals who may be reading this book either have tried or have thought about trying some of the "diet pills".

The proper use of prescription antiobesity drugs in the United States is clearly limited. Antiobesity drugs should only be given as part of a complete weight-loss program under medical supervision. It is, I believe, the feeling of most experts in this field that amphetamines should not be used in the treatment of obesity under any circumstances. In fact, efforts are currently underway to totally eliminate the availability of amphetamines in medicine (with a few limited exceptions).

If anti-obesity drugs are prescribed, they should be used as a short-term aid to initial weight loss, while other aspects of the anti-obesity program are being implemented. These other aspects include dietary teaching, learning of coping skills (behavior modification), increasing exercise, etc. If this isn't done, it is very likely that weight will be quickly regained after the drug therapy is discontinued.

The antiobesity drugs most commonly prescribed in the United States include mazindol (e.g., Mazanor, Sanorex), phentermine (e.g., Adipex, Fastin, Ionamin, Oby-Trim, Teramine) and phenylpropanolamine (e.g., Anorexin, Dexatrim, Dieutrim). Phenylpropanolamine is also found in many over-the-counter cold remedies, as well as in non-prescription forms strictly for obesity.

It is unclear how these drugs promote weight loss. It is likely that they have different mechanisms of action. A recent study took advantage of the different mechanisms of action by combining lower doses of two of these drugs rather than a higher dose of a single one (69). The combination of the two drugs was as effective as either drug by itself. Subjects receiving the combination lost an average of 18.5 pounds, while those receiving placebo lost 9.7 pounds over the 16-week study period. As expected, drug side effects were less frequent with the combination regimen than with either drug alone. It is noteworthy that of the 81 volunteers who began the study, 37 dropped out, 18 for reasons related to drug treatment.

Antiobesity drugs are usually prescribed short-term, and in fact, many investigators have observed that these drugs lose their efficacy with prolonged administration. The observation has been made, however, that fenfluramine may remain effective (compared to placebo) for more than 1 year in *selected* individuals (70). For instance, whereas 19 out of 21 patients regained weight while taking placebo, 8 of 21 taking fenfluramine maintained their weight loss. However, 7 others did regain weight, and 6 patients had to be taken off the drug.

As has been emphasized throughout this book, evaluation of the efficacy of a regimen is only half the story. The other half, of course, relates to any side effects of the therapy. In this regard, the track record of the most commonly used antiobesity drugs is somewhat worrisome. For instance, there have been several recent reports of young adult patients having strokes while taking Dexatrim and Dietac (phenylpropanolamine/caffeine combination) (71,72). Although these anecdotal reports certainly cannot prove a cause-and-effect relationship between these drugs and the occurrence of the stroke, they certainly do raise that possibility. The fact that strokes are extremely rare in young adults lends further support to this hypothesis, as does a recent experiment wherein 18% of rats given a high dose of phenylpropanolamine/caffeine had strokes (73).

The Bottom Line

As is true of many other antiobesity therapies, antiobesity drugs only work while they are being taken, and are effective in a minority of obese patients. When such patients stop taking the drug, weight is usually regained. In view of this fact, it seems unreasonable to take antiobesity drugs, unless this is part of a comprehensive program. Such a regimen, which will involve habit retraining, increases the likelihood that weight will not be regained once ingestion of the drugs ceases. The interested reader is referred to two recent reviews on this topic for further information (74,75).

Surgical Therapy

Although widely viewed as therapy of last resort, it is estimated that over 100,000 patients have undergone surgical therapy for obesity. The major impetus for the performance of obesity surgery is the realization that massive obesity markedly increases morbidity and mortality (28,76). Assessing the proper role of surgery in the treatment of morbid obesity has been difficult due to the paucity of controlled trials.

Most reliable centers which offer obesity surgery offer it only to selected individuals. The usual criteria include:

(1) "morbid" obesity, defined as at least double ideal body weight or 100 pounds overweight,

(2) stable psychological status and sincere motivation to lose weight, as well as realistic expectations from the surgery (e.g., the surgery does not solve all the person's problems, and the weight-losing effects of the surgery *can* be defeated if the patient does not comply with the prescribed dietary instructions after surgery)

(3) relatively good health (diabetes, hypertension and gallbladder problems do not usually preclude surgery, but severe heart, kidney or liver disease do)

(4) the patient must have demonstrated previous serious attempts at weight loss without success

(5) some centers will not perform the surgery on individuals more than 50 years of age

Many different operations have been tried, but none has been found to be entirely satisfactory. Only the 3 most common ones—intestinal bypass, gastric bypass, and gastric stapling—will be discussed here. In addition, a new procedure for removing fat from certain locations in the body—called suction lipectomy— will be briefly discussed.

Intestinal (Jejunoileal) Bypass

Intestinal bypass was the first obesity operation to achieve popularity, but was supplanted by the gastric operations in the late 1970s. In fact, a surgeon recently told me that he believes that doing the intestinal bypass operation today would constitute medical malpractice. Although jejunoileal bypass is effective in promoting weight loss (an average 100-pound loss within 5 years after surgery), side effects and complications are also substantial (77). For instance, diarrhea persisted in 58% of the study patients, and various fluid, electrolyte, vitamin and mineral deficiencies were observed. Most important of all, however, is that progressive liver damage occurred in almost one-third of the patients, and 7% developed severe (potentially life-threatening) liver damage (77,78). The authors of this study stated that the above findings have led them to abandon the intestinal bypass surgery in favor of the gastric bypass.

The issue of whether individuals who have had the intestinal bypass surgery should undergo another surgery to reverse the bypass is unclear at the present time. This decision will depend on individual desires and circumstances. Patients who are contemplating this should seek the opinion of a qualified surgeon.

Gastric Bypass

In this operation, a small pouch (two ounces or less) is made in the upper part of the stomach. This pouch then bypasses the rest of the stomach and part (duodenum) of the small intestine; the food from the pouch then empties into another portion (jejunum) of the small intestine. The small pouch and the attendant delay in stomach emptying produce a sensation of fullness, which reminds the patient to eat smaller amounts and to eat them more slowly. If the patient does not respect this cue, nausea and vomiting are likely to occur.

Gastric Stapling (Gastroplasty)

There are several gastric stapling procedures, but perhaps the most popular one is the vertical-banded (Mason) gastroplasty. This procedure also results in the formation of a small pouch, but once the food passes through the pouch, it travels the same path as food in a normal person. Therefore, this operation is viewed as being more "physiologic" than the gastric bypass, because the path of food travel is unaffected. The small size of the pouch and the small exit ("stoma") from the pouch significantly decrease the amount of food that can be ingested at one sitting and slow down the passage of food. This accomplishes the same objective that the gastric bypass operation achieves, i.e., providing feedback to the patient regarding speed and quantity of food consumption.

Weight loss with either gastric operation is similar, but gastroplasty appears to cause fewer complications (79,80). Complications of either operation include reflux gastritis and esophagitis (heartburn), perforation (formation of a hole), dilation of the pouch or stoma, ulcer of the stoma, stomal obstruction, staple line disruption and excessive vomiting (81). Stoma ulcer and vomiting are two problems which occur less frequently with the gastric stapling procedure.

It must be emphasized that *surgery does not eliminate the need for dietary discretion*. In fact, gastric surgery introduces several restrictions which must be carefully observed. For instance, a clear liquid diet is recommended for the first 6 weeks after the stapling procedure. The liquids must be sipped, not gulped, and no more than one to two ounces can be ingested at one sitting. After the six week period, patients must still eat small amounts, chew the food carefully, and avoid drinking liquids with the meal. High-calorie liquids are discouraged, because if they are taken frequently, they can defeat the purpose of the surgery and prevent weight loss.

The major benefit of the operation is weight loss. This can lead to a fall in serum cholesterol and triglyceride levels, and may eliminate the need for high blood pressure or diabetes medications (82-85). While total cholesterol and triglycerides decreased in patients who had had surgery, HDL (the "good" cholesterol) increased (83). Other complications of the obese state, such as arthritis, difficulty breathing, and premature cardiovascular death, are expected to be ameliorated, although there is little direct proof of these benefits at this time. Another potential benefit is the increase in the social activities of obese patients who lose weight.

Several complications of gastric reduction surgery are also observed. Mortality from the operation itself and during the immediate postoperative period ranges from 0 to 4% (86). Nausea, vomiting, dehydration, stretching of the pouch, and failure to lose weight are all potential complications. Various vitamin deficiencies, osteoporosis, and hair loss have also been reported (87,88). The incidence of gallstones increases after gastric bypass surgery (89), but probably not after gastric stapling.

Suction Lipectomy

The selective removal of fat from certain areas of the body has been an unattainable goal until recently, when suction lipectomy became available. Exercise may be of help in slimming down the waist or removing "saddle bag" deformities of the thighs, but often, these unsightly localized fat deposits remain despite all efforts to remove them.

Suction lipectomy, which involves suctioning small amounts of fat from certain areas of the body, has received much attention recently in both the lay and scientific press (90-92). The procedure, which is primarily performed by plastic surgeons, usually begins by marking off the area to be suctioned while the patient is standing. In the operating room, the surgeon then makes a small incision (which is usually hidden in a skin crease) through which a long hollow tube (cannula) is passed. Tunnels of fat are then suctioned through the cannula, and the overlying skin is then smoothed out and bandaged so that the suctioned area does not fill with body fluids. It is recommended that no more than 6-8 pounds of fat be removed in one operation, but the operation can be repeated several times to remove more fat.

It should be emphasized, however, that this operation is not intended for obese individuals. The ideal candidate should be under 40 years of age, is no more than 30-40 pounds overweight, and has good skin elasticity and bulges which have been refractory to dieting and exercise. As was true of the obesity operations described above, the potential patient must also have realistic expectations of the surgical results.

Complications include excessive fluid loss, burning and tearing sensations in the operated area, which sometimes last for months, unusual skin pigmentation, and numbness or swelling of the area. Obviously, it is also possible that the desired cosmetic results will not be achieved, and sometimes, a wavy skin indentation may be seen. Finally, the procedure is unlikely to be paid for by most insurance companies; thus, the cost of $1000 to $4000 must be kept in mind. This cost may decrease as more physicians learn how to perform the technique, but bad results may also occur more frequently as less experienced practitioners perform the procedure.

Finally, since the procedure has been performed only in the last few years, its long-term effects are totally unknown. For instance, it is not known if fat cells removed are gone for good or if they will reaccumulate. The exact role of the surgery remains unclear, but most physicians are proceeding slowly to delineate it.

POPULAR WEIGHT REDUCTION PLANS AND FAD DIETS

Many popular weight-loss diets have come and gone in the past decade. It would be impossible to review all such diets, and apologies are made to the reader whose favorite diet is not included here. The interested reader, however, is referred to an excellent book by *Consumer Guide* entitled *Rating the Diets* (92a). This book evaluates over 100 diets in an objective fashion. It also discusses diet clubs, diet pills and surgery. The evaluations are usually fairly objective, although on occasion somewhat inconsistent. For instance, while (correctly) berating the high-fat, high-protein, low-carbohydrate Atkins' Diet (p.123), they (improperly, in my opinion) accord two stars in evaluating the Dieting by the Stars diet (p.108), which has a similar composition. On the whole, however, *Rating the Diets* is highly recommended.

Several general observations can be made about popular weight reduction plans, especially those which are touted as "breakthroughs". In general, it appears that the "breakthroughs" of yesteryear weren't breakthroughs after all, because if they had been, there would be no need for more breakthroughs this year. Upon closer inspection, it is obvious that the fad diets sport differences in inconsequential details, such as the packaging, but that the basic faddish elements are nearly the same. Most dietary fads have been fashioned by advertising specialists, not by scientists or biologists. The content or details of the fad are unimportant; the package is everything. If this were not so, how could the *Beverly Hills Diet* have sold so well?

Most of the time, fad diets are neither effective nor potentially dangerous to health. To remind the reader, however, that diets can, on occasion, be hazardous and even fatal, the liquid protein diets will be discussed first. Although not much used anymore, the history of these diets is interesting and quite informative for our purposes. An evaluation of some current popular diets will follow the discussion on the liquid protein diets.

Liquid Protein Diets

Liquid protein diets (LPD) achieved great popularity in the late 1970s after a book entitled *The Last Chance Diet* was published in 1976, extolling their virtues (93). It was estimated that more than 100,000 people used LPDs as their sole source of nutrition for at least one month in 1977 (94). This diet did in fact represent the "last chance" for at least 60 of these people who died while following the LPD. Needless to say, these diets quickly disappeared from the dieting scene, but one wonders if any of the entries in the current diet scene might also be dangerous to their adherents. What is also somewhat disconcerting is that the mechanism by which liquid protein diets contributed to the death of their followers remains unknown. This is of more than academic importance because there are several similarities between LPDs and the supplemented fasts described above, and some authors have argued that supplemented fasting may also be dangerous.

There are some obvious differences, however, between the LPDs of the late

1970s and the PSMF as practiced by medical obesity specialists today. First of all, the LPDs utilized a "notoriously poor quality protein" (95) made from collagen and gelatin derived from cow hides and other sources of connective tissue. Secondly, many of the LPDs neglected vitamin and mineral supplements, and in fact, lack of potassium supplementation was implicated as one of the potential causes of death in individuals taking the LPDs. Finally, many of the individuals taking the LPDs were totally unmonitored by medical personnel familiar with LPDs. Although monitoring would not have helped in all cases (in fact, some individuals died while they were physically in the hospital), it may have helped in some cases.

Many reports of deaths in individuals taking LPDs appeared in the late 1970s and early 1980s (96-106). It may be of interest to review one of these case reports (97):

> A 38-year-old woman was admitted to a hospital in October, 1977, complaining of fainting spells. In February of 1977, she had weighed 337 pounds and against her physician's advice, began following *The Last Chance Diet*. She took 600 calories daily of beef-hide extract, as well as multivitamin, calcium, folic acid, and potassium supplements (24 mEq/day). She felt well during the 8 months on this diet, and lost 139 pounds. Serial laboratory tests were essentially within normal limits.
>
> Two days prior to admission, she had an episode of dizziness while driving, followed by a fainting spell a few minutes later. During the ensuing few hours, she felt unwell and vomited several times. Although she felt well on the next day, she was found unresponsive at home on the following day. By the time she reached the hospital, she was awake and alert. Her physical examination was essentially normal, except for a nodule in her thyroid gland. Her EKG showed normal rhythm but a low voltage and a prolonged QTc (0.56 sec) (a finding noted in other patients who have died while taking LPDs). Other laboratory tests in this patient were essentially normal.
>
> Shortly after arrival in the emergency room, an episode of ventricular tachycardia (a dangerous irregularity in the heart rhythm) occurred, with loss of consciousness after 1 minute. Electrical cardioversion (electrical shock to the chest to end the bad rhythm) was required. The patient was given a bolus of 100 mg of lidocaine and started on a continuous drip of 4 mg/min (to hopefully prevent recurrence of the bad rhythm). The patient had recurrent episodes of ventricular tachycardia and required intubation (a tube to help her breathe). Numerous electrical cardioversions and multiple drugs, as well as a pacemaker, were used in efforts to control the recurrent ventricular tachycardia. Approximately 12 hours after admission, the patient had a cardiac arrest from which she could not be resuscitated.
>
> Autopsy showed the heart and its arteries to be grossly normal. However, microscopical sections of the heart revealed decrease in the size and protein content of the muscle fibers.

As was true in this case, several of the individuals who died did so in the hospital and in spite of the best efforts of modern medicine to prevent the death. Some dieters died a few days after stopping the LPD and resuming normal eating habits.

In addition to this point, several important observations may be made from an analysis of the papers referenced above:

1) No deaths were recorded in subjects who had followed the diet for less than two months.

2) Ventricular arrhythmias, as in the case described above, were documented in about one-half of the patients who died.

3) Approximately one-half of the patients were under medical supervision while on the diet.

4) Approximately two-thirds of the patients had underlying diseases that may have contributed to their death; the other third did not. The fact that arrhythmias were not present in patients before the diet was initiated and disappeared after the diet was stopped suggests that the diet itself was responsible for the arrhythmias (and consequently, the sudden deaths).

5) Many of the patients who were medically supervised had normal EKGs; therefore, the normality of the EKG did not preclude fatal complications. Some patients did have abnormal EKGs—usually a prolonged QTc and low voltage of the QRS complex.

6) Although some patients have had hypokalemia (low potassium in the blood), many had totally normal laboratory tests.

Although the mechanism of the sudden death observed in adherents to the LPD remains unclear, several investigators have proposed abnormalities of heart muscle function as a possibility (108,109). This hypothesis is also supported by autopsy studies of many of the LPD victims; their hearts often showed loss of protein and energy content which could explain the sudden death. What is perhaps most disconcerting is the fact that it remains to be proven that liquid protein diets (or *any* kind of diet) is/are effective in *maintenance* of weight reduction. This makes the above deaths all the more tragic. Thus, these "unnecessary deaths are a somber reminder of the tragic consequences that can occur when therapy outstrips its research base" (95).

The liquid protein diet is rarely used today and was discussed more for illustrative purposes. The diets which are evaluated below are commonly used by the dieting public. In fact, all of the diets discussed below have at one time been on the New York Times Bestseller list, and some are on it as this chapter is written (December, 1985).

Many of these popular diets have been previously considered in the popular (110,111) as well as the scientific literature (112-116). All of these articles have pointed out the fallacies of various fad diets, yet these plans continue to be as popular as ever. Interestingly, not even 1 of 11 popular diets provided 100% of the U.S. RDAs for the 13 vitamins and minerals studied. Three of the diets (Beverly Hills, Richard Simmons and Stillman) supplied less than 70% of the RDAs for more than half the vitamins and minerals evaluated.

Some selected popular diets are discussed below in more detail. The discussion is unfortunately limited by the lack of literature which has studied these plans. However, some of the claims are so outrageous that just a modicum of understanding of the physiologic processes of the human body is sufficient to dismiss them entirely. No diet is a better example of this concept than . . .

The Beverly Hills Diet

This diet recommends that for the first 10 days, the dieter eat nothing but fruit (pineapples, bananas, watermelon, mangoes, etc.), all in a very regimented order, and without substitutions. You are not allowed to eat different types of food at the same time—you even have to wait two hours between two different types of fruit. Essentially no protein is ingested until the 11th day, and an adequate amount of protein isn't eaten until the 19th day of this plan.

The Beverly Hills Diet book rivals the *Life Extension* book for the greatest number of scientifically incorrect statements in one book, as pointed out recently in the scientific press (117,118). The author has neither nutritional nor medical training. This, however, does not seem to deter her from making the most nonsensical statements in her book. The most ridiculous of all statements was pointed out at the beginning of this chapter. Other scientifically preposterous proclamations include:

> "the idea of eating a 'balanced' meal is as absurd as wearing two skirts or two pairs of shoes at the same time" (p.14)
> "most enzymes can't work simultaneously"(p.16)
> "God created us with the thymus gland, which excretes the enzyme necessary to digest milk"(p.37)
> "The harder the cheese, the harder it is to digest"(p.38)
> "it [cheese] makes anything else you eat after it fattening because anything you eat after the cheese will get trapped in your stomach right along with the cheese"(p.38)

I had initially intended to go through the whole book and delineate the fallacies. I had also intended to comment on each of the fallacies. I have found, however, that I do not have the intestinal fortitude for either task. I will leave it to the enlightened reader to make the above search. Failing that, the reader may wish to consult reference 117.

The Cambridge Diet

The Cambridge Diet, a very-low-calorie but supplemented liquid formula diet, is said to have been used by more than three million overweight Americans. This diet has also attracted attention in the medical literature (119-121). This diet is similar to the protein-supplemented modified fasts (PSMF) discussed earlier in this chapter. Various diets are available, ranging from 330 to 800 calories, although the 330-calorie diet remains the most popular. This version contains 33 g of high quality protein and 44 g carbohydrate. The brochure contains several testimonials from users of this diet who (incredibly) lost 20 pounds in the *first 72 hours* of the diet.

What's unique about Cambridge is the way in which it is distributed. The diet supplies are provided by lay persons known as "counselors". Criteria for the selection of counselors are unclear; it appears, however, that nutrition training is not a prerequisite. This mode of distribution is the major criticism leveled at the diet in the scientific press (119). These authors, and others, have recommended that such low-calorie diets be distributed and monitored solely by physicians and dietitians. This would facilitate the proper selection, monitoring, and discontinuation (if necessary) of the diet.

Although Cambridge Plan International recommends that the dieter "Consult your doctor before starting this diet", it is likely that most participants do not follow this advice. Consequently, most participants are likely to be following a very low calorie diet without any meaningful medical supervision. Further advice recommends that the "formula is designed for use as a sole source of nutrition for periods of not to exceed four consecutive weeks at any one time". It is unknown if compliance with this advice is adequate, and whether interspersing a week or two of a regular diet would be sufficient before resuming another four-week cycle.

In a survey of 400 college women, 191 (48%) reported following a weight reduction program since their enrollment at the university (121). The 191 dieters used the following for weight control: hypocaloric diets (47%); Cambridge (19%); exercise (19%); drugs (7%); weight loss clinics (4%); and low carbohydrate diets (4%). The subjects on the Cambridge diet reported spending an average of $18 per week for the formula. They followed the diet for about 2 weeks, during which time they lost an average of 10 pounds. Subjects reported nausea, fatigue, thirst, excessive urination, diarrhea and hunger, which they rated as mild. Despite reporting these side effects, 48% rated the diet as good and 62% said they would recommend the diet.

In defense of the diet, Alan Howard, Ph.D., the developer of the diet, stated that only six reports of death in Cambridge dieters had been reported to the FDA by the end of 1982, and that this is no greater than would be expected by chance alone. The critics responded that this defense is valid only if there has been complete reporting of deaths in users of the diet. Since many physicians may not know that their deceased patients have been using the Cambridge diet, they would be unlikely to report the association.

A recent independent study of 27 dieters on the Cambridge diet in which the participants were closely monitored suggests that the diet, at least when used for 4 weeks, is safe (122). It should be noted, however, that this is a very small sample from which sweeping conclusions cannot be made. Furthermore, many people on liquid protein diets who died were under medical supervision; thus, medical supervision obviously does not preclude death on hypocaloric diets.

In the final analysis, it is probably fair to say that hypocaloric diets of *any* type can be dangerous, and that we do not yet know what aspect of hypocaloric diets makes them potentially lethal. Lesser degrees of caloric restriction as well as medical supervision decrease, but do not eliminate, the risk of such diets. Thus, as is true of many things in life, it is probably not the diet but how it is used that determines its potential for morbidity and mortality.

Herbalife

This company sells several products which contain herbs and are meant to be used in weight reduction. One of these, Herbalife Slim and Trim Formula, used to contain mandrake and pokeroot, two very toxic herbs (123). In fact, mandrake was once used by American Indians as a suicide drug (123). These toxic components were removed from the preparation after the FDA took action against the company (124). More recently, California's attorney general filed a consumer protection lawsuit against Herbalife (125). According to the complaint, Herbalife misrepresented the abilities of several of its products to curb appetite, promote weight loss, etc. The case is still pending at this time.

Testimony on Herbalife is also being heard by the Permanent Subcommittee on Investigations, Senate Governmental Affairs Committee (126). In fact, the American Dietetic Association, which represents the nation's 50,000 dietitians, recently submitted a statement to the committee in which they took exception to testimony by Dr. David Katzin, representing Herbalife. It appears that Dr. Katzin made reference to an ADA diet which does not exist, in an attempt to lend legitimacy to the Herbalife diet.

F-Plan Diet

While the United States seems to be the country of origin of most diet books, the F-Plan Diet is an import from England (127). A bestseller in 1982 in Europe, this book crossed the Atlantic in 1983 and has been on the New York Times bestseller list for 19 weeks. Fortunately for its readers, this book preaches a sensible diet plan, based on high fiber intake (that's where the F in F-Plan comes from).

As was pointed out in Chapters 11 and 12 of this book, a high-fiber, high-complex-carbohydrate diet is the way to go, and the F-Plan capitalizes on this. The F-Plan Diet is a low-fat diet, and may be marginal in protein content. Protein content should not be a problem, however, since dairy and meat dishes are allowed, though in small amounts.

This diet is conceptually similar to the Pritikin diet, though not as restrictive as the latter. The F-Plan is also the direction in which national dietary recommendations are being focused, and rightly so. A high-fiber diet is especially useful in promoting weight loss because the quantities of food which can be taken are large, while the caloric content is low. It is also a diet which is high in nutrients, and which the obese person (or formerly obese) can continue for the rest of his life.

The Setpoint Diet

This popular diet is quite unique in that it was developed under the auspices of a large corporation (General Foods) and was advertised in medical journals before it became widely available to the general public in book form in September, 1985 (128). It is also unique in that the Setpoint diet plan is based on a substantial (but far from unanimous) body of medical literature. Finally, it is one of the few mass-market paperback books which advises a sensible diet-and-exercise plan which can be followed for the rest of one's life without endangering it.

The Setpoint Diet plan is based on the theory that each person's body automatically adjusts weight to a particular level, or "setpoint". The body's defense of this setpoint will resist any attempts to change it, such as dieting efforts. The existence of this setpoint is the reason (says the theory) that dieting attempts are doomed to failure. The only way to achieve a lower weight is by resetting the setpoint. The setpoint is reset by pursuing moderate regular (almost daily) exercise.

To speed weight loss along, however, the plan also includes a sensible balanced low-calorie diet in which essentially all foods are allowed, but in moderation. Depending on the specific circumstances and goals of each individual, several calorie levels, ranging from 1200 to 2400 calories per day, may be ingested. The key to achieving the low-calorie diet is portion control. The structure of the diet plan itself is very reminiscent of the American Diabetic Association's exchange diet. The Setpoint Diet provides all the protein, vitamins, minerals, and other nutrients necessary for optimal health. The very reasonable goal of this diet is a weekly weight loss of 1-3 pounds.

Dr. Leveille, the developer of the diet, is the director of nutrition and health sciences at the General Foods Corporation and has good credentials, with both an M.S. and a Ph.D. in nutrition and biochemistry from Rutgers University. I am afraid, however, that he has allowed his evangelistic zeal for the "setpoint theory" to cloud his scientific objectivity. He presents the setpoint theory as a *proven* entity rather than as an attractive scientific theory, which has both proponents and opponents. In doing so, he makes no mention of many articles which disagree with this point of view. Although 70 references are included at the end of the book, they are not specifically cited in the text, making it difficult, if not impossible, to evaluate the specific data upon which the author bases his statements. It would have been helpful to specifically cite such references, especially in a book that has been advertised in medical journals and ostensibly meant for medical professionals.

One of the central concepts of the Setpoint Diet deals with the basal metabolic rate (BMR). The BMR is the amount of energy which the body needs just to "stay alive"—for respiration, heartbeat, etc. The BMR accounts for a substantial amount of energy—more than half the caloric expenditure of the average person. In refrence to the BMR, the Setpoint Diet book states, for example, that, "Your skinny neighbor may actually be burning more calories all day long—whether he is napping or mowing the lawn—than you are when you do the exact same things for the exact same amounts of time". Although some obesity experts would agree with this view, many investigators have shown, in fact, that "obese subjects tend to have higher resting energy expenditure than subjects of the same age, sex, and height who are not obese" (quoted from ref. 129, who lists references 130-138 in support of this statement). Indeed, ref. 129 itself also showed that "the greater the percentage fat, the greater the metabolic rate".

Other inaccurate statements include (p.3) that, "The only way you can lose weight and keep it off is to lower your setpoint. Just lowering your caloric intake isn't enough". At worst, this statement simply isn't true; at best, it implies that we currently understand the mechanisms by which people gain and lose weight, which also is not the case. The author also promises to "solve, once and for all, your chronic weight problem" (p.3), as if there is proof that no cases of obesity would be refractory to this plan. Another overoptimistic statement: "Experts don't agree on exactly how exercise works to lower the setpoint, but all studies show that it does". This is a rather strange statement because "setpoint" is a rather nebulous concept, and there isn't even a consensus that it exists. Even if it does exist, however, there is certainly far from consensus that exercise lowers it. Although it may be argued that the only way one would be able to motivate a large number of individuals to follow the plan is by overstating the theory as if it were proven fact, this does not seem scientifically reasonable.

As pointed out in a recent review article on this topic (139), some observations on energy-obesity relationships are not in dispute. Metabolic rate does increase with intake of meals, and the thermic response to protein is higher than that to carbohydrate or fat. Secondly, BMR decreases as caloric intake decreases, as in dieting. We also know that two people of the same age, sex, body composition and pattern of activity may differ by 40% in energy expenditure (140), the reasons for which are unclear. One should not lose sight of the fact, however, that this field is characterized more by controversy than by consensus, as recently pointed out (141):

> "My conclusion . . .was, I hoped, sufficiently cautious to warn readers that evidence currently available is inadequate to provide an answer. A score card on the published literature would show about 50 per cent for and 50 per cent against a role in human beings . . ."

The book is, however, full of good information, and the diet-and-exercise plan is an excellent one. Dr. Leveille correctly points out, for instance, that "no diet, including the Setpoint Diet, can promise you a weight loss of more than 5 pounds of *fat* per week". He also accurately states that the "very act of dieting can make it increasingly difficult to lose weight". As is also pointed out, "The cornerstones of the diet [and this should apply to *any* diet] are balance, variety, and moderation".

In the final analysis, whether the setpoint theory is correct or not is a moot issue, because the recommendations of a diet-and-exercise plan are sound. Emphasizing a high-carbohydrate, low-fat diet is also reasonable. For many reasons which are well presented in the book, an exercise plan does facilitate initiation and maintenance of weight loss, and has other benefits. Thus, the Setpoint Diet book is highly recommended to the reader, who may follow the detailed dietary plans with confidence. As is always true, consultation with a physician and/or nutrition professional is prudent prior to beginning a weight-loss diet.

The Hilton Head Metabolism Diet

This is another diet book that has recently made the national bestseller list (142). Interestingly, the concepts espoused by the author of this book are strikingly similar to those embraced in the Setpoint plan discussed above. The Hilton Head book, at least by copyright date, predated the Setpoint plan by 2 years. The basic premise is that "You are overweight because of your failure to burn calories efficiently through metabolism" (p.3). He calls this inefficient burning *metabolic suppression*, a term not used in the scientific literature. Both diets focus on the energy *expenditure* side rather than the energy *intake* side of the equation. These diets are reacting to the traditional assessment that obesity is due to excessive intake rather than inadequate expenditure of calories.

The author, a Ph.D. in clinical psychology, states that "An overwhelming number of recent studies" (p.7) support his view. No studies, however, are cited in the book, making it difficult to assess the "overwhelming" literature upon which he bases his hypothesis. He also states, incorrectly (as pointed out in the above discussion on Setpoint), that the BMR of obese individuals is "usually at the lower end of the average range", and that "their thermostats are defective" (p.11). His plan, however, will enable the reader to "fix your thermostat so that you burn more calories" (p.12).

Dr. Miller then goes through much the same discussion that the Setpoint book did, dealing with other factors (age, gender, body composition, heredity, etc.) that affect BMR. He then provides a formula which I haven't seen previously scientifically verified to calculate fat weight (p.32). This formula involves multiplying the waist measurement (in centimeters) by 0.592 and thigh measure by 0.36. The two amounts are added together and 53.11 is subtracted from the total. That result is multiplied by 2.2, and this answer represents fat weight in pounds.

Despite the above criticisms, the dietary and exercise recommendations of the Hilton Head Diet are sound. The caloric content of the diet consists of 15% protein, 55% carbohydrate, and 30% fat (very similar to the recommendations of the American Heart Association and other national organizations). An abundance of breads, cereals, fruits and vegetables are reasonably recommended, and the lowest daily caloric intake which is endorsed is 800. Dr. Miller argues that overdieting can slow your metabolism excessively. In fact, after two weeks on the Low-cal (of 800 calories) phase, he insists that you switch to the Booster phase, during which the dieter will increase his intake by 300 calories to 1100 calories, to "stir up" the metabolism. If you have more weight to lose, you can alternate two weeks of Low-cal with one week of Booster until you are within a few percent of your goal weight. You then transcend into the Reentry phase, during which you will be gradually increasing calories from 1100 to 1500, and then to your maintenance number of calories.

Dr. Miller tells you that "Because of the Metabolic effect [of his diet], it [your maintenance number of calories] will be much higher than it was before your diet" (p.41). This, of course, is great news to the dieter, but I am unaware of any evidence to back up this statement. But, perhaps there is a catch to this that Dr. Miller hasn't told us about, and perhaps it's found in the next chapter, where we are told that "a moderate, consistent exercise plan . . . will stimulate your metabolism and keep it stimulated" (p.46). He has also invented a fourth meal, called the *metabo-meal*, which also is supposed to stimulate the metabolism. The author recommends that this meal be eaten in the late evening, between 9:00 PM and 10:30 PM. He also cautions you *never* to skip a meal, and to eat everything as prescribed in the book. Alcoholic beverages and table salt are verboten, as are canned fruits and vegetables.

The exercise plan consists of two 20-minute periods of continuous exercise, which are supposed to follow any two of the four daily meals by about 30 minutes. Exercise may be walking, bicycling (outdoor or stationary), swimming, rebounding (on a trampoline-like exerciser), rowing or dancing. The author states that these are not meant to be aerobic exercises in that you are not required to increase your heart rate to a certain training level. For instance. a leisurely 3 mile per hour walking and an 8-9 mph cycling speed is advised. When you get within 10 pounds of your goal weight, Dr. Miller recommends "Muscle Firmer" exercises. These should be done three times per week, instead of one of the regular exercise periods on the appropriate days. These include calisthenic-like exercises such as jumping jacks, push-ups, heel raises, leg lifts, etc.

In summary, a diet-and-exercise plan that emphasizes carbos and restricts fats is very reasonable. Unfortunately, there's a lot of hype associated with this diet, which dilutes its effectiveness. In addition, eliminating canned vegetables makes no sense, and proscribing all alcohol, though certainly not unhealthy, may be unnecessarily restrictive. The various dietary phases (e.g., Low-cal, Booster, Reentry) represent, in my opinion, more magic than science, and a continued low-cal (approximately 1200-1500 calories/day) diet seems more reasonable.

Diets Don't Work

Finally, in a book section on dieting, we have to discuss at least one *no-diet* book. Several have been published in the past few years (e.g., *Dr. Rader's No-Diet Program for Permanent Weight Loss*), but the current favorite is probably *Diets Don't Work* (143). Mr. Schwartz believes in the psychological approach to weight loss, "It's not the weight that's the real problem—it's the mentality behind it. Get rid of the mentality and the weight comes off by itself" (p.21). In this book, he asks you to fill out answers (lots of blank space is included in the book) to questions about why you overeat, under what circumstances you do so, why you want to lose weight, why you haven't been successful in doing so in the past, etc.

He points out (as has been appreciated by behavior modification experts for quite some time) that thin people eat as a result of a major *internal* cue—hunger. Obese individuals, on the other hand, eat because of *external* cues, e.g., as a reward for being good, as a consolation if things aren't going well, etc. The first 140 pages of the book is devoted to this psychoanalytic approach to obesity. In the third section of the book, entitled "The Thin Life", the reader will make a "breakthrough into being a thin person and seeing everything around you from that perspective" (p.143). Exactly how this transition will occur is not quite clear in this book, but the reader is assured that if he *really* wants to be thin, he will be. There's something to be said for positive thinking, and this book may be helpful in enabling the obese person discover the reasons for why he overeats. I doubt, however, and most behavior modification programs would support this doubt, whether positive thinking and introspective understanding of the mechanisms underlying obesity are sufficient to enable one to lose weight. As a component of a comprehensive weight-loss program, however, the behavioral concepts discussed in this book merit some attention.

EPILOGUE ON OBESITY AND ITS TREATMENT

The obese person looking for an easy fix has no doubt been disappointed by the foregoing comments. It seems that there's no free lunch, and that to achieve something, you've really got to work for it, you really have to pay your pound of flesh. There are many groups out there willing, ready and able to help would-be dieters achieve their weight-loss goals. Many of these groups are described and evaluated in the *Rating the Diets* book (92a) referred to previously. The interested reader is encouraged to consult this resource for this information, and I wish the reader GOOD LUCK.

Finally, to leave on a humorous note, I have reprinted, with permission, a tongue-in-cheek essay on "How To Write Your Own Diet Book".

How to Write Your Own Diet Book

A *New York Times* editorial last summer marked the decline in American literary taste: The most popular books on the paper's best-seller list were guides to losing weight and volumes of cat cartoons. At present, cat books have gained the greater share of the market, but more diet manuals are surely waiting in the wings. Because no diet works for long, millions of people are caught in the lose-gain trap. And writing a diet book with a new angle, however strange, can be the surest way to a publishing fortune.

What counts in this kind of work is the formula, and diet books follow a pattern as rigidly as Gothic romances or spy stories. We plowed through as many diet books as we could stand (at 20 or so, we hit our limit) in an effort to divine their guiding principles. From this arduous labor we devised a 10-point plan for writing a successful diet book—a set of instructions that, needless to say, we hope fewer and fewer writers will follow.

1. *Tell them who you are.* It helps to be a physician—like Dr. Atkins and Stillman, and the late Dr. Tarnower—or an osteopath like Robert Linn, the liquid protein man. But laymen, too, can cut themselves into the deal. Consider *The Amazing Diet Secret of a Desperate Housewife* and *The Hollywood Emergency Diet*. (The actor who wrote the latter, the advertisement boasts, "is not a scientist or a doctor. He's not even a college graduate.") Nathan Pritikin, who has made a fortune on his diet-and-exercise plan, began as an inventor in Chicago. And Judy Mazel, author of *The Beverly Hills Diet*, explains herself thus: "I do not purport to be a medical doctor . . . If medical experts had conclusively proven the causes of fat, we'd all be thin. I have simply pulled together scattered facts and synthesized them . . ."

2. *Pick a catchy title.* This is essential. In 1958, Richard Mackarness pub-

lished a high-fat, low-carbohydrate diet with the bland title *Eat Fat and Grow Slim*. It went nowhere. Just three years later, Herman Taller, M.D., published a similar diet plan called *Calories Don't Count*. It stayed on the best-seller lists for the better part of a year. Drama is everything. Robert Linn's liquid protein diet sold well over a million paperback copies as *The Last Chance Diet*—even though the title became funereally apt when deaths were attributed to liquid protein diets.

3. *Get 'em into the tent.* Dieting is a drag. To be motivated, your readers need both a carrot and a stick. Tell them that they had better listen to you if they don't want to die young. Sound the familiar warning that extra weight leads to heart disease, cancer, lumbago, diabetes, gout and arthritis, and throw in one or two diseases they've never heard of. Then turn around and play the sympathetic friend. Promise to help them with a plan—based on newly discovered scientific principles—that makes it easy to lose and will improve their sex lives simultaneously.

4. *Present . . . The Master Plan.* This takes ingenuity. As a general rule of thumb, the diet should be as unnatural and unbalanced as possible: There is, by now, no other way to make it seem special. A tried-and-true method is to tell people to eat only certain food groups and exclude others. The most serviceable villains are carbohydrates—bread, sugar, even fruits and vegetables. A bolder approach is to base a diet on a single food. Eggs and grapefruit are now hallowed by tradition; one recent count turned up no less than 51 diets based on these two staples. People get sick of eggs and grapefruits, and will certainly lose weight if that's all they eat; but they may also become sick of your diet altogether. Your readers may also suspect that you think they're simple-minded.

Judy Mazel has cleverly surmounted these obstacles in *The Beverly Hills Diet*. Her rigid six-week plan is based largely on single-food days, but the food-of-the-day *varies* in a programmed way. Watermelon, grapes, pineapples and other fruits predominate. Such a diet, of course, can lead to diarrhea, which Mazel applauds. "If you have loose bowel movements, hooray! Keep in mind that pounds leave your body in two main ways—bowel movements and urination. The more time you spend on the toilet, the better. On watermelon days especially, you can expect to urinate a lot. That's the idea."

5. *Break out the textbooks*. However unbalanced your diet is, you shouldn't be hard put to find some scientific-sounding rationale for it. Old diet books are a good place to look, also any book on folk medicine. Low- carbohydrate diets have been recycled, with the same justification, for a century. If you can't find a ready-made reason for your gimmick, look through some articles on nutrition and metabolism, take a few quotes out of context, and make something up. Inspiration comes from unlikely places: Mazel found hers in a book on enzymes that she picked up in a health-food store, where she went to buy cashew nuts. Don't be shy about theorizing. Remember that human nutrition is still very poorly understood.

6. *Pad, pad, pad.* You don't really have much to tell your readers, so fill up the book with recipes, anecdotes, homilies and reprints of government nutrition tables (which aren't copyrighted). One famous author broke up his diet book into 25 short chapters, each with its own title page. Like fiber, this adds bulk.

7. *Foretell the future.* Your readers know that weight lost is quickly regained. Tell them that you know this too, and have designed your diet to help them change their eating habits permanently—even if the plan is so bizarre that only a monomaniac could stick to it for more than a week.

8. *Contemplate exercise.* But ignore it as much as possible; don't make yourself a bore by pushing sweat.

9. *Blame the victim.* Most of your readers will get nothing whatever from your book. Absolve yourself of any responsibility. Follow Robert Linn's example. In *The Last Chance Diet*, he claims that "the program cannot fail. Only you can fail." End of discussion.

10. *Cover yourself.* Somewhere, in large type or small, advise the reader to consult her or his physician before going on your diet.

From *The Dieter's Dilemma*, by William Bennett, M.D., and Joel Gurin. © 1982 by William Bennett and Joel Gurin. Reprinted by permission of Basic Books, Inc., Publishers.

REFERENCES

1. National Institutes of Health: Health implications of obesity. Volume 5, number 9, 1985
2. Truswell AS: Pop diets for weight reduction. Br Med J 285:1519, 1982
3. Bray GA: Definition, measurement, and classification of the syndromes of obesity. Int J Obesity 4:1, 1978
4. U.S Department of Health Education and Welfare: Obesity in America (Bray GA, ed.). NIH publication #80-359, 1980
5. Dahms WJ, Glass AR: Correlation of percent with body specific gravity in rats. J Nutr 112:398, 1982
6. Szeluga DJ, et al: Nutritional assessment by isotope dilution analysis of body composition. Am J Clin Nutr 40:847, 1984
7. Whyte R, et al: The measurement of whole body water by $H_2^{18}O$ dilution in newborn pigs. Am J Clin Nutr 41:801, 1985
8. Lukaski HC, Johnson PE: A simple, inexpensive method of determining total body water using a tracer dose of D_2O and infrared absorption of biological fluids. Am J Clin Nutr 41:363, 1985
9. Presta E, et al: Measurement of total body electrical conductivity: a new method for estimation of body composition. Am J Clin Nutr 37:735, 1983
10. Lukaski HC, et al: Assessment of fat-free mass using bioelectrical impedance measurements of the human body. Am J Clin Nutr 41:810, 1985
11. Owen GM: Measurement, recording and assessment of skinfold thickness in childhood and adolescence: report of a small meeting. Am J Clin Nutr 35:629, 1982
12. Cronk CE, Roche AF: Race- and sex-specific reference data for triceps and subscapular skinfolds and weight stature. Am J Clin Nutr 35:347, 1982

13. Siervogel RM, et al: Subcutaneous fat distribution in males and females from 1 to 39 years of age. Am J Clin Nutr 36:162, 1982
14. Mitchell CO, Lipschitz DA: The effect of age and sex on the routinely used measurements to assess the nutritional status of hospitalized patients. Am J Clin Nutr 36:340, 1982
15. Ashwell M, et al: Female fat distribution — a simple classification based on two circumference measurements. Int J Obes 6:143, 1982
16. Borkan GA, et al: Assessment of abdominal fat content by computed tomography. Am J clin Nutr 36:172, 1982
17. Tokunaga K, et al: A noel technique for the determination of body fat by computed tomography. Int J Obes 7:437, 1983
18. Fanelli MT, Kuczmarski RJ: Ultrasound as an approach to assessing body composition. Am J Clin Nutr 39:703, 1984
19. Conway JM, et al: A new approach for the estimation of body composition: infrared interactance. Am J Clin Nutr 40:1123, 1984
20. Frisancho AR, Flegel PN: Elbow breadth as a measure of frame size for U.S. males and females. Am J Clin Nutr 37:311, 1983
21. Garn SM, et al: The bony chest as a frame size standard in nutritional assessment. Am J clin Nutr 37:315, 1983
22. Katch VL, Freedson PS: Body size and shape: derivation of the "HAT" frame size model. Am J Clin Nutr 36:669, 1982
23. Katch VL, et al: Body frame size: validity of self-appraisal. Am J Clin Nutr 36:676, 1982
24. Obesity. A report of the Royal College of Physicians, London, England. Published in the Journal of the College 17:6, 1983. Also quoted in Lancet 1:177, 1983
25. Peckham CS, et al: Prevalence of obesity in British children born 1946 and 1958. Br Med J 286:1237, 1983
26. Build and Blood Pressure Study, 1959. Society of Actuaries, Chicago, 1959
27. 1979 Build Study, Society of Actuaries and Association of Life Insurance Medical Directors of America, 1980.
28. Lew EA, Garfinkel L: Variations in mortality by weight among 750,000 men and women. J Chron Dis 32:563, 1979
29. Gordon T, Kannel WB: Obesity and cardiovascular disease. The Framingham study. Clin Endocrinol Metab 5:367, 1976
30. Sonne-Holm S, et al: Risk of early death in extremely overweight young men. Br Med J 287:795, 1983
31. Weltman A: Unfavorable serum lipid profiles in extremely overfat women. Int J Obes 7:109, 1983
32. Khoury P, et al: Weight change since age 18 in 30- to 55-year-old whites and blacks. Associations with lipid values, lipoprotein levels and blood pressure. JAMA 250:3179, 1983
33. Bonham GS, Brock DB: The relationship of diabetes with race, sex, and obesity. Am J Clin Nutr 41:776, 1985
34. Simopoulos AP, Van Itallie TB: Body weight, health and longevity. Ann Int Med 100:285, 1984
35. Hubert HB, et al: Obesity as an independent risk factor for cardiovascular disease: a

26-year followup of participants in the Framingham Heart Study. Circulation 67:968, 1983

36. Andres R: Effect of obesity on total mortality. Int J Obes 4:381, 1980

37. Pugliese MT, et al: Fear of obesity. A cause of short stature and delayed puberty. N Engl J Med 309:513, 1983

38. Golden N, Sacker IM: An overview of the etiology, diagnosis, and management of anorexia nervosa. Clin Peds 23:209, 1984

39. Crisp AH: Anorexia nervosa. Br Med J 287:855, 1983

40. Lacey JH: Bulimia nrevosa, binge eating, and psychogenic vomiting: a controlled treatment study and long term outcome. Br Med J 286:1609, 1983

41. Anonymous: Binge and purge: Road back from bulimia. U.S. News and World Report, October 8, 1984, pp. 62

42. Bliss EL, Branch CH. Anorexia Nervosa: Its History, Psychology and Biology. New York: Paul B. Heuber, 1960

43. Casper RC, et al: Bulimia: Its incidence and clinical significance in patients with anorexia nervosa. Arch Gen Psych 37:1030, 1980

44. Feigner JP, et al: Diagnostic criteria for use in psychiatric research. Arch Gen Psych 26:57, 1972

45. Isner JM, et al: Anorexia nervosa and sudden death. Ann Intern Med 102:49, 1985

46. Rigotti NA, et al: Osteoporosis in women with anorexia nervosa. N Engl J Med 311:1601, 1984

47. Szmuckler GI, et al: Premature loss of bone in chronic anorexia nervosa. Br Med J 290:26, 1985

48. Hsu LK: Outcome of anorexia nervosa. Review of the literature (1954 to 1978). Arch Gen Psych 37:1041, 1980

49. Garrow JS, et al: Factors determining weight loss in obese patients in a metabolic ward. Int J Obes 2:441, 1978

50. Warwick PM, et al: Individual variation in energy expenditure. Int J Obes 2:396, 1978

51. Garrow JS: Luxuskonsumption, brown fat, and human obesity. Br Med J 286:1684, 1983

52. Ackerman S: The management of obesity. Hosp Prac :117, 1983

53. Gotto AM, et al: Obesity — A new approach to an old problem. Heart & Lung 9:719, 1980

54. Howard AN, Baird IM: A long-term evaluation of very low calorie semi-synthetic diets: an inpatient/outpatient study with egg albumin as the protein source. Int J Obes 1:63, 1977

55. Howard AN, et al: The treatment of obesity with a very-low-calorie liquid formula diet: an inpatient/outpatient comparison using skimmed-milk protein as the chief protein source. Int J Obes 2:321, 1978

56. Scheen AJ, et al: Hormonal and metabolic adaptation to protein-supplemented fasting in obese subjects. Int J Obes 6:165, 1982

57. Stokholm KN, et al: Very-low-calorie diet in the treatment of massive obesity: preliminary experience. Int J Obes 4:213, 1980

58. Contaldo F, et al: Protein-sparing modified fast in the treatment of severe obesity: weight loss and nitrogen balance data. Int J Obes 4:189, 1980

59. Wadden TA, et al: Very low calorie diets: Their efficacy, safety and future. Ann Intern Med 99:675, 1983
60. Bistrian RR, et al: Nitrogen metabolism and insulin requirements in obese diabetic adults on a protein-sparing modified fast. Diabetes 25:494, 1976
61. Bistrian BR, et al: Effect of a protein-sparing diet and brief fast on nitrogen metabolism in mildly obese subjects. J Lab Clin Med 89:1030, 1977
62. DeHaven J, et al: Nitrogen and sodium balance and sympathetic-nervous-system activity in obese subjects treated with a low-calorie protein or mixed diet. N Engl J Med 302:477, 1980
63. Rosen JC, et al: Mood and appetite during minimal-carbohydrate and carbohydrate-supplemented hypocaloric diet. Am J Clin Nutr 42:371, 1985
64. Bogardus C, et al: Comparison of carbohydrate-containing and carbohydrate-restricted hypocaloric diets in the treatment of obesity. Endurance and metabolic fuel homeostasis during strenuous exercise. J Clin Invest 68:399, 1981
65. Dietz WH, Wolfe RR: Interrelationships of glucose and protein metabolism in obese adolescents during short-term hypocaloric dietary therapy. Am J Clin Nutr 42:380, 1985
66. Fisler JS, et al: Nitrogen economy during very low calorie reducing diets: quality and quantity of dietary protein. Am J Clin Nutr 35:471, 1982
67. Chan J, Bartter FC: Weight reduction. Renal mineral and hormonal excretion during semistarvation in obese patients. JAMA 245:371, 1981
68. Drenick EJ, Johnson D: Weight reduction by fasting and semistarvation in morbid obesity: long-term follow-up. Int J Obes 2:123, 1978 Liquid Protein Diets
69. Weintraub M, et al: A double-blind clinical trial in weight control. Use of fenfluramine and phentermine alone and in combination. Arch Intern Med 144:1143, 1984
70. Douglas JP, et al: Long-term efficacy of fenfluramine in treatment of obesity. Lancet 1:384, 1983
71. Johnson DA, et al: Stroke and phenylpropanolamine use. Lancet 2:970, 1983
72. Bernstein E, Diskant B: Phenylpropanolamine, a potentially hazardous drug. Ann Emerg Med 11:311, 1982
73. Mueller SM, et al: Cerebral hemorrhage associated with phenylpropanolamine in combination with caffeine. Stroke 15:119, 1984
74. Sullivan AC, Comai K: Pharmacological treatment of obesity. Int J Obes 2:69, 1978
75. Douglas JG, Munro JF: The role of drugs in the treament of obesity. Drugs 21:362, 1981
76. Drenick EJ,et al: Excessive mortality and causes of death in morbidly obese men. JAMA 243:443, 1980
77. Hocking MP, et al: Jejunoileal bypass for morbid obesity. Late follow-up in 100 cases. N Engl J Med 308:995, 1983
78. Alpers DH: Surgical therapy for obesity. N Engl J Med 308:1026, 1983
79. Herbst CA, Buckwalter JA: Weight loss and complications after four gastric operations for morbid obesity. South Med J 75:1324, 1982
80. Linner JH: Comparative effectiveness of gastric bypass and gastroplasty: a clinical study. Arch Surg 117:695, 1982

81. Priddy ML: Gastric reduction surgery: A dietitian's experience and perspective. J Am Diet Assoc 85:455, 1985

82. Halverson JD, et al: Altered glucose tolerance, insulin response, and insulin sensitivity after massive weight reduction subsequent to gastric bypass. Surgery 92:235, 1982

83. Gleysteen JJ, Barboriak JJ: Improvement in heart disease risk factors after gastric bypass. Arch Surg 118:681, 1983

84. Herbst CA, et al: Gastric bariatric operation in insulin-treated adults. Surg 95:209, 1984

85. Olsson SA, et al: Effect of weight reduction after gastroplasty on glucose and lipid metabolism. Am J Clin Nutr 40:1273, 1984

86. Anonymous: Gastric operations for obesity. The Med Letter 26:113, 1984

87. MacLean LD, et al: Nutrition following gastric operations for morbid obesity. Ann Surg 198:347, 1983

88. Schilling RF, et al: Vitamin B_{12} deficiency after gastric bypass surgery for obesity. Ann Intern Med 101:501, 1984

89. Wattchow DA, et al: Prevalence and treatment of gallstones after gastric bypass surgery for morbid obesity. Lancet 1:763, 1983

90. Anonymous: Lipectomy: 'Magic bullet' for fat removal? Am Med News, 5/27/83, pp.15

91. Fuerst ML: Suction-assisted lipectomy attracting interest. JAMA 249:3004, 1983

92. Anonymous: Fat suction. Lancet 2:192, 1985

92a. Berland T: Rating the Diets. Publications International, Consumer Guide, 1983

93. Linn R, Stuart SL: The Last Chance Diet. Secaucus, NJ, Lyle Stuart Inc., 1976

94. Schucker RE, Gunn WJ: A national survey of the use of protein products in conjunction with weight reduction diets among American women. Centers for Disease Control, Atlanta, GA, 1978, p.73

95. Van Itallie TB: Liquid protein mayhem. JAMA 240:144, 1978

96. Singh B, et al: Liquid protein diets and Torsade de Pointes. JAMA 240:115, 1978

97. Michiel JR, et al: Sudden death in a patient on a liquid protein diet. N Engl J Med 298:1005, 1978

98. Felig P: Four questions about protein diets. N Engl J Med 298:1025, 1978

99. Brown JM, et al: Cardiac complications of protein-sparing modified fasting. JAMA 240:120, 1978

100. Isner JM, et al: Sudden unexpected death in avid dieters using the liquid-protein-modified-fast diet. Circulation 60:1401, 1979

101. Lantigua RA, et al: Cardiac arrhythmias associated with a liquid protein diet for the treatment of obesity. N Engl J Med 303:735, 1980

102. Letters to the editor: Cardiac arrhythmias during liquid protein diet. N Engl J Med 304:297, 1981

103. Sours HE, et al: Sudden death associated with very low calorie weight reduction regimens. Am J Clin Nutr 34:453, 1981

104. Van Itallie TB, Yang MU: Cardiac dysfunction in obese dieters: a potentially lethal complication of rapid, massive weight loss. Am J Clin Nutr 39:695, 1984

105. Felig P: Editorial retrospective. Very-low-calorie protein diets. N Engl J Med 310:589, 1984

106. Letters to the editor: Very-low-calorie protein diets. N Engl J Med 311:129, 1984
107. Editorial: The very low calorie diet. Lancet 2:500, 1984
108. Russel D, et al: Skeletal muscle function during hypocaloric diets and fasting: a comparison with standard nutritional assessment parameters. Am J Clin Nutr 37:133, 1983
109. Russell D, et al: Metabolic and structural changes in skeletal muscle during hypocaloric dieting. Am J Clin Nutr 39:503, 1984
110. Anonymous: Fad diets: The public eats them up. Moneysworth, Winter, 1983 issue, pp.16
111. Meyer A: Latest diet craze — not for everyone. USN & WR, 10/8/84, pp.57
112. Dwyer J: Twelve popular diets. Brief nutritional analyses. Psych Clin North Am 1(3):621, 1978
113. Volkmar FR, et al: High attrition rates in commercial weight reduction programs. Arch Intern Med 141:426, 1981
114. Truswell AS: Pop diets for weight reduction. Br Med J 285:1519, 1982
115. Gotto AM, Goodrick GK: Evaluating commercial weight-loss clinics. Arch Intern Med 142:682, 1982
116. Fisher MC, Lachance PA: Nutritional evaluation of published weight reducing diets. J Am Diet Assoc 85:450, 1985
117. Mirkin GB, Shore RN: The Beverly Hills Diet. Dangers of the newest weight loss fad. JAMA 246:2235, 1982
118. Editorial: Head for the hills: It's another fad diet! Mod Med, 3/82, pp.217
119. Wadden TA, et al: The Cambridge Diet. More mayhem? JAMA 250:2833, 1983
120. Howard AN: The Cambridge Diet. JAMA 252:897, 1984
121. Arrington R, et al: Weight reduction methods of college women. J Am Diet Assoc 85:483, 1985
122. Kreitzman SN, et al: Safety and effectiveness of weight reduction using a very-low-calorie formulated food. Arch Intern Med 144:747, 1984
123. Larkin T: Herbs are often more toxic than magical. FDA Consumer 17(8):6, 1983
124. Letters: Herbalife complains. FDA Consumer 18(9):2, 1984
125. Updates: California sues Herbalife. FDA Consumer 19(6):4, 1985
126. Anonymous: ADA submits statement on weight-loss products. J Am Diet Assoc 85:983, 1985
127. Eyton A:The F-Plan Diet Plan. Bantam Books, 1982
128. Leveille GA: The Setpoint Diet. Ballantine Books, New York, 1985
129. Garrow JS, Webster J: Are pre-obese people energy thrifty? Lancet 1:670, 1985
130. Kaplan ML, Leveille GA: Calorigenic response in obese and non-obese women. Am J Clin Nutr 29:1108, 1976
131. Pittet P, et al: Thermic effect of glucose in obese subjects studied by direct and indirect calorimetry. Br J Nutr 35:281, 1976
132. Shetty PS, et al: Postprandial thermogenesis in obesity. Clin Sci 60:519, 1981
133. Sharief NN, Macdonald I: Differences in dietary-induced thermogenesis with various carbohydrates in normal and overweight man. Am J Clin Nutr 35:267, 1982
134. Morgan JB, et al: A study of the thermic responses to a meal and to the sym-

pathomimetic drug (ephedrine) in relation to energy balance in man. Br J Nutr 47:21, 1982

135. Ravussin E, et al: Twenty-four hour energy expenditure and resting metabolic rate in obese, moderately obese and control subjects. Am J Clin Nutr 35:566, 1982

136. Nair KS, et al: Thermic response to isoenergetic protein, carbohydrate or fat meals in lean and obese subjects. Clin Sci 65:307, 1983

137. Blaza S, Garrow JS: Thermogenic response to temperature, exercise and food stimuli in lean and obese women, studied by 24h direct calorimetry. Br J Nutr 49:171, 1983

138. Welle SL, Campbell RG: Normal thermic effect of glucose in obese women. Am J Clin Nutr 37:87, 1983

139. Garrow JS: Luxuskonsumption, brown fat, and human obesity. Br Med J 286:1684, 1983

140. Warwick PM, et al: Individual variation in energy expenditure. Int J Obes 2:396, 1978

141. Himms-Hagen J: Thermogenesis in brown adipose tissue. N Engl J Med 312:1062, 1985

142. Miller PM: The Hilton Head Metabolism Diet. Warner Books, New York, 1983

143. Schwartz B: Diets Don't Work. Breakthru Publishing, Houston, 1982

CHAPTER 14

Summary—Putting It All Together

Whereas Section One of this book has discussed some of the principles by which scientific inquiry is conducted, Section Two has reviewed the scientific data on cholesterol and fats, carbohydrates, vitamins, salt and other minerals, and fiber and vegetarian diets. More than 1000 articles have been referenced in the preceding 13 chapters of this book, and even the medical reader may feel overwhelmed by the quantity of the material which has been presented. The reader may also wonder whether there isn't a specific diet which in a sense "summarizes" the concepts presented in the previous 13 chapters, and in fact, there is.

This diet consists of low-fat, low-cholesterol, low-sodium foodstuffs which are high in carbohydrates, especially the complex variety. Although some question has been raised previously about actual differences between simple and complex carbohydrates in terms of their usefulness in the diabetic diet, complex carbohydrates are still better in general because simple carbohydrates tend to be empty calories, usually devoid of nutrients and fiber. Complex carbohydrates, on the other hand, such as fruits, vegetables, cereals, breads and legumes, often contain many nutrients and fiber. This diet has been referred to as the HCF (high carbohydrate and fiber) diet. While emphasizing the complex carbohydrate components of the diet, intake of red meat and whole-fat dairy products is decreased or eliminated. Instead, fish, poultry and low-fat dairy products should be encouraged, although an ovolactovegetarian diet devoid of fish and poultry can also satisfy these dietary goals.

Specifically, this diet should consist of no more than 30% of total calories as fat, with no more than 10% coming from saturated fat. Since 10-15% protein is adequate for most individuals, the balance of 55-60% must be made up of carbohydrate. No more than one-quarter of this amount (13-15% of the total dietary calories) should be made up of simple carbohydrates (sugars). These recommendations are very similar to those recently made by the American Heart Association, in an effort to decrease average serum cholesterol in the United States, and consequently, the risk of heart disease.

Even if the reader cannot immediately tailor his diet according to the plan described above, modifying the diet slowly in this direction will still be beneficial. For instance, someone who is used to whole milk may find nonfat milk unpalatable. A sudden switchover may be extremely unpleasant and difficult to adhere to, but a gradual change may be better tolerated. This also applies to the fat (especially saturated) content of the diet. To eliminate all saturated fat from the diet overnight may be an unrealistic goal, but a slow but steady decrease should be achievable. For instance, initially, one may eliminate bacon and sausage from the diet and substitute margarine for butter. Gradually, other sources of saturated fat can be decreased or eliminated.

The HCF diet has been alluded to in several preceding chapters, and has been essentially spelled out in Chapter 7 in the discussion about "diets for diabetics". The HCF diet is both preventive of and therapeutic for most diseases which can at least be partially treated with nutrition. These include, among others, obesity, diabetes mellitus, hypertension, and elevated cholesterol. Some have also suggested that this diet may decrease the risk of cancer, although this is speculative at the present time. The fact that the same diet can be taken by a 50-year-old hypertensive, hypercholesterolemic executive and his 17-year-old currently-healthy son will facilitate compliance. In addition, if the teenager follows this diet, he may never develop the conditions which his father developed and to which he is genetically predisposed.

Some individuals have argued that widespread adoption of this diet is premature, and that the studies to *prove* its value haven't been done yet. Although this is true, it is unlikely that such studies will ever be done. Thus, someone waiting for the "definitive data" will undoubtedly be doomed to inaction. In the meantime, what really needs to be considered is the potential benefit of implementing this diet now, versus the potential costs, both financial and in terms of side effects.

The potential benefits have been amply demonstrated in previous chapters. It has been shown that lowering serum cholesterol (with drugs, in the case of the Lipid Research Clinics Study) decreases risk of cardiac disease and death. Many studies have shown that decreasing dietary saturated fat and cholesterol can decrease serum cholesterol in most, though not all, individuals. Some dietary intervention trials have also shown benefits of the low-fat diet.

Additional advantages of the HCF diet have been reviewed in other chapters. The HCF diet can promote weight loss, improve diabetic control, decrease blood pressure, improve bowel function and perhaps decrease the risk of colorectal, and possibly other forms of, cancer. In view of these proven and/or potential benefits, it seems reasonable for such a diet to be recommended unless there are side effects which outweigh the benefits.

To my knowledge, no significant side effects have been observed with the HCF diet. As mentioned previously, the HCF diet can increase intestinal gas production, but this is usually temporary. Some have suggested that the HCF diet can decrease absorption of certain minerals, e.g., zinc or calcium, but at present, this is more of a theoretical than a practical concern. Most patients who are used to a meat-and-potatoes diet may find the HCF diet hard to follow, but if a slow changeover is made, this should not prove to be an insurmountable obstacle.

In conclusion, there are many reasons to recommend adoption of the HCF-type diet as our "national" diet, and no reasons not to. This type of diet is becoming national policy in many countries, and some nutrition experts have suggested that the 25% decrease in cardiovascular mortality which has been observed in the United States over the past decade may be partially due to adoption of this diet. It is hoped that this salutary trend in cardiovascular mortality will continue as use of this diet becomes more widespread.

APPENDIX A

Essentials of the Scientific Method

Many claims are made in talk shows, magazine articles, health food stores, diet books and other forms of the mass media. These claims are often stated as facts, although it stands to reason that proponents of various diets and nutritional programs (with vested economic interest) may make claims that are either untrue or inaccurate. I have no vested interest in any of the regimens discussed herein, and a "magic" diet is not offerred in this book. It is hoped, however, that the knowledge gained from reading this book will help the reader tailor an adequate diet for himself.

It is my opinion that in order to properly evaluate and render an informed objective opinion on these controversial topics, it is necessary to examine the scientific literature; that is the primary goal of this book. The purpose of this appendix is to explain the basic tenets of the scientific method, and perhaps more importantly, discuss some of the pitfalls commonly encountered in the popular (and sometimes also in the scientific) literature. This discussion of the scientific method is not meant to be comprehensive; rather, it is meant to highlight certain aspects of the method which are especially germane to this book.

Loosely described, the scientific method depends upon *observation*, which leads to the formation of an *hypothesis*. The hypothesis is tested via *experiments*, after which a *conclusion* is reached. The conclusion will either support or refute the initial hypothesis. Often, the conclusion leads to the modification of the initial hypothesis; the modified hypothesis can then be tested in a future experiment. Obviously, this is a very simplistic view. In reality, many experiments are done, some of which may contradict one another, and hypotheses are not very easily proved or disproved. Understanding this framework, however, should serve the reader well while reading this book.

STUDY DESIGNS

As mentioned above, experimentation is an important way of evaluating hypotheses. Not all experimental designs are equally reliable, and the reader
. . . . ave at least a rudimentary understanding of various study des'

a) *Prospective study*—two groups of subjects, which are treated differently (or are different to begin with, e.g., smokers vs. nonsmokers) are observed over a period of time in order to determine if their outcomes are different (e.g., death from lung cancer). If a difference in outcome is observed, it may be concluded that their initial differences (smoking habits) accounted for the final differences (incidence of lung cancer). Ideally, the only difference between the groups should be smoking habit—all other parameters should be as similar as possible. If not, one might ascribe the difference in lung cancer rates to the wrong reason. If, for instance, it turned out that the smokers also happened to drink more coffee, it might be the coffee intake that caused the difference in lung cancer rates rather than smoking (this is just a hypothetical example—it is *quite clear* that smoking causes lung cancer).

b) *Retrospective study*—two groups of subjects with different outcomes are examined for differences that may have existed between them in the past. For instance, one can determine if people dying of heart disease in 1984 were more likely to have had heart attacks in the past compared to people who didn't die of heart disease in 1984. The study is retrospective in the sense that the investigator is looking at what happened in the past in order to draw conclusions about the present. Retrospective studies are much easier and cheaper to carry out, but they are less reliable than prospective studies.

c) *Placebo-controlled study*—one group of subjects is receiving inactive drugs ("sugar pills") while the other group is receiving the real treatment. Essentially all placebo-controlled studies are double-blind (see below).

d) *Double-blind study*—neither the subject nor the investigator know which subject is receiving which treatment. Therefore, bias due to the expectations of the subject or investigator is minimized. Bias is not always eliminated because patients often figure out whether they are taking the real or placebo treatment (1).

e) *Crossover study*—during the first half of the experiment, one-half of the subjects get treatment A while the other gets treatment B. Both A and B can be real treatments or drugs; alternatively, one may be a placebo. During the second portion of the experiment, the two subject groups switch treatments. Thus, every subject receives both treatments, i.e., each patient is his own control, which is the best way to compare two treatments. The only difference between the two groups is the order in which the subjects were exposed to the treatments. By changing this order, this source of bias is also eliminated.

f) *Randomized*—subjects are enrolled in the two treatment groups at random. This increases the likelihood, but doesn't guarantee, that significant differences between the two groups won't appear. Thus, differences in age, sex, weight, extent of disease, etc., which could affect the outcome of the experiment, are less likely.

Further discussion of scientific study designs is beyond the scope of this brief appendix. The interested reader may consult a basic text (2) or some review articles (3-3b) for further detail. In addition, several recent papers delineate some innovative research designs (4-7).

Although certainly not perfect (8,9), the best study design is a prospective, randomized, double-blind, placebo-controlled, crossover study (10). The investigator should always strive for such a study, although they are not always practical, or even feasible. Indeed, it is often necessary to reconcile the need for such trials with the difficulty of enrolling patients in a trial wherein their treatment will be essentially decided by the flip of a coin (recently discussed in refs. 11,12). If insufficient numbers of patients are enrolled, the confidence in the results will be decreased. This realization has lead to proposals (13) to modify the classical randomized study design. It remains true, however, that if some type of randomized and controlled design is not used, the problems delineated below can invalidate an otherwise well-performed study.

The concepts and definitions discussed above may understandably seem arcane and abstract to the reader. The paragraphs below, which discuss pitfalls which may trap the uncritical reader, will hopefully bring these concepts to life.

For instance, although it does sound trite, the true scientist is a seeker of truth and cares not whether an hypothesis that he proposes is proven correct or incorrect—either answer is *scientifically* equally satisfying. In actuality, however, many non-scientists and some scientists may become enamored with an hypothesis and lose their objectivity, and even without intending to, such an individual may not do service to both sides of an argument. This difficulty is exacerbated if the individual has financial ties to the hypothesis (e.g., an individual who advocates cytotoxic testing also happens to own or have a financial interest in the lab which does such testing). This is why randomized, double-blind, placebo-controlled studies are emphasized in this volume. Such studies are most objective because neither subject nor investigator bias can influence the results.

Lack of objectivity does not apply only to the performance of experiments. The point has been made previously that utilization of the scientific literature is one way of maintaining a reasonable balance in the evaluation of various claims, although the presence of a voluminous bibliography does not always guarantee scientific quality. On occasion, one sees very biased, selectively-documented articles or books, more commonly in the popular press but also in the scientific literature. The Pearson and Shaw book on life extension (see Chapter 5) is one example of this practice. One-sided literature reviews can easily be used to "prove" almost any hypothesis; such selective literature citations are very misleading and do not constitute acceptable scientific practice. Such practice is reminiscent of the adversary relationship in the courtroom wherein each attorney presents only evidence beneficial to his client. Although one-sided presentation of the evidence is encouraged in the courtroom, it is to be decried in scientific proceedings.

MEDICAL DOGMA

Although much of this book focuses on demystifying poorly-documented popular regimens, the reader should not assume that science itself has been free of such dogma. A large body of medical knowledge has been passed on uncritically to each new generation of medical students, and this medical "knowledge" is subject to scrutiny in this book along with the popular regimens (see two recent editorials on this topic (14,15)). A professor once told me: "You will learn a lot of facts in medical school. We know that half will be true, and half false. The only problem is that we don't know which half is which".

An excellent example of erroneous medical dogma is the teaching up until recently that since diabetes is due to insufficient carbohydrate metabolism, a *low* carbohydrate diet is indicated in the management of this disorder. Because this made a lot of sense, it was accepted uncritically and was taught to countless medical students (see p.146). However, when experiments were finally performed, this was shown to be incorrect. Once this was realized, the recommendation shifted toward a high-carbohydrate diet in the management of this disease, with an emphasis on complex carbohydrates, because, we were told, complex carbohydrates were more slowly digested than simple sugars. Before the ink on this pronouncement was dry, further experiments showed that some complex carbohydrates are absorbed as if they were pure sugar, whereas some simple carbohydrates act like the prototypical complex carbohydrates. This topic is discussed in more detail in Chapter 7.

Another example of medical dogma at its best is the management of heart attack victims, a topic perspicaciously discussed by Mitchell in a recent review article (16). Strict bed rest for six to eight weeks following a heart attack used to be recommended. When Sam Levine challenged this dogma in 1944, he was vilified as an unethical heretic, but when clinical trials were done in the early 1970s, it was shown that bed rest was not only unnecessary but actually detrimental to recovery (17).

It would be wishful thinking to believe that medical dogma is no longer generated today. It is very easy to fall into that trap, and only continuous vigilance will ensure that plausible but untested notions be recognized in their proper light. At the same time, it should be noted that the heretics of today may be proven right tomorrow, so that *implausibility* of an idea does not guarantee its erroneousness (see p. 47). Albert Einstein's theory of relativity certainly stretched the minds of the late 19th century physicists who heard it, although this theory has been amply proven since. The conclusion here should be, then, that plausibility or implausibility do not necessarily coincide with scientific truth, and that in order to establish the latter, unbiased controlled studies must be done. In the absence of such studies (or until they are done), we should be humble and honest enough to admit that what we think we know, and what we teach to our students, is simply an educated guess.

CAVEATS OF THE SCIENTIFIC METHOD

An important point to consider when reviewing the scientific literature is biologic variability, one of the basic properties of living creatures. Biologic variability is especially important in man, due to his physical complexity. Biologic variability is one of the basic tenets of Darwin's theory of evolution and natural selection ("survival of the fittest"), because nature "selects" among the biologic variants. This rather noble concept has its mundane applications; one of these is that identical drugs, nutrients and treatments affect various individuals differently, sometimes *very* differently. Biologic variability is one reason why anecdote cannot be used to prove hypotheses. Although this concept of biologic variability is intellectually recognized by many scientists and nonscientists as well, it often seems readily forgotten when results of experiments are interpreted.

Another common mistake in the popular nutritional literature is the presentation of anecdotal evidence as proof of an hypothesis. There are several reasons why anecdotal evidence cannot be useful as proof. One was mentioned in the paragraph above—namely that of biologic variability. For instance, an individual with high blood pressure might decrease his sodium intake on the advice of his physician. If his blood pressure does not change significantly, he might erroneously conclude that reduction of dietary sodium is of no value in the control of high blood pressure. However, the most he can reasonably conclude (if he indeed reduced his sodium intake significantly and for an appropriate length of time) is that sodium reduction is of no value in the control of *his* blood pressure. As a matter of fact, this example is not hypothetical—approximately two-thirds of hypertensive individuals do not seem to respond to dietary sodium restriction, while the other third does.

Another reason that anecdotal evidence cannot be used to prove an hypothesis is that almost by definition, anecdotal evidence is uncontrolled. For instance, the person with the severe cold says that vitamin C helped him recover from the cold. The question is, What would have happened in the absence of the vitamin C? Since colds tend to get better spontaneously, how do we know what would have happened if vitamin C wasn't administered? Perhaps a personal example will clarify this. I recently saw a 4 year-old with conjunctivitis whose mother requested eyedrops "that always clear his infection right up". She had been seeing another physician who was in the habit of prescribing medication even when it might not be necessary. I explained that her son's conjuctivitis was most likely due to a virus, that I had been seeing lots of it lately, that I had cultured several patients' eyes and no bacteria had grown. I further opined that it would most likely get better on its own within a couple of days. The mother was unconvinced, and persisted in her request. Since the side effects of the eyedrops were minimal, I cultured the eye and gave her the drops, but I asked her to perform a little (admittedly anecdotal) experiment. She was to put the eyedrops as directed in the *right eye only* and leave the left eye untreated.

As you might guess, the culture grew no bacteria, and both eyes cleared simultaneously within 48 hours. Had the mother not done this experiment, she would have been convinced that it was the medication that cured her son's eye infection (as she had concluded all the previous times that he had conjuctivitis). I am sure that many doctors have received the credit for similar cures, cures that would have occurred in the absence of both the doctor and the medication (see discussion below on the placebo effect).

The third reason why anecdotal evidence cannot be used as proof of hypotheses is that of bias. Even without consciously intending to, individuals who are undergoing a treatment are much more likely to see benefit from that treatment compared to doing nothing. For instance, as discussed in Chapter 7, many people erroneously believe that they have "hypoglycemia", and attribute it to various foods. They state in testimonials that whenever they eat food X, they get certain very debilitating symptoms. However, when such individuals were given food X in a blind fashion (without knowing what they ate), most had no symptoms. This does not imply that these individuals were faking or malingering—it just goes to show the tremendous power of the human mind, and explains why scientists are skeptical of anecdotal, uncontrolled data.

There is a legitimate use of anecdote (or case reports, as they are known in medical journals) and that is to *suggest* hypotheses or cause-and-effect relationships. For instance, an alert physician notices that a patient taking a new drug develops hepatitis, and proposes that the hepatitis might be due to the drug. As a *stimulator* of hypothesis, the case report is quite valuable; as *proof* of hypothesis, it is without merit.

Another caveat which should be observed by the reader relates to the interpretation of scientific data. First, it must be remembered that studies which deal with animals, though often necessary, are not directly applicable to human conditions. Indeed, many experiments utilize genetically abnormal animals which have been specifically bred to simulate certain human diseases (so-called animal "models"). The ob/ob mouse and the obese Zucker rat are two such models of human obesity.

Second, the type(s) and number of patients studied should be noted by the reader. For instance, many studies are initially carried out in animals, and later repeated in human males. Females are often initially excluded due to concerns about possible effects of the treatment on the fetus if the woman is pregnant. If a positive effect of a treatment is found in such a study involving only males, the question often arises as to whether such a result can be applied to women as well.

If children weren't studied, can the results be applied to them? If sodium restriction lowers blood pressure in hypertensive patients, will it also do so in people with normal blood pressure? In some cases, such generalization is probably safe, although usually, the conclusions should be restricted to the types of patients studied. In addition to sex and age, socioeconomic status and other demographic characteristics of the study group should be as similar as possible to the "population at large" if the investigator wants to apply his results to the general population.

Finally, sample size (the number of subjects enrolled in the study) should be sufficient so that confidence can be placed in the results. If the sample size is small, the study may not show a statistically significant effect of the active treatment. If the treatment does in fact have an effect, this type of error (concluding that it does not have an effect) is called a type II or *beta* error, as is well explained in a recent article (17a). This can be a serious error. For instance, a recent study concluded that hospital care is no better than home care for uncomplicated heart attacks (17b). If this conclusion is erroneous, and is acted upon by keeping heart attack victims at home, much harm can be done.

PLACEBO EFFECT

One topic, alluded to above, which bears careful discussion in this appendix, is the placebo effect. It is interesting to note that although it has been estimated that 80% of the treatments currently used in medicine are no better than placebo, the topic of the placebo effect is barely discussed in any medical school curriculum. When the placebo effect is discussed, it is usually to say something like, "The frequency with which placebos are used varies inversely with the combined intelligence of the doctor and his patient" (18). Thus, there is significant misunderstanding of the placebo effect, even among physicians (e.g., the belief that pain relieved by placebo must not be real, and using the placebo to catch "fakers").

Placebo has gotten a bad name among some scientists and clinicians, who are enamored only of active drugs and treatments. These individuals should heed the comment that, "The doctor who fails to have a [beneficial] placebo effect on his patients should become a pathologist or an anesthetist" (18a). This correspondent concluded: "if the patient does not feel better for your consultation you are in the wrong game, call it placebo or what you like".

Placebo, a Latin term meaning "I shall please", has been with us since time immemorial. Whether it's recognized or not, the placebo still constitutes a significant portion of all medical (and even more so, of quasi-medical) practice. We, as medical professionals, must recognize the healing powers of the caring physician and the act of prescription, and the authority of and the confidence in the white coat and the trappings of science. More importantly, nontraditional healers unable to use real drugs are still able to offer the caring touch, the confidence in their healing powers. Indeed, it has been suggested that these nontraditional practitioners, who are undistracted by active drugs, are able to concentrate more effectively on the placebo aspects of their contact with the patient.

The major factor which aids the placebo in demonstrating its effects is the inherent recuperative powers of the human organism and the tendency of the vast majority of diseases to be self-limited. Even in diseases that aren't self-limited (e.g., cancer), the power of the placebo has been demonstrated (please see the vitamin C and cancer controversy in Chapter 8).

The power of the placebo is surprising. Wolf, in a classic paper on the placebo effect (19), gives the following example. When syrup of ipecac (a substance used to induce vomiting) was given to a group of individuals, gastric motor activity was interrupted, followed by vomiting. The experiment was repeated on the nauseated subjects one at a time. The patients were given more ipecac, but were told that it was a new medicine which was sure to correct the nausea and vomiting. Within 15 minutes, nausea disappeared and gastric motor activity resumed (20).

It is not only *substances* that have placebo effects. Like the administration of drugs, surgery can yield very impressive placebo effects. For instance, in the 1930's, John Douglas reported an 80% 5-year cure rate in 68 patients with duodenal ulcer who had been treated with gastroenterostomy (21), a procedure which would today be considered malpractice. It would be interesting to speculate on which of our current drugs and surgeries will be found to be no better than placebo and considered malpractice in the future!

The physiological mechanism of placebo has received considerable attention, and along with the therapeutic use of placebos, has been recently reviewed (22,23). Some have suggested that placebos relieve pain via the endogenous (in the body) production of endorphins, proteins which have been shown to have impressive pain-relieving qualities. Even if this is true (and many scientists do not believe it to be), this does not explain the other, non-pain-related effects of placebos. It seems that explaining the varied effects of placebos with *one* mechanism is unlikely.

EVALUATING CAUSE-AND-EFFECT RELATIONSHIPS

Perhaps the most confusing aspect of reading a scientific report is the determination of whether a cause-and-effect relationship exists. Much scientific research is aimed at this question. Does a fatty diet cause heart disease? Does a high salt intake cause high blood pressure? Does eating fried foods cause cancer?

Does cigarette smoking cause lung cancer? In order to answer such questions, the central question that the scientist must ask himself is, What kind of evidence do I need in order to establish a cause-and-effect relationship between two events?

In science, one often starts with the observation of a *relationship* or an *association*. For instance, one may note that event B (e.g., lung cancer) is associated with environmental feature A (e.g, smoking). How can we pass from this irrefutable observed *association* to a verdict of causation? In a paper that continues to be the definitive work on this topic, Bradford Hill, a British statistician, listed the following aspects of an association which suggested that causation was at play:

1) *Strength*—for instance, it was noted that chimney sweeps had a risk of scrotal cancer *200 times higher* than that of workers not exposed to that environment. The strength of this association very strongly suggests causation, but absence of such excess risk does not imply lack of causation.

2) *Consistency*—has the association been repeatedly observed by different investigators, in different places, at different times? Essentially all studies have shown that smoking is associated with approximately a 30-fold increase in the risk of lung cancer; although this is not as impressive as a 200-fold difference, the consistency of the smoking studies is convincing.

3) *Specificity*—if the association is limited to specific workers and to particular types and sites of disease, there is a strong argument in favor of causation (e.g., the chimney sweeps and scrotal cancer example).

4) *Temporality*—which came first, the disease or the supposed cause? An excellent example of this is the observation that individuals with very *low* cholesterol levels (as well as those with high cholesterol levels) have a higher cancer mortality than individuals with intermediate cholesterol levels. Some have proposed that lowering one's cholesterol excessively can therefore increase the risk of dying from cancer. An equally reasonable hypothesis is that individuals who are dying of cancer tend to have lower cholesterol levels. In other words, does low cholesterol cause cancer, or is it the other way around?

5) *Biological gradient*—otherwise known as dose-response relationship. For instance, the fact that the risk of lung cancer increases linearly with the number of cigarettes smoked daily supports the causation interpretation.

6) *Plausibility*—it is helpful if the suspected mechanism of causation is biologically plausible, although causes are often determined before they can be explained biologically. Thus, absence of plausibility should not rule out a cause-and-effect relationship.

7) *Coherence*—on the other hand, the interpretation of the relationship should not seriously conflict with the general understanding of the disease.

8) *Experiment*—for instance, does cessation of the smoking habit decrease the risk of lung cancer? If it does (which it does) that is supportive of a causal interpretation, and is probably the most important factor in concluding that a

cause-and-effect relationship exists. The recently published Lipid Research Clinics study (see Chapter 6) is an excellent example of this.

9) *Analogy*—this really belongs under *coherence*. Hill gives us an example: in view of the well-established teratogenic (producing birth defects) effects of rubella and thalidomide, we would surely be ready to accept slighter but similar evidence that another drug or viral disease can also cause birth defects.

These are nine guidelines which Hill believes to be (and are widely accepted) as supportive of causation. It should be recognized, however, that not all nine of these are *required* in order for a cause-and-effect relationship to be inferred. It will serve the reader well to consider these, and other points discussed in this appendix, when a causal relationship is proposed.

THE BOTTOM LINE

The scientific method in general, and specific abuses of the method which are illustrated in the rest of this book, have been described. The ideal prospective, double-blind. placebo-controlled, randomized, crossover trial has been introduced, realizing that such a design is not always possible. The reader is encouraged to mentally review this appendix when questionable claims are presented to him. Although the concepts may seem arcane at this time, they are referred to repeatedly in this book.

REFERENCES

1. Brownell KD, Stunkard, AJ: The double-blind in danger: Untoward consequences of informed consent. Am J Psych 139:1487, 1982. Also discussed in Med Tribune 24:1, 1983.

2. Colton T: Statistics in medicine (ed.1). Boston, Little, Brown and Co., 1974.

3. Goldberg RJ: Clinical uses of the epidemiologic approach. Hosp Prac 18(8):177, 1983

3a. Larkin T: Evidence vs. nonsense: A guide to the scientific method. FDA Consumer, June, 1985, pp.27

3b. Pocock SJ: Current issues in the design and interpretation of clinical trials. Br Med J 290:39, 1985

4. Kolata G: A new kind of epidemiology. Science 224:481, 1984

5. Mayer JD: Medical geography. An emerging discipline. JAMA 251:2680, 1984

6. Gurling HMD: Genetic epidemiology in medicine—recent twin research. Br Med J 288:3, 1984

7. Hrubec Z, Robinette, CD: The study of human twins in medical research. N Engl J Med 310:435, 1984

8. Dudley HAF: The controlled clinical trial: an outsider looks in. Br Med J 287:957, 1983

9. Multiple authors (letters to editor): Bias in treatment assignment in controlled clinical trials. N Engl J Med 310:1610, 1984

10. Louis TA, et al: Crossover and self-controlled designs in clinical research. N Engl J Med 310:24, 1984

11. Taylor KM, Margolese RG, Soskolne, CL: Physicians' reasons for not entering eligible patients in a randomized clinical trial of surgery for breast cancer. N Engl J Med 310:1363, 1984

12. Angell M: Patients' preferences in randomized clinical trials. N Engl J Med 310:1385, 1984

13. Ellenberg SS: Randomization designs in comparative clinical trials. N Engl J Med 310:1404, 1984

14. Linzer M: Doing what "needs" to be done. N Engl J Med 310:469, 1984

15. Ralph JC: Early eating habits of infants. Ped News 17:28, 1983

16. Mitchell JRA: "But will it help *my* patients with myocardial infarction?" The implications of recent trials for everydat country folk. Br Med J 285:1140, 1982

17. Bloch A, et al: Early mobilization after myocardial infarction. Am J Cardiol 34:152, 1974

17a. Detsky AS, Sackett DL: When was a 'negative' clinical trial big enough? How many patients you needed depends on what you found. Arch Intern Med 145:709, 1985

17b. Hill JB, et al: A randomized trial of home-versus-hospital management for patients with suspected myocardial infarctions. Lancet 1:837, 1978

18. Platt R: Two essays on the practice of medicine. Lancet ii:305, 1947.

18a. Blau JN: Clinician and placebo. Lancet 1:344, 1985

19. Wolf S: The pharmacology of placebos. Pharmacol Rev 11:689, 1959

20. Wolf S: The relation of gastric function to nausea in man. J Clin Invest 22:877, 1943

21. Douglas J: Discussion of papers on mortality and late results of operations for gastric and duodenal ulcers. Ann Surg 92:631, 1930

22. Vogel AV, Goodwin JS, Goodwin JM: The therapeutics of placebo. Am Fam Phys 22(1):105, 1980.

23. Editorial: Shall I please? Lancet ii:1465, 1983

24. Hill AB: The environment and disease: Association or causation? Proc Royal Soc Med 58:295, 1965

APPENDIX B

Glossary

Aggregation (platelets)—"sticking together" of platelets, which causes blood to clot

Amenorrhea—absence of menstrual periods

Amylase—a starch-digesting enzyme made by the pancreas and salivary glands (glands which make saliva)

Anemia—low amount of red blood cells (and hemoglobin) in the blood

Animal model—an strain of animal that is bred to simulate a human disorder, so that experiments can be done with it, e.g., the ob/ob mouse is supposed to simulate human obesity, and the Dahl rat simulates hypertension

Anticoagulant—"blood thinner", a drug given to decrease blood clotting

Antioxidant—a compound which prevents free radical activity

Arrhythmia—abnormal heart rhythm

Atherogenesis—process by which atherosclerosis occurs

Beta carotene—a plant substance that can be converted to vitamin A in the human body, thought to maybe decrease the likelihood of developing cancer

Biochemistry—the study of chemical reactions, in living things, which produce energy, growth, etc.

Body mass index—a measure of fatness

Canthaxanthin—a carotenoid related to beta carotene; the main ingredient of "tanning pills"

Carbohydrate—a group of organic substances composed of carbon, hydrogen and oxygen, and divided into *simple* (sugars) and *complex* (e.g., cereals, breads, legumes, fruits and vegetables)

Carotenoids—a group of plant-derived substances which can be converted to vitamin A in the human body

Chemotherapy—drug treatment for cancer

Cohort—a group of people who are followed in a scientific study (see Appendix A)

Colorectal cancer—cancer of the colon or rectum

Coronary—pertaining to the heart, e.g., coronary artery

Crossover study—see Appendix A

de novo—made "from scratch" rather than from another substance

Diastolic blood pressure—the lower of the two numbers in the blood pressure measurement (e.g., the 90 in $^{140}/_{90}$). See also *systolic*

Diet-heart hypothesis- also known as the lipid hypothesis, namely, the hypothesis which states that diet, especially saturated fat and cholesterol, can increase the chance of heart and blood vessel disease

Digestion—the breakdown of food to its components. Protein is broken down to amino acids; carbohydrates to glucose; and fats to triglycerides and fatty acids

Disaccharide—a type of sugar molecule

Diverticulosis—a condition characterized by multiple outpouchings from the large bowel. These outpouchings can become inflamed, a condition known as diverticulitis

Double-blind—see Appendix A

Dysplasia—abnormal development of cells, which is considered precancerous

Dyspnea—difficulty breathing

Edema—swelling of (usually) the legs, due to retention of water (sometimes due to heart disease)

Efficacy—how well a drug or treatment works

Epidemiology—the study of populations (large groups of people) in order to draw associations between traits of the population and their common diseases

Etiology—cause

Fibrocystic breast disease—very common breast disease characterized by formation of cysts and swelling of parts of the breast

Free radicals—highly reactive chemicals formed in all living things which are hypothesized to cause various types of damage

Gastric carcinoma—stomach cancer

Gastritis—inflammation of the stomach lining; can be caused by alcohol, various drugs (e.g., aspirin, and related drugs)

Gastrointestinal (GI) tract—tract from mouth to anus, responsible for digestion and absorption of food, and for elimination of wastes

Hematologic—pertaining to the blood

Homeopathy—a system of medical care that treats disease with minute doses of a remedy that would, in healthy persons, produce symptoms of the disease

Hypercholesterolemia—high blood level of cholesterol

Hyperkalemia—high blood potassium

Hyperkinesis—hyperactivity (as in kids)

Hyperlipidemia—high blood level of either (or both) cholesterol and triglycerides

Hyperlipoproteinemia—high blood levels of lipoprotein(s). See Ch. 5

Hyperosmolarity—high concentration of substances in the blood

Hypertension—high blood pressure

Hypoglycemia—abnormally low blood sugar; often (incorrectly) used as a synonym for reactive hypoglycemia, which requires, in addition to a low blood sugar, specific symptoms, appropriate timing, and several other criteria; see Ch. 6 for complete definition

Hypotension—low blood pressure

Idiopathic—of unknown cause

Incidence—the number of new cases of a disease or condition appearing during a certain period of time (e.g., one year). See also *prevalence*

Intestinal mucosal cells—cells lining the gastrointestinal tract

Intravenous—by vein, usually refers to fluids or drugs given by this route

in vitro—referring to experiments done in the laboratory

in vivo—referring to experiments done in a living organism

Lipase—a fat-digesting enzyme produced by the pancreas

Lipids—synonym for "fats" (often those measured in the blood—like cholesterol and triglycerides

Macrobiotic—a term descriptive of a very restricted diet, containing chiefly whole grains, considered by its advocates to promote health

Malabsorption—poor absorption, usually in the gastrointestinal tract

Median—can be used interchangeably with "average" (although the terms are not synonymous)

Megavitamin—greater than RDA amounts of vitamins; usually defined as *10 times* greater than RDA amounts

Meningitis—an often-life-threatening infection of the membranes around the brain

Morbidity—disease

Mortality—death

Obesity—condition characterized by an excessive amount of body fat

Oncologist—doctor specializing in the field of cancer

Osteoporosis—a thinning of the bones, usually in women, predisposing them to fractures of the bones

Pancreas—organ which secretes amylase, insulin, and other important substances

Pathogenesis—the process by which disease occurs

Peripheral vascular disease—atherosclerosis of the arteries of the extremities (usually legs)

Pharmacopeia—a book describing drugs and medicinal preparations

Pharmacology—the study of drugs

Phaseolamin—a substance found in kidney beans which inhibits the action of amylase, a starch-digesting enzyme

Physiology—the study of the function of various organs in the body

Placebo—an inactive pill or treatment given to a group of people (usually) to help compare the real effects of a treatment or medication

Postprandially—after a meal

Prevalence—number of cases of a certain disease or condition present in a population at a point in time (usually expressed as number of cases/100,000 people

Prospective study—see Appendix A

Prostacyclin—a prostaglandin with effects opposite to thromboxane

Prostaglandins—a group of hormones made in the body, each of which has certains biological activities

Randomized study—see Appendix A

Reactive hypoglycemia—see definition for "hypoglycemia"

Retinoids—group of substances related to vitamin A

Retrolental fibroplasia—disease of the eyes of babies, due to exposure to high oxygen concentrations, and which can cause blindness

Retrospective study—see Appendix A

Serum glucose—sugar level in the blood

Systolic blood pressure—the higher number of the two numbers. See also *diastolic blood pressure*

Tachycardia—fast heart rate

Thrombophlebitis—clot formation in, and subsequent inflammation, of veins, usually in the legs

Thrombosis—clot formation

Thromboxane—a prostaglandin compound which enhances the aggregation (stickiness) of platelets (blood cells responsible for blood clotting); also causes vasoconstriction (clamping down) of arteries and veins

Vasoconstrictor—substance with a tendency to constrict blood vessels

Vasodilator—substance with a tendency to dilate blood vessels

Vasospasm—spasm of the arteries

Index

314   *Popular Nutritional Practices: A Scientific Appraisal*

bulimia 264
burns, and aloe vera 45
bypass surgery, and Pritikin 118
calcium 174,198-201
    and hypertension 226,233
    and vegetarian diets 252
cancer 23,82
    alternative approaches 31
    and low cholesterol diet 124-126
    and obesity 262
    PS 92
    and selenium 202
    terminal 24
    and vitamin C
canthaxanthin 44
capsaicine, capsicum 45
carbohydrate,
    metabolism 141
    types 139
carotene 98PS
carotenoids 161-167
    clinical uses—dermatology 163-164
    clinical uses—prevention of cancer 164-165
    side effects 165-166
    recommendations 166-167
carcinogens, natural 52
catecholamines 73-74
cavities, and fluoride 210
cellulose 140,240
cerebellar ataxia 73
cervical dysplasia, and folic acid 182
    and vitamin C 184
CHD 104-130
chelation therapy 117
chemotherapy 24
chicken soup, dangers 18
Chinese restaurant syndrome 57
chiropractic 18,30,36,45-46
    dangers 46
cholera, and niacin 177
cholesterol 104-130
    and bran 242
    and fiber 240
    and garlic 45
    PS 85,92,94
    and zinc
cholestyramine 110
    and regression of CHD 116
choline 72-73
Christian science 32-34

chromium 211
clairvoyant diagnosis 30
clinical trials, alternative medicine 30
clofibrate 129
cobalamin 180
coffee, and cholesterol 127
cold, and vitamin C 185
colon cancer, and fiber 241
    and calcium 165
conversion reaction, and hypoglycemia 153
cost-benefit analysis 19
coumarins, natural 38
CPR, 93PS
cyanide 26
cystic fibrosis 92PS
cytotoxic testing 60,65-66
Datura 42
dental cavities 143
depression 73,74
    and hypoglycemia 154
diabetes 142,144
    and chromium 211
    dietary recommendations 145,149-150
    and fiber 239,242-243
    and hypertriglyceridemia 128
    and obesity 261
    and smoked foods 58
Diapid 97PS
diet and exercise 283,284
diet clubs 275
dieting 267-269,274-288
    balanced diets 267
    psychologic approach 285
    very-low-calorie diets 268-269
diets,
    elimination 36,63,64,66,77-78,79
    exchange, in diabetes 149
    HCF 145
    natural 25
    Pritikin 118
digestion 19
digitalis 37
disaccharides 139
disease, psychosomatic 31
diuretics, and magnesium 227
diverticulosis, and fiber 239,244
DMSO 36
dogma, and diabetes 146
dopamine 73-74,90PS
drugs, and HDL 115